"*DBT Principles and Strategies in the Multidisciplinary Treatment of Eating Disorders* provides a fabulous platform to launch a fully multidisciplinary approach to utilizing Dialectical Behavior Therapy for eating disorders care. Kalata and Miller provide in-depth application of therapeutic concepts that maintain the scope of practice for each discipline of eating disorder professionals in an easy to understand and utilize format. With multidisciplinary practice as the state of the art in eating disorders care, this book is a must-have guide."

Leah L. Graves, *RDN, LDN, hon CEDS-S, FAED*

DBT Principles and Strategies in the Multidisciplinary Treatment of Eating Disorders

DBT Principles and Strategies in the Multidisciplinary Treatment of Eating Disorders is an in-depth exploration of DBT strategies and principles that can be applied by all members of a client's multidisciplinary team, including dietitians and psychiatric providers. While previous DBT-related texts focus on therapists, counselors, and social workers, this book's discipline-specific and cross-discipline examples and dialogue, as well as thoughtful descriptions of DBT principles and strategies create an accessible text carefully designed to benefit a wide variety of audiences.

By showing the multidisciplinary application of DBT tools and techniques, this book gives providers of all disciplines a shared language and framework that can assist with multidisciplinary case conceptualization, treatment planning, and therapeutic interventions, rather than leaving providers operating in discipline-specific silos that are often atheoretical or eclectic in terms of their framework for conceptualizing and providing care. Exercises embedded throughout the text focus on helping providers implement what they are learning in their day-to-day clinical practice. The book is replete with activities that are focused specifically on assisting providers in implementing DBT strategies, like diary cards, chain analyses, exposure-based procedures, and cognitive modification procedures. Lastly, there is an emphasis on how DBT concepts and methods can be applied in different settings, especially in inpatient, residential, and partial hospitalization settings.

DBT Principles and Strategies in the Multidisciplinary Treatment of Eating Disorders is an accessible, practical guide for eating-disorder professionals of all disciplines who would like to integrate DBT principles and strategies into patient care.

Alyssa H. Kalata, Ph.D, is a licensed psychologist with significant experience as a provider, supervisor, administrator, and public speaker in the realm of behavioral healthcare.

Elysse Thebner Miller, MPH, RDN, LDN, CEDS-S, is a registered dietitian with fifteen years of clinical and supervisory experience treating eating disorders across the lifespan in inpatient and outpatient settings.

DBT Principles and Strategies in the Multidisciplinary Treatment of Eating Disorders

Alyssa H. Kalata and
Elysse Thebner Miller

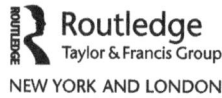

Routledge
Taylor & Francis Group

NEW YORK AND LONDON

Designed cover image: Larisa Rusina © Getty Images

First published 2025
by Routledge
605 Third Avenue, New York, NY 10158

and by Routledge
4 Park Square, Milton Park, Abingdon, Oxon, OX14 4RN

Routledge is an imprint of the Taylor & Francis Group, an informa business

ISBN: 9781032801292 (hbk)
ISBN: 9781032797229 (pbk)
ISBN: 9781003495604 (ebk)

DOI: 10.4324/9781003495604

Typeset in Times New Roman
by Newgen Publishing UK

Contents

Chapter 1

Introduction

The Purpose of this Book

In the three decades since the Cognitive-Behavioral Treatment of Borderline Personality Disorder (Linehan, 1993) text was released, researchers and clinicians have taken Dialectical Behavior Therapy (DBT) and adapted it successfully for numerous disorders, populations, and settings. Although the gold standard in eating disorders treatment is to provide multidisciplinary care, non-therapist providers have historically been viewed as ancillary in the context of providing DBT in the treatment of eating disorders. The purpose of this book is to explore how DBT can be adapted in a way that shifts dietitians, psychiatric providers, medical providers, case managers, culinary staff, nurses, and mental health technicians from adjunctive roles to integral ones in the provision of DBT-based treatment.

It may seem controversial to some to train non-therapist providers in principles and strategies drawn from a psychotherapeutic treatment, however there is ample evidence that non-therapist providers can be successfully trained to use psychotherapeutic interventions to good effect, while also remaining within their scope of practice. One of the most notable examples of this is the use of Motivational Interviewing by providers from a multitude of disciplines, including dietitians, medical providers, and nurses (e.g. Smart, Clifford, & Morris, 2014). We strongly believe that when all treatment team members operate from a shared theoretical framework, case conceptualization, treatment planning, and therapeutic interventions are enhanced, and the likelihood of providing efficacious treatment is increased.

The principles and strategies described in this book are drawn primarily from standard DBT, although principles and strategies from Radically Open Dialectical Behavior Therapy (RO DBT) (Lynch, 2018) are incorporated as well. We recognize that this is possibly another controversial decision, yet it is one we felt was in the best interest of the audience for whom this book is intended. The reality for the majority of providers of eating disorder treatment is that they will see patients with a wide range of eating disorder diagnoses,

DOI: 10.4324/9781003495604-1

in addition to a broad array of diagnostic comorbidities. While some of these patients may neatly fall into a group that would benefit from standard DBT only or RO DBT only, the diagnostic comorbidities and clinical complexity of the patients most providers treat requires incorporating components of both approaches to some extent. It is often not pragmatic to be a purist when translating academic research into clinical practice.

For Whom Is This Book Written?

This book is written for any provider working with a patient diagnosed with a primary eating disorder. While our focus throughout the book will be on therapists, counselors, dietitians, psychiatric providers, and medical providers, we will also highlight the roles of case managers, nurses, mental health technicians, and culinary staff in providing care within a DBT framework. It is important to note that this book assumes that the reader has foundational eating disorders knowledge as relevant to the reader's specific discipline.

For What Patient Populations Is This Book Intended?

The patient populations to which information in this book most applies are patients diagnosed with Anorexia Nervosa (AN), Bulimia Nervosa (BN), Binge Eating Disorder (BED), and Other Specified Feeding and Eating Disorder (OSFED), and particularly patients with one of these diagnoses where other comorbidities that DBT has been shown to be effective in treating are present, like Borderline Personality Disorder (BPD) or Substance Use Disorder (SUD). While many of the principles and strategies of DBT can be applied to good effect in the treatment of Avoidant/Restrictive Food Intake Disorder (ARFID), for patients diagnosed with this disorder who do not have other diagnostic comorbidities for which DBT has been found to be effective, there are existing CBT-based protocols that are more targeted in their approach in the treatment of ARFID specifically.

The Structure of This Book

In each section of this book, we have attempted to do three things. First, each section aims to teach about a set of DBT principles or strategies from a multi-disciplinary lens. DBT as it was originally designed was intended to be a treatment that was implemented by therapists, however key figures within the DBT community like Charlie Sweson and Suzanne Witterholt have illustrated ways in which providers from other disciplines can implement DBT principles and strategies in their work to good effect. We expand upon the foundation they have established through both broadening the scope of providers included in this discussion, as well as through providing examples of the application of DBT principles and strategies specifically in the context of multidisciplinary eating disorders care.

Second, numerous examples of patient and provider dialogue are given in an attempt to bring DBT to life. You will follow one specific patient (Megan, who will be introduced shortly) throughout the entire text. In following one patient throughout your reading, we hope you are able to immerse yourself in her story and make the connections between all the principles and strategies within DBT, rather than learning about them in a more piecemeal fashion. Additionally, we incorporate other patient examples when relevant. We felt that it was important to include these additional examples in order to show cross-diagnostic application of DBT principles and strategies, in addition to illustrating how care may need to be adapted based on various sociodemographic factors, like age and gender.

Finally, wherever possible we have attempted to include provider exercises for you to complete. When it comes to providing patient care, DBT tends to favor the approach of doing, rather than talking about. This principle applies not only to patient care, but to provider learning as well. As both a learner and as a trainer, I (AHK) have found engaging in experiential activities to be the single most valuable tool for clinical growth once someone has a base knowledge of the topic at hand. These provider exercises are included throughout this book as a way of encouraging you to not just read about DBT, but to thoughtfully put DBT principles and strategies into practice when providing patient care.

Important Caveats and Considerations

There are a couple of important caveats we would like our readers to keep in mind as they work through this text. First, there has yet to be a randomized controlled trial comparing treatment outcomes for teams where therapists are the only treatment team members applying DBT principles and strategies versus teams where all treatment team members are applying DBT principles and strategies. This book is based on our anecdotal experiences as supervisors and treatment providers in a program where all treatment team members received training in DBT principles and strategies and applied this training in their work with patients and their families and supports. It is our hope that this text might serve as a catalyst for a randomized controlled trial that could provide quantitative data either confirming or disconfirming the validity of our anecdotal experience.

Second, for therapists and counselors who may have come across this text, it is recommended if you are going to provide DBT, that you are aiming to remain as adherent to standard DBT or existing adaptations of DBT that have empirical support, unless a compelling reason can be made for deviation from existing treatment protocols. As such, if you have not read the Cognitive-Behavioral

Treatment of Borderline Personality Disorder (Linehan, 1993) text and the DBT Skills Manual (Second Edition) (Linehan, 2015) at minimum, it is recommended that you start with these books prior to reading this text. In writing this book, we made our best efforts to balance writing a comprehensive text with writing a book that was pragmatic and accessible. In striking this balance, it is important to note that all DBT strategies are not covered within our text. Particularly in situations where applicability of a given strategy was primarily within the scope of therapists and psychiatric providers only, we have made the decision to exclude these strategies in order to ensure that our focus remains on strategies that a broader array of providers can use.

Chapter 2

Empirical Literature Supporting the Use of DBT in the Treatment of Eating Disorders

DBT was originally developed to treat Borderline Personality Disorder and highly suicidal and self-injurious individuals by addressing difficulties in emotion regulation (Linehan, Armstrong, Suarez, Allmon, & Heard, 1991). As of 2020, 53 randomized controlled trials had been conducted examining the efficacy of DBT (Harned, 2020). Studies have found that DBT is effective in treating a wide range of diagnoses beyond Borderline Personality Disorder (e.g. Substance Use Disorders, complex PTSD). DBT has also been shown to be effective for individuals spanning a wide range of ages in a broad range of treatment settings and levels of care.

DBT has also been shown to be effective in the treatment of eating disorders. As with Borderline Personality Disorder, many of the behaviors seen in individuals diagnosed with an eating disorder, such as bingeing, purging, restricting, and exercising, are thought to aid in regulating emotions (Bankoff, Karpel, Forbes, & Pantone, 2012). While DBT is a treatment that focuses on dysregulation in multiple areas, the focus on targeting emotion dysregulation is at the very core of the treatment. It is also worth noting that there is a significant overlap between individuals diagnosed with an eating disorder who are also diagnosed with a comorbidity for which DBT has been found to be efficacious.

Looking at Borderline Personality Disorder specifically, around 34% of individuals who meet criteria for Borderline Personality Disorder also met criteria for an eating disorder (Zanarini, et al., 2004). When looking at specific eating disorders, around 3% of individuals diagnosed with Anorexia Nervosa, Restricting Type, 21% of individuals diagnosed with Bulimia Nervosa, and 9% of individuals diagnosed with Binge Eating Disorder also meet criteria for Borderline Personality Disorder (Cassin & von Ranson, 2005). Additionally, the rates of suicide attempts and non-suicidal self-injury (NSSI) in individuals diagnosed with an eating disorder are also notably elevated. According to one study, 15.7% of individuals diagnosed with Anorexia Nervosa, Restricting Type, 44.1% of individuals diagnosed with Anorexia Nervosa, Binge/Purge Type, 31.4% of individuals diagnosed with Bulimia Nervosa, and 22.9% of individuals

DOI: 10.4324/9781003495604-2

diagnosed with Binge Eating Disorder have made a suicide attempt (Udo, Bitley, & Grilo, 2019). Up to 72% of individuals diagnosed with an eating disorder also engage in non-suicidal self-injury (NSSI), with estimates ranging from 13.6% to 42.1% for individuals diagnosed with Anorexia Nervosa, Restricting Type, 27.8% to 68.1% for individuals diagnosed with Anorexia Nervosa, Binge/Purge Type, and 26% to 55% for individuals diagnosed with Bulimia Nervosa (Claes & Muehlenkamp, 2014).

The overlap between eating disorders and substance use disorders is also substantial. Up to 50% of individuals with an eating disorder will abuse a substance and 35% of individuals who abuse substances will also meet criteria for an eating disorder (National Center on Addiction and Substance Use, 2003). Looking at eating disorders by subtype, Bulimia Nervosa tends to have the highest association with comorbid substance use, followed by Binge Eating Disorder. It appears that substance use in individuals diagnosed with Anorexia Nervosa may also be more common than initially thought, although when examining subtypes of Anorexia Nervosa, this increase is likely accounted for by individuals diagnosed with Anorexia Nervosa, Binge/Purge Type. Examining the literature as a whole it appears as though purging behavior specifically, regardless of diagnosis, may be most related to increased rates of substance use.

The first study examining the effectiveness of DBT in the treatment of eating disorders was conducted by Telch, Agras, and Linehan (2001) and focused on the use of DBT in the treatment of women diagnosed with Binge Eating Disorder. The study found significant improvements in binge eating and eating disorder psychopathology in comparison to controls, with binge abstinence rates of 89% at the end of treatment and 56% at six-month follow-up for the DBT condition. No differences were found between the treatment condition and control condition on measures of weight, affect regulation, or mood. A subsequent randomized controlled trial comparing DBT-BED (DBT for Binge Eating Disorder) to active comparison group therapy found that DBT-BED had fewer treatment dropouts and greater initial improvement in symptoms, as measured by abstinence from binge episodes (64% for DBT-BED versus 34% of active comparison group therapy at posttreatment). However, the differences in abstinence rates between groups narrowed substantially at subsequent follow-ups, with DBT-BED maintaining a 64% abstinence rate and active comparison group therapy achieving an abstinence rate of 56% (Safer, Robinson, & Jo, 2010). The most recent randomized controlled trial was conducted with individuals labeled as overweight who were also diagnosed with binge eating disorder and compared a DBT group to a waitlist control group (Rahmani, Omidi, Asemi, & Akbari, 2018). Individuals in the DBT group showed greater improvements in symptoms of binge eating disorder and their ability to regulate emotions and also demonstrated greater reductions in body mass index (BMI) than individuals in the control group. Remaining research has been limited to pilot studies (e.g.

Chen, et al., 2008; Masson, et al., 2013) and quasi-experimental research (e.g. Lammers, et al., 2020), which has continued to suggest that DBT is an effective treatment for Binge Eating Disorder. Further research continues to be needed, particularly research focused on comparison to other empirically-supported treatments for Binge Eating Disorder.

Around the same time the application of DBT in the treatment of Binge Eating Disorder was being studied, a randomized controlled trial of DBT in the treatment of Bulimia Nervosa was also conducted (Safer, Telch, & Agras, 2001). The study found significant decreases in bingeing and purging behavior in the DBT condition in comparison to waitlist controls. As with the study examining the effectiveness of DBT in the treatment of Binge Eating Disorder, no significant differences were found between conditions on measures of affect regulation and mood. Since this time, only one additional randomized controlled trial has been conducted, which focused on a modified version of DBT, called appetite focused DBT (DBT-AF) (Hill, Craighead, & Safer, 2011). The study found that those receiving treatment displayed fewer symptoms of Bulimia Nervosa than controls. Ultimately, all participants received treatment and 61.5% of participants achieved sufficient symptom reduction to no longer meet full or subthreshold criteria for Bulimia Nervosa and 26.9% achieved full abstinence from binge/purge episodes over the past month. The remaining studies have been limited to case studies (e.g. Salbach-Andrae, et al., 2008), open trials (Murray, et al., 2015), and pilot studies (e.g. Fischer & Peterson, 2015), all of which have demonstrated promising preliminary results.

Unfortunately, no randomized controlled trials have been conducted examining the application of standard DBT in the treatment of Anorexia Nervosa. Research to date has been limited to a pre-post open trial (Kröeger, Schweiger, Sipos, Kliem, Arnold, Schunert, & Reinecker, 2010) and case studies (Salbach-Andrae, Bohnekamp, Pfeiffer, Lehmkuhl, & Miller, 2008), although both studies found promising results in terms of remission rates. However, an adaptation of standard DBT, called Radically Open DBT (RO DBT), has been studied. The initial research on RO DBT was focused on the use of RO DBT as a treatment for treatment resistant depression and maladaptive overcontrol features. Given that maladaptive overcontrol behaviors are common and pervasive in individuals diagnosed with Anorexia Nervosa, subsequent research has begun to examine RO DBT as a treatment for this specific eating disorder. The first study exploring the efficacy of RO DBT in the treatment of Anorexia Nervosa was conducted by Lynch and colleagues in 2013. In the study, 47 individuals diagnosed with Anorexia Nervosa, Restricting Type who were being treated in an inpatient setting received RO DBT. The overall response rate was 90%, with 35% of participants achieving full remission and 55% of participants achieving partial remission. Subsequent research on the effectiveness of RO DBT in the treatment of Anorexia Nervosa, although promising, has been limited to case series' (e.g. Baudinet, et al., 2020; Chen, et al., 2015; Isaksson, et al., 2021).

The growing body of research on the application of DBT in the treatment of eating disorders has also allowed for various systematic reviews and meta-analyses to be conducted. The first systematic review by Bankoff, Karpel, Forbes, and Pantalone (2012) looked at thirteen peer reviewed articles published between 2000 and 2011 that examined treatment efficacy of DBT in any form for individuals diagnosed with Bulimia Nervosa, Binge Eating Disorder, or Anorexia Nervosa, with or without a diagnosis of comorbid Borderline Personality Disorder. Nine studies were reviewed to determine the efficacy of DBT as a treatment for eating disorders, with eight of the nine studies finding that DBT reduced the frequency of eating disorder behaviors. Although results varied widely, abstinence and remission rates from the studies examined were also promising. Four studies were also reviewed to determine the efficacy of DBT for comorbid eating disorders and Borderline Personality Disorder. All four studies found that DBT reduced the frequency of eating disorder behaviors and abstinence and remission data for eating disorders were also promising. All thirteen studies found reductions in overall psychopathology, including self-injurious behaviors and symptoms of mood and anxiety disorders. Lastly, a number of studies examined found positive results in terms of treatment dropout, which is particularly notable given the ambivalence that many patients with eating disorders experience around pursuing treatment and recovery.

A subsequent meta-analysis conducted by Lenz and colleagues (2014) examined the effectiveness of DBT for treating eating disorder episodes as well as treating co-occurring symptoms of depression among people diagnosed with eating disorders. Nine studies from peer-reviewed publications that utilized either between-group or single-group designs were included in the analyses. Patients were a mix of individuals diagnosed with Binge Eating Disorder, Bulimia Nervosa, Anorexia Nervosa, and Eating Disorder Not Otherwise Specified. Settings in which the studies were conducted also varied, with six studies being conducted in an outpatient level of care, two studies being conducted at inpatient facilities, and one study being conducted at a partial hospitalization level of care. The meta-analysis found a large effect size for between-group studies and a very large effect size for single-group studies in terms of decreases in eating disorder episodes. Positive results were also found in terms of reducing co-occurring symptoms of depression, with between-group studies yielding a medium effect size and single-group studies yielding a very large effect size.

Two other systematic reviews and meta-analyses have been conducted more recently. Rozakou-Soumalia, Dârvariu, and Sjögren (2021) conducted a systematic review and meta-analysis examining the effectiveness of DBT in targeting eating disorder symptoms, emotion dysregulation, and general psychopathology. Eleven studies were included and participants in the studies were primarily diagnosed with either Binge Eating Disorder or Bulimia Nervosa, although one study included participants with Anorexia Nervosa. The quality assessment of the overall meta-analysis was assessed as intermediate, due to some of the included studies having some risk of bias. Greater improvements were found in measures of eating disorder psychopathology, objective binge episodes, BMI, emotion regulation, and depressive symptoms for individuals who received DBT in comparison to individuals assigned to control groups.

Buerger and colleagues (2021) specifically examined the effectiveness of third-wave interventions for adolescents and young adults with eating disorders. Twelve studies, two of which were randomized controlled trials and the remainder of which were uncontrolled pre-post studies, were included in the systematic review and meta-analysis. Eleven of the twelve studies included in the systematic review and meta-analysis either utilized DBT as a sole intervention or as a component of the treatment intervention utilized in the study. Although moderate effects in terms of changes in Eating Disorders Examination (EDE) scores were found, the authors cautioned that the low quality of research to date coupled with the significant variation in terms of elements of DBT utilized in this research should limit any conclusions made about the effectiveness of DBT as a treatment intervention for adolescents and young adults diagnosed with eating disorders.

Finally, of particular note for clinicians working with child, adolescent, and young adult populations, recent research has begun to explore outcomes associated with blended FBT-DBT approaches in the treatment of eating disorders. Murray and colleagues (2015) examined the efficacy of a blended FBT-DBT approach for adolescents diagnosed with Bulimia Nervosa being treated at a partial hospitalization level of care. Results of this open pilot trial demonstrated significant improvements in general eating disorder psychopathology, objective binge episodes, and self-induced vomiting. A significant increase in parental efficacy was found as well. A second study by Johnston and colleagues (2015) examined the effectiveness of an intensive outpatient program that combined FBT with DBT skills training groups. This pilot study found significant decreases in eating disorder psychopathology and significant improvements with regard to weight restoration. Sixty-four percent of participants were weight restored at one-year follow-up and eating disorder psychopathology also continued to improve. A third study by Pennell and colleagues (2020) examined treatment outcomes for adolescents who completed a DBT-informed partial hospitalization program that integrated FBT into treatment as well. Findings of the study demonstrated improvements in weight restoration and decreases in bingeing and purging behaviors. Finally, a pilot study by Peterson and colleagues (2019) examined the effectiveness of a DBT skills group as adjunct to FBT for adolescents diagnosed with a restrictive eating disorder. Large effect sizes were found for increases in adaptive skills and decreases in maladaptive coping, small to medium effects sizes were found for decreases in binge eating and improvements in weight restoration, and small effect sizes were found for decreases in global eating disorder psychopathology, restraint, and symptoms of depression. Although more methodologically rigorous studies are needed to examine the effectiveness of a blended FBT-DBT approach, results from these initial studies show promise.

Chapter 3

Bringing DBT to Life

In our collective years of experience providing supervision, consultation, and training focused on DBT principles and strategies, we have found that for many providers, it is hard to understand DBT concepts without consistently and directly linking them to patient care. We have observed that providers are able to make incredible growth with regard to patient care when they are able to see what DBT actually looks like in an interaction between patient and provider. As such, we will be introducing a patient whom you will be following throughout this book as we demonstrate how to apply specific DBT principles and strategies. The patient we describe below is a fictional one, however one who bears resemblance to many of the patients with whom we have both worked.

Bringing DBT to Life – Patient Vignette

Megan is a 24-year-old, Caucasian, cisgender female from Youngstown, Ohio, who spent her early childhood in a small suburban home with her mother, father, and three siblings. She recalls both her parents as being hard-working, lower middle class individuals who frequently worked overtime in order to make ends meet. While she had a good relationship with her mother, she remembers her mother often dieting, avoiding "fattening foods," and taking diet pills. She recalls regular verbal conflict between her parents, which often worsened in intensity in the context of her father consuming alcohol. Much of her father's commentary was about her mother's weight and appearance, as well as being "an emotional trainwreck." Verbal conflicts eventually escalated into physical conflicts, including a particularly salient instance in which Megan witnessed her older brother being struck violently by her father as he tried to intervene during a physical altercation. As a result of their ongoing verbal and physical conflicts, Megan's mother made the decision to divorce her husband when Megan was eight years old.

After her parents' divorce, Megan's mother relied greatly on her parents to watch Megan and her siblings, as working as many hours as possible became

DOI: 10.4324/9781003495604-3

necessary to support her family. In the context of these roles, Megan's grandparents were responsible for the majority of decisions around meals and snacks, in addition to fulfilling other parental duties. Megan's grandparents also relied on other family members to provide support. Megan's uncle was one of the individuals who was asked to provide supervision on occasion and in this context, he became the perpetrator of multiple instances of childhood sexual abuse toward Megan specifically. Megan remembers attempting to speak with her oldest brother about what was happening, however he accused Megan of lying about her experience. The instances of abuse stopped when Megan's uncle took a job in another state.

Megan recalls her older brothers picking on her due to her weight, which included some name calling and comparing her to her peers. Megan also remembers her pediatrician referencing the growth charts around age 10, stating Megan would "benefit from watching what she eats." Around age 11, Megan noticed her weight increased further leading up to puberty. At this time, her grandparents began to cut her portions and encourage more physical activity. Over the next year or two, Megan remembers losing weight and receiving a lot of positive feedback from her peers, teachers, and family. Taking this as a challenge, Megan started to overly fixate on her weight and food consumption, tracking everything she ate in her journal, with the goal to be "as skinny as possible." She describes her obsession with tracking as "almost ritualistic" and compulsive. She began to weigh herself multiple times per day, a behavior that has continued to the present day. She recalls hiding Halloween and Easter candies and other "junk foods," feeling she would be shamed by her brothers if they found out. She continued to focus on cutting back on food through early high school, believing she would only attain new friendships in a smaller body. She recalls excelling at school at this time, pushing herself for "a perfect grade, anything less was unacceptable." Around the same time she started to experience periods of overeating that escalated quickly, occurring multiple times a week. The binges would always occur following periods of significant restriction during which Megan would aim to consume less than 500 calories a day. Megan recalls extreme efforts, such as stealing food and taking food out of garbage cans, to satisfy her binges. She chose to not disclose this behavior to anyone due to the immense shame she experienced. She also started stealing her grandfather's vodka when she could, finding relief and escape in inebriation, similar to what she noticed with binge eating and purging. Concurrently, a peer of Megan's suggested she start to self-induce vomiting so she could eat freely and "not worry about gaining weight."

Megan experienced another instance of sexual assault in tenth grade, in the context of attending a house party. While at the party, she consumed multiple alcoholic beverages, to the point her memory became somewhat impaired. After assisting her in walking to a spare bedroom where she planned to lie down for a bit, one of the partygoers sexually assaulted her and then left the party. Megan blames herself for the assault.

Megan continued to cycle through periods of restriction, binge eating and purging until her eleventh-grade teacher became aware via concerns expressed by a friend of Megan. Megan entered residential treatment in April of that year for her eating disorder and initially responded well with "full intention of actually recovering," but eventually struggled with an increase in depression and suicidality as eating disorder behaviors improved. Additionally, she began engaging in self-injurious behavior by cutting with a razor on her inner thighs, typically occurring two to three times per week. She always cuts in the same place with the same implement.

Megan cycled between levels of care and other facilities when treatment wasn't effective. She recalls brief periods of reprieve from eating disorder behaviors where she remembers being "committed to recovery," however notes these were times when she eventually turned back to alcohol or self-injurious behaviors. Her passive suicidality and hopelessness remained pervasive as she spent her late teens and early twenties in and out of treatment centers. She has had two inpatient admissions for brief psychiatric stabilization following two suicide attempts of high lethality, the second requiring brief intubation. She recalls that these attempts were premeditated with extensive planning.

Despite multiple instances of treatment throughout her adolescent and adult life to date, Megan was slowly able to complete her Pharmacy Technology diploma through her local community college. Her employment has been sporadic since receiving her diploma and has included work both in pharmacies and grocery stores. In terms of interpersonal relationships, she has a small number of friendships, largely with individuals she has known since middle school. She cites "trust issues" as the main barrier to establishing new relationships. She is currently single and does not have a history of any significant romantic relationships. Her interest in recreational activities is relatively limited, although she does enjoy spending time outdoors, reading books, and caring for animals.

At present, we find Megan in her eighth eating disorder treatment center on residential level of care, an admission that follows an unexpected encounter with the perpetrator of her childhood sexual abuse at a family reunion. Following this encounter, Megan began to engage in significant restriction that led to rapid weight loss, in addition to returning to purging behaviors in the absence of binge eating. Megan reported that she had been engaging in infrequent self-injurious behaviors via cutting approximately one to two times per month. She stated that her symptoms of depression are at "baseline," and expressed hopelessness that they will ever improve. Megan reported that she has been abstinent from alcohol for the past year and a half. Finally, with regard to symptoms related to trauma, Megan reported that she is not experiencing any currently, although said it's possible that she's "numbed" herself out to the point it wouldn't be possible to experience them even if they were present. She considers herself "treatment savvy" at this point and expects treatment to go a certain way, noting, "I'll do most of what you say to get through the program as quickly as possible to return to my eating disorder. I'll probably find loopholes in the system as I go along… I always do." Megan also offers she likes to know when her providers plan to see her for a session as "spontaneity doesn't work" and she has a hard time set-shifting if her schedule goes awry.

Diagnostically, Megan meets criteria for the following: Anorexia Nervosa, Binge Eating and Purging Subtype, Alcohol Use Disorder, Moderate, in Sustained Remission, Major Depressive Disorder, Recurrent, Moderate, Posttraumatic Stress Disorder, and features of Borderline Personality Disorder.

Provider Exercise – Your Initial Thoughts About Megan

What are your thoughts about Megan's case? Consider taking notes in the space below about your initial impressions, recommendations for treatment, case conceptualization, and potential treatment interventions. In completing this exercise and then reflecting upon it after completing this text, we hope you are able to see both ways in which your current approach to case conceptualization and treatment planning dovetails with DBT principles and strategies, as well as ways to enhance your work through information you will learn in reading this text.

Chapter 4

The "Spirit" of DBT

Before entering into a detailed discussion of strategies drawn from DBT, we thought it important to start with a discussion of the "spirit" of DBT. Embracing the "spirit" of DBT is a great starting point for non-therapist providers to begin to engage with the principles of DBT, without becoming overwhelmed by specific terms and jargon or lack of knowledge about psychotherapy more broadly. Furthermore, we would argue that a provider who embraces the "spirit" of DBT while still learning about specific strategies is likely to be more effective than a provider who knows an assortment of strategies drawn from DBT but lacks a larger framework and DBT-consistent mindset. Metaphorically, if I'm attending a book club meeting and haven't read the book, but have an hour to read something before going to the meeting, I'd rather have an opportunity to read an overarching summary of the book over reading random paragraphs selected from different chapters in the book. Understanding overall themes and sentiments is likely to be more useful than granular details without context.

DBT as a Principle-Driven Treatment

It is important to know that DBT is a principle-driven treatment, rather than a protocol-driven treatment. This means that although there are manuals that describe DBT as a treatment, DBT treatment done well is not "manualized." Focusing on therapists specifically, there are tools that can be used to measure adherence to treatment, however paths achieving the threshold of adherence within a given session can look quite different. Two therapists might approach the same session using different therapeutic styles and with some variation in treatment interventions, yet through operating from the same set of principles they both could meet the threshold for an adherent session. This is in stark contrast to session-by-session manualized protocols that offer little room for deviation from content or process.

What is the benefit of operating from a principle-driven standpoint, particularly in the treatment of eating disorders? It is important to remember that DBT

DOI: 10.4324/9781003495604-4

adapted for the treatment of eating disorders is an adaptation from the original treatment, as is DBT being applied at higher levels of care, as is DBT being utilized with children or adolescents. This means that DBT being used to treat a child with an eating disorder in a residential setting is an adaptation upon an adaptation upon an adaptation! There is no way to rigidly apply standard DBT, nor any of its adaptations in a situation such as this one.

However, there is a much more compelling rationale than simple necessity for principle-driven rather than protocol-driven care. Working with patients in general, let alone patients diagnosed with eating disorders who often present with complex comorbidities, will often lead you into uncharted territory. Humans are complex beings. When operating from a protocol-driven framework, there is only if-then decision-making, which can only respond to a certain degree of complexity and which rarely comes accompanied with a Plan B or Plan C option if Plan A isn't working. Operating from a principle-driven framework allows us to respond to the individualized nature of patient care, and also opens up the possibility of there being multiple "right" solutions to any given patient scenario.

The Dialectical Worldview

In order to be able to strive toward living into the "spirit" of DBT, it is first important to understand the dialectical worldview, as this is the framework from which DBT-informed providers think about the nature of reality and human behavior. The dialectical worldview is made up of three principles: the principle of interrelatedness and wholeness, the principle of polarity, and the principle of continuous change (for additional perspectives on the dialectical worldview, readers are encouraged to review Linehan, 1993, pp. 31–35).

The principle of interrelatedness and wholeness takes a systems view of reality. In order to understand the parts of a system, you must also understand the system itself, as well as the ongoing transactions between the system and its parts. As an example of this principle in action at a macro level, we might look at the transaction between diet culture and an individual patient. Diet culture is one of many complex factors that may play into the development of eating disorders and how a patient interacts with diet culture can have an impact not only on that individual, but may have transactional impacts on their family members, their peers, corporations, and diet culture as a whole. For example, a patient who embraces a diet culture mentality may express this through their posts on social media. A positive response from their followers on social media not only impacts the patient, in that they may be likely to post similar content in the future and may find that the response further reinforces their diet culture mentality, but it may impact the thoughts and behaviors of their social media followers as well, perpetuating diet culture at a more systemic level. Transactions between a patient and diet culture can also work out in ways that are more positive. For example, one of my (AHK) favorite group topics to cover, particularly with adolescents, is media literacy. In exploring the messages they receive from advertising, television, movies, and so forth, and who benefits from these messages, I have found that many patients choose to engage with media through a more critical lens moving forward, and that some have even chosen to take actions advocating for systemic change. In this example, e-mails and phone calls to corporations advocating for changes to their media portrayals may lead to changes around the extent to which they choose to convey diet culture messages moving forward, which in turn can have impacts on an individual patient. As an example of the principle of interrelatedness and wholeness at play at a more micro level, I think about the involvement of families and supports in eating disorders treatment. All patients come from a context and either will return to that context after treatment (for patients who are being treated at a higher level of care) or will remain in that context as they receive treatment. While our work with our patients individually can certainly impact their thoughts, feelings, and behavior, there is a compelling argument for working to directly impact our patients' families and supports as well when we are considering human behavior from the framework of the principle of interrelatedness and wholeness. Through impacting how our patients' families and supports respond in their interactions with our patients, we are indirectly influencing our patient's behavior as well.

The principle of polarity views reality as being composed of opposing forces, referred to as the thesis and antithesis, that are integrated to create a synthesis, which in turn has its own new opposing forces. There is benefit for patients and providers alike to embrace the principle of polarity in the treatment of our patients' eating disorders. There are a number of common dialectical "failures" expressed as eating disorder symptomatology, like cycles of binging, purging, and restricting, or black-and-white thinking. Many of the therapeutic strategies you will learn throughout this book focus on helping patients to think and act more dialectically, which aligns with the principle of polarity. From a provider standpoint, the principle of polarity can help us to better understand our patients. Through this principle, we can see both the function and dysfunction of our patients' eating disorder behaviors. For example, if purging has the immediate effect of reducing anxiety for a patient, it can make sense that they have relied on purging as a coping mechanism and simultaneously, purging for most people is not a sustainable or values-consistent way to manage anxiety. The principle of polarity can also help us to see both the valid and invalid in our patients' eating disorder thinking. For example, a patient who is undergoing weight restoration is indeed experiencing body changes, so is not incorrect in thinking and perceiving that their body is changing, and the thoughts and perceptions around these body changes can be quite distorted in comparison to reality. Finally, the principle of polarity can help us as providers to be more flexible in our approach to treatment. At times as providers, we can become entrenched in the belief that our course of action is the only "right" way to approach treatment when there are other courses of action that may be equally as valid. The principle of polarity sets the stage for being curious about what you might be missing in terms of understanding your patient and how that missing information impacts your approach to treatment.

Finally, the first two principles necessitate that the principle of continuous change exists. If the world is comprised of parts that are transacting with the whole in an ongoing way and if the nature of reality is such that it is dynamic rather than static, then an unavoidable byproduct of the first two principles of the dialectical worldview is that the world is in a state of continuous change. Marsha Linehan describes a tension that emerges for patients in this context where there is both a desire for self-preservation and a simultaneous desire for self-transformation. The tension between these two poles is particularly salient when working with patients diagnosed with eating disorders. There is often both a desire on the part of our patients to hold on to their eating disorder at all costs, while at the same time a desire to be relieved from the anguish caused by their eating disorder. Successful treatment often involves repeated iterations of a negotiation of where a patient can maintain the status quo and where the patient has the capacity and willingness to make change, out of which emerges a new status quo from which self-preservation and self-transformation are negotiated yet again.

Provider Exercise – Reflecting on the Dialectical Worldview

What are your initial reactions to the dialectical worldview? In what ways is it consistent with your perspectives about the nature of reality and in what ways does it differ? Now that you have learned about the dialectical worldview, do you think that this will impact how you conceptualize and/or treat your patients? If yes, in what ways? Make some notes on your initial reflections about the dialectical worldview below and consider discussing your initial thoughts and reactions with a trusted colleague.

DBT Assumptions

Another important element in embodying the "spirit" of DBT involves embracing the DBT assumptions. In short, the DBT assumptions are a list of statements that reflect core beliefs about patients, providers, and DBT as a treatment. What you may notice in reviewing the DBT assumptions is that many of them are borne out of the dialectical worldview. The assumptions listed below are based on the original DBT assumptions (Linehan, 1993), with some additions and adaptations based on the work of Lucene Wisniewski (Wiśniewski, 2018).

Assumption #1: Patients are doing the best they can. When we take into account a patient's makeup in terms of biology, temperament, history, abilities, comorbidities, and so forth, DBT operates under the assumption that when all of these things are considered, our patients are doing the very best they can in that exact moment. It can be hard to hold this assumption to be true when we are working with a patient who is refusing to even pick up a utensil in the context of a meal or who says they are too depressed to get out of bed and go to a group, yet we believe that even in these circumstances our patients are doing the very best they possibly can. Eating disorders are often disorders of ambivalence and shifting degrees of motivation. It can be easy to forget that decreasing ambivalence and increasing motivation often requires a "perfect storm" of hopeful emotions and thoughts, skills and planful behaviors, and environmental factors reinforcing positive change to all align! For many of our patients who have sought out a higher level of care, they have come to this level of treatment because their very best efforts in lower levels of care were still not sufficient to create change. Thus, it is critical to avoid sending the invalidating message that their current efforts at change are not the extent of effort they have the capacity to bring. When we take the time to explore in-depth with a patient the factors that have blocked adaptive responding, you will often find they have made efforts beyond what you can even imagine to try to make change in those moments.

Assumption #2: Patients want to improve. We operate under the assumption that any patient who is in treatment, regardless of their stated reason for being there, wants something to be different in their lives. This can be hard to believe when a patient is simultaneously stating that they never want to give up their eating disorder, yet we believe it is not only possible but actually helpful to hold both sides of this dialectic. There are so many reasons our patients may struggle around willingness to let go of their eating disorder, including fears of who they would be without it or how they would tolerate their emotional distress, hopelessness about their ability to make sustained change, concerns about their ability to fulfill the functions their eating disorder has served with more adaptive behaviors, and so on. To paraphrase Marsha Linehan, to assume that our patients aren't improving to the extent that we might want or at a pace that we find to be more tolerable because they simply don't want to is faulty logic at best, and a further barrier to helping us to help them be more motivated to change at worst.

Assumption #3: Patients need to do better, try harder, and be more motivated to change. Assumption #3 provides the necessary opposite side of the dialectic of assumption #1, and honors the tension within assumption #2. While we can honor and wholeheartedly believe that our patients are doing the very best they can at any given moment, it is also necessary that they do better, try harder, and be more motivated to change, and as providers, we have tools that can help. Among the many things we can offer our patients, we can teach them new skills, cheerlead them on in exceeding what they thought to be possible, and help them connect with their values and goals in the service of enhancing their motivation. Metaphorically, I (AHK) relate the combination of assumption #1 and assumption #3 to my experience in running road races. I do not find running to be enjoyable in the slightest. I've often found myself running at a pace that I truly believed to be the maximum pace I could run at that given moment – in other words, me trying the very best that I can – only to find that as I take in other things going on in my environment (e.g. another runner passing me, people cheering and waving encouraging signs, a high-energy song coming on my playlist), I all of a sudden have the capacity to do better and try harder. Assumption #1 and assumption #3 can comfortably coexist.

Assumption #4: Patients may not have caused all of their own problems, but they have to solve them anyway. Eating disorders are biologically-mediated, brain-based illnesses. With this in mind, our patients, as well as their families and supports, did not cause their eating disorder. Yet our patients are the only people with the power to implement the solutions necessary for eating disorder recovery. I've (AHK) had patients wish aloud that there was some way I could swap their brain out and give them a reboot of sorts. If only I was so lucky to possess such a power! The reality is that the tools we can offer our patients only go so far without their buy-in and associated efforts.

Assumption #5: For many patients, their current lives are unbearable. It is absolutely critical as providers that we do not minimize our patients' pain. Many patients with eating disorders present as suffering less than they actually are. At the same time, many of our patients must feel their suffering is truly understood before they can summon the motivation and energy to make difficult changes. Understand and acknowledge that for many of your patients, they are truly in a living hell.

Assumption #6: Patients must learn new behaviors in all relevant contexts. One of the challenges that goes along with eating disorder treatment in general, but particularly eating disorder treatment at higher levels of care, is that our patients must learn to emit adaptive behaviors and effectively utilize skills across all relevant contexts in their lives. Treatment at an inpatient or residential level of care bears little resemblance to the environment a patient will ultimately return home to. A critical component of treatment for our patients is figuring out ways for them to practice adaptive behaviors and skills in all contexts that they will routinely encounter in their lives. As we will discuss much later on in this book, thoughtful exposures and other homework assignments play a critical role in helping our patients to emit adaptive behaviors across all contexts.

Assumption #7: The most caring thing a provider can do is help patients to change in ways that bring them closer to their own ultimate goals. While this assumption might seem to be quite self-evident, there are nuances within it that are important to highlight. First, there are times when helping a patient to make change does not actually feel particularly caring, whether it is watching a patient sob through an entire meal or become angry at you for setting and holding firm to a boundary. Helping patients make significant and lasting change in the context of eating disorder treatment means being willing to do things that won't always feel good to you or to your patient. Second, it is important to be cognizant of your patient's ultimate goals. This is important to highlight because in eating disorders work, sometimes it can be hard to find our patient's life worth living goals buried beneath the heap of goals set by their eating disorder.

Assumption #8: Patients cannot fail in treatment. As we will discuss more thoroughly in the next two assumptions, if a patient drops out of treatment, doesn't make progress in treatment, or actually becomes more ill in the context of treatment, this is because the treatment has failed, the patient's providers have failed, or both. When patients don't make progress in treatment or become more ill in the context of treatment, the story that providers often tell places the blame on the shoulders of the patient. We have all probably heard our colleagues say or have said ourselves things along the lines of, "They just weren't ready to change" or "They weren't really motivated for treatment" about our patients. "Readiness" and "motivation" are never the sole determinants of patient progress or lack thereof in treatment. However, even if these variables were the only things that accounted for patient change, the onus is on providers and the treatment itself to provide mechanisms by which readiness and motivation can be enhanced.

Assumption #9: DBT providers can fail. This assumption is often an emotionally evocative one for providers, and if you are striving to become the best provider you can be in the treatment of eating disorders, it is critical to give this assumption consideration. I (AHK) would argue that DBT does not make the assumption of intentional or calculated failure on the part of providers and there are ways in which providers can engage in behaviors that result in a failure of treatment. Some examples that come to mind are failing to make adequate efforts toward maintaining adherence to DBT principles and strategies, incorporating other treatments lacking in empirical support while also attempting to maintain adherence to DBT principles and strategies, or rigidly applying DBT strategies in a way that appears to adhere to the protocol of DBT while falling short of aligning with the spirit of DBT.

Assumption #10: DBT can fail even when providers do not. As with any treatment, medical or psychological, DBT is imperfect. There is no treatment that I (AHK) can think of that is guaranteed to work for 100% of patients 100% of the time. You can provide patient care in a way that is fully consistent with DBT principles and that appropriately applies DBT strategies in the right contexts and your patient may not improve and may actually worsen. For some patients, DBT simply isn't the right fit for them. For other patients, DBT very much might be the right fit, yet still missing some yet-to-be-discovered components that would be needed to make it an effective treatment for your patient. There will be times where you put your very best effort forth and treatment still comes up short.

Assumption #11: Clarity, precision, and compassion are of the utmost importance in the conduct of DBT. This assumption summarizes many elements of DBT that make it such an artful and effective treatment. DBT done well is thorough in our assessment of the problems our patients face, thoughtfully targeted in the specific interventions that are chosen for specific problems, and both these things are done with a backdrop of unrelenting compassion for our patients.

Assumption #12: Behavioral principles are universal, affecting providers no less than patients. As much as we may not like to admit it, providers are subject to principles of reinforcement, shaping, extinction, and punishment just as much as our patients are! For example, if I (AHK) have a patient who used to complete their therapy homework every week and discuss it with me at the beginning of session, but for the past month has told me they haven't done their homework when I ask about it in session, the behavior of asking for completed therapy homework assignments could become extinguished. Similarly, if I have a patient who refuses to talk or becomes angry with me any time I try to discuss an eating disorder behavior that has occurred, but who engages warmly and deeply in discussion about difficulties she is having with her husband, you might be able to see how this dynamic could shape what I choose to bring up in session if I'm not being mindful of the behavioral principles at play. This assumption can help you stay aware of behavioral principles on a moment-to-moment basis and whether your responses in the context of these behavioral principles are effective or maladaptive.

Assumption #13: Providers need support. We would argue that all healthcare providers, regardless of area of focus, need support in doing their work and two elements of eating disorders care make this support particularly crucial. First, eating disorders have a notably elevated mortality rate, both due to medical and psychiatric reasons, that is often painfully accompanied by patient ambivalence around seeking treatment, staying in treatment, and pursuing recovery. Having these two realities in play simultaneously is a recipe for provider burnout, particularly in the absence of support from other providers who understand what this experience is like. Second, it is difficult to provide effective eating disorder care when existing in silos. Good eating disorders treatment requires a true multidisciplinary team, rather than a group of treatment providers operating independent of each other. You enter risky territory if you don't have an understanding of how your patient is doing from a psychological, medical and nutritional standpoint. For example, if I (AHK) am working with a patient who is denying all eating disorder behaviors, however that patient's laboratory tests suggest that behaviors are occurring, that is critical information for me to be aware of. Doing this work requires support and requires teamwork.

Provider Exercise – Reflecting on the DBT Assumptions

As you reviewed the DBT assumptions, what thoughts and emotional reactions did you have? Are there specific DBT assumptions that resonated with you? Are there specific DBT assumptions that you disagree with? How do you envision the DBT assumptions influencing how you provide patient care? Are there ways you would like to intentionally incorporate the DBT assumptions into your work? Make some notes on your initial thoughts about the DBT assumptions below and consider discussing your initial thoughts and reactions with a trusted colleague.

DBT Provider Characteristics

There are three dialectics that are present when considering a provider's over-arching stance with regard to DBT (readers are encouraged to review Linehan, 1993, pp. 108–111). The first of these dialectics is acceptance versus change. As we will allude to at various points throughout this text, eating disorders are disorders that are often characterized by ambivalence. In order for a provider to be effective working with an individual diagnosed with an eating disorder, they must have the capacity not only to acknowledge this ambivalence, but be willing to wholeheartedly embrace it. This is the antidote to the "just eat a sandwich" mantra or other invalidating messages our patients have heard as solutions to their eating disorder. By accepting where our patients are, we acknowledge that their eating disorder behaviors serve very real and very critical functions in their day-to-day lives. Imagine how hard it might be to give up a set of behaviors that regulated unpleasant affect, communicated your needs to others, quieted an unrelenting negative internal dialogue, or made up what you perceived to be the very core of your identity. By taking the stance of acceptance, we acknowledge that our patients have needs that their eating disorder has served the function of fulfilling. On the other side of the dialectic, we know that eating disorder behaviors are not a sustainable solution in terms of meeting these needs. With the exception of Opioid Use Disorders, Anorexia Nervosa is the most lethal mental illness. For our patients, they cannot work to fulfill needs if they are dead. Taking up the side of change, we recognize that patients have entered into treatment for a reason. Sometimes this reason is internally motivated and some-times it is externally motivated, and there is a reason nonetheless. Something has to change, and we can provide our patients with solutions that meet similar functions that their eating disorder behaviors serve.

One of the contexts in which we have found wholeheartedly embracing the acceptance and change dialectic is when we have worked with individuals who have a more chronic illness course. There can be an overwhelming sense of urgency around the need for change for these individuals, particularly if they enter treatment in a medically or psychiatrically compromised state. Yet change is not something that can be forced, no matter the urgency of the situation. Opening up the possibility for change paradoxically begins with deeply and wholeheartedly accepting your patient and the situation at hand before beginning to seek a path forward.

The second dialectic present within a DBT provider's overarching stance toward treatment is that of unwavering centeredness versus compassionate flexibility. Unwavering centeredness involves believing in yourself, in the patient, in the patient's team of providers, and in the treatment you are providing. Staying the course in eating disorders treatment is oftentimes challenging. When a patient is becoming increasingly unstable due to an increase in eating disorder behaviors or when a parent or family member is anxious or frustrated and expressing to you that they feel treatment isn't working, it can be tempting to make a significant change in your approach to treatment, even if you believe that treatment as you are providing it is working. Unwavering centeredness is knowing your true north and moving toward it, regardless of the chaos that might be surrounding you. On the other side of the dialectic is compassionate flexibility, which involves being willing to let go of a strongly held perspective or opinion in the service of better meeting the needs of your patient or their supports. This doesn't mean that you stop going toward your true north, but perhaps you consider a different path in getting there. I (AHK) think that imagery can be a powerful teaching tool, so I like to use a scene from the movie "The Matrix" as another way to think about the dialectic of unwavering centeredness versus compassionate flexibility. There is a scene in "The Matrix" where Neo, the protagonist in the movie, is in a gunfight with the antagonist of the movie, Agent Smith. As Agent Smith fires dozens of bullets in Neo's direction, time slows and Neo flexibly bends his body around the bullets, all while keeping his feet firmly planted in the exact place they started! Thinking from a more clinical angle, a couple of examples come to mind. When working with a patient who is diagnosed with a more chronic form of Anorexia Nervosa, it may be quite likely that your patient is literally not able to focus simultaneously on weight restoration while also eating a socially normative, diverse array of foods. In honoring this dialectic, you may hold firm that 100% weight restoration is a non-negotiable goal (unwavering centeredness), while allowing your patient to have some choice in the process of moving that direction, perhaps through allowing unusual food choices (compassionate flexibility). As another example, in working with a patient on an outpatient basis, I may have the goal of the patient being able to complete 100% of the nutrition their body needs at each meal and snack, yet the patient might be clear in their unwillingness to do so at this present time. A way to strike the balance in these circumstances might be to find a goal that both you and the patient can agree upon that represents significant enough clinical progress, like eating 80% of the nutrition prescribed by their meal plan (compassionate flexibility), while also being entirely transparent that the end game is to get them to meet 100% of their nutritional needs on a consistent basis and incrementally adjusting the goal to move in this direction (unwavering centeredness). When we are too rigid as providers, we risk losing patients entirely, yet when we are too flexible, we can find ourselves in situations where our patients aren't progressing. Being strategic about the balance between unwavering centeredness and compassionate flexibility helps to avoid either outcome.

The final overarching dialectic embraced by DBT providers is nurturing versus benevolent demanding. Nurturing involves things like coaching, educating, and cheerleading our patients, all in a compassionate, validating, and supportive manner. The path to recovery is often long, challenging, and painful. Our patients deserve the same support, compassion, and patients that we would offer someone who was learning to walk after a severe accident. On the other side of the dialectic, benevolent demanding acknowledges that each of our patients has existing capacities and strengths that they can leverage in the treatment and recovery process. It is important not to fragilize our patients by stepping in to do things they are capable of doing themselves. To share another visually-oriented metaphor, balancing nurturing with benevolent demanding is like helping someone get over a tall wall. Faced with a wall where you can't even grab the top, you need someone or something to give you a bit of a height boost. At the same time, once you are able to grab the top of the wall, it's also critical that you use your strength to pull yourself up and over. This dialectic is often particularly relevant in the context of family and couples' work. For example, if I (AHK) am working with a patient who has difficulty having conversations with her family about what she needs, I am not doing this patient any favors by having those conversations on her behalf in a family therapy session. On the other side of the dialectic, I am also not doing her any favors if I expect her to have those difficult conversations on her own, without any preparation or support. Striking a balance here could involve giving my patient space during an individual session to role-play the conversation with her family, and then being present as she has the conversation with her family members, providing encouragement and coaching when needed.

Provider Exercise – Examining Where You Fall With Regard to Overall Provider Characteristics

For each of the dialectics below, put an "X" where you would say you land in terms of each dialectic and write a brief explanation for why you placed yourself there. If you would like to add a few additional fun twists to this exercise, try the following: (1) Consider whether you would have placed yourself at a different place on the dialectic at a different point in your professional career. Reflect on the factors that you believe accounted for any shifts in where you would have placed yourself before and where you place yourself currently, (2) Share this exercise with a trusted colleague and ask for their feedback about where they would put you on each of the dialectics. Have a conversation with them about the factors that led them to select that specific placement, and/or (3) Reflect on where you are currently with each of these dialectics and whether there are any shifts you think it could be beneficial to make in the service of providing optimal patient care.

Dialectic #1: Acceptance versus Change

I--I
Acceptance   Change

Why did you select this particular location on the dialectic?

Dialectic #2: Unwavering Centeredness versus Compassionate Flexibility

I--I
Unwavering Centeredness   Compassionate Flexibility

Why did you select this particular location on the dialectic?

Dialectic #3: Nurturing versus Benevolent Demanding

I--I
Nurturing   Benevolent Demanding

Why did you select this particular location on the dialectic?

Other Thoughts on the "Spirit" of DBT

There are a few other things we believe go into the "spirit" of DBT that aren't necessarily neatly captured in prior writing on the subject, but that we have found to be important in our efforts to implement DBT principles and strategies in our own work and in our work with teams. First, if you want to embody the "spirit" of DBT, you must actively apply DBT principles, procedures, and skills in your own personal life. For the first two years of being part of a full-model outpatient DBT program, I (AHK) completed my own diary card (a tool we will discuss a bit later in this text) on a daily basis. Not only did this help me to make some positive changes in my own life, it also gave me a better understanding of what it might be like for my patients to complete a diary card on a daily basis, including barriers that they encountered in the process. Relatedly, when I facilitate DBT skills groups, I complete the same homework assignments that I give to patients in groups. Doing so sends the message that everyone needs and benefits from skills, as well as helps me in coming up with real-life examples of skills in action. There is a big difference between simply teaching about skills based on lecture points in a book and teaching about skills with the backing of your own lived experience.

Second, it is important to strike a balance between confidence in your work and belief in the treatment you are providing with a healthy dose of vulnerability and humility. The most effective DBT providers we have worked with not only demonstrate openness to feedback and new information, they actively seek it. It is possible to both deeply believe in something while simultaneously treating it as a loosely held hypothesis that can be disconfirmed. One approach we have taken to ensuring that we maintain open minds is to notice any time we are holding on to a belief or perspective strongly and ask the question, "What's being left out?" When it comes to something as complex as patient care, there is never a point where there is no additional information to be taken in or considered. Relatedly, the "spirit" of DBT requires that you are constantly making efforts to learn and to refine your craft, layering in new skills and adding nuance to old ones over the course of time.

Third, the "spirit" of DBT involves a willingness to strive for an egalitarian stance, both between patient and provider, as well as amongst providers themselves. Taking an egalitarian stance between yourself and your patient does not mean compromising your boundaries or professionalism, but rather acknowledging that we are just as human as our patients and that our patients are deserving of being treated as such. This mindset acknowledges the inevitable power differential between provider and patient and seeks to minimize it. It also allows for providers to bring more of their authentic selves in the work they do with patients. When it comes to an egalitarian stance between providers, this involves also trying to minimize power differentials that can arise within the workplace, whether differentials by role within an organization or differentials based on credentials, experience, and so forth. Some of the most sage wisdom I (AHK) have seen shared in the context of a treatment team came from the mouths of interns, and some of the most problematic behaviors I have seen have come from providers who used their advanced degrees or years of expertise as tools to get others to agree to their perspectives. We all have something to learn from each other and DBT encourages the openness and humility needed to take advantage of those opportunities.

Fourth, above all else, compassion. Seek to maintain a compassionate stance toward your patients, toward the providers with whom you work, and with yourself. A word that we have heard all too many times attached to patients is the word "manipulative." If you have a moment, try doing a quick internet image search for the word "manipulative" and notice the emotional reactions you have to the pictures that come up. If you were seeking help for a psychiatric illness, is this how you would want your provider to feel about you? For us, this underscores why it is just so critical to keep compassion at the forefront of our minds and ever-present in our words and actions.

Finally, we wanted to highlight that tapping into the "spirit" of DBT can occur without having any formal training in DBT. This is especially important as we consider the highly intricate nature of DBT, which can limit its accessibility. We observed our own multidisciplinary DBT consultation team gradually and organically incorporate the principles of DBT into their work, which in turn improved case conceptualization, increased compassion, and decreased provider burnout. We have seen dietitians, medical providers, psychiatric providers, nurses, case managers, and other frontline staff embody the framework of DBT and coalesce around a common language and therapeutic bend. Focusing on the "spirit" of DBT also allows for basic foundational tenets of DBT to be woven into client care and clinical supervision, as providers work to master knowledge of specific DBT skills and strategies. Our hope for readers of this text is that you will learn a number of tools that can assist you in improving your patient care, rather than having the expectation that after reading this text, you will have the necessary knowledge, ability, and resources to conduct "adherent" DBT.

Chapter 5

The Multidisciplinary Team in DBT-Based Eating Disorders Treatment

One common error we have seen providers who are new to the treatment of eating disorders make is attempting to treat an eating disorder in the absence of a multidisciplinary team. The bare minimum array of multidisciplinary team members when providing outpatient eating disorders treatment includes an individual therapist, a dietitian, a medical provider, and a psychiatric provider. Other providers that should also be considered on a case-by-case basis include family/couples' therapists, group therapists, expressive arts therapists (e.g. individuals capable of doing art therapy, music therapy, and so forth), movement-focused therapists, occupational therapists, case managers, dentists, and specialty medical providers. Any member of a patient's multidisciplinary team should have specialty training in working with individuals diagnosed with eating disorders.

The array of multidisciplinary team members when providing eating disorders treatment at higher levels of care includes all types of providers that would be included at an outpatient level of care, and may also include culinary specialists, dietetic technicians, teachers, tutors, vocational specialists, recreational therapists, nurses, and mental health technicians. As with outpatient providers, these individuals should have specialty training in the treatment of eating disorders as well.

The last thing we feel is important to highlight about multidisciplinary teams in eating disorders treatment is that it is not only critical for patients to have a multidisciplinary team in place, but that the multidisciplinary team communicates regularly and is on the same page with regard to the treatment plan. Eating disorders work is fraught with situations in which, in the absence of good multidisciplinary treatment planning and collaboration of care, providers on the multidisciplinary team could be actively working against each other with regard to their approach to patient care. For example, a patient may be seeing a dietitian who is working diligently on targeting weight restoration for a client, however the patient's psychiatric provider is prescribing medications that have appetite suppressing effects. Or an adolescent patient may have a family therapist who is working with the patient's parents to assume more responsibility in preparing

DOI: 10.4324/9781003495604-5

and supervising the patient's meals, while at the same time, the parents' couple's counselor is encouraging them to let their child have increased autonomy. These two examples underscore the importance of the necessity of ongoing multidisciplinary collaboration in providing effective eating disorders care.

Bringing DBT to Life – Megan's Multidisciplinary Team

Let's take a look at all the individuals who are part of Megan's team when she enters Residential treatment and a general description of the roles these individuals have in her care. As you read through further chapters in this text, you'll learn more about the specifics of the care that each of these individuals provides.

Psychotherapist (Serena). Serena is a Licensed Clinical Social Worker (LCSW) who has been treating eating disorders for around four years. She conducts individual therapy sessions a couple of times per week with Megan utilizing the principles and strategies that we will cover throughout this text. However, in short, Serena's sessions with Megan focus on targeting eating disorder behaviors and other high-priority target behaviors through assessing relevant emotions, thoughts, behaviors, bodily sensations, and environmental events preceding and following these behaviors and tailoring treatment interventions based on insights gained through the assessment process. Serena is also responsible for conducting family sessions with Megan's mother that focus on topics like psychoeducation, communication, and structuring the home to be conducive to recovery. Finally, Serena conducts a few of the groups that Megan attends each week, two that are DBT skills groups and one that is a group focused on body image. Although Serena has been doing eating disorders work for a few years, she still has numerous growth edges, the most notable of which is that she can sometimes be too focused on validation and acceptance in her individual therapy sessions.

Art Therapist (Vivian). Vivian is a Board Certified Registered Art Therapist (ATR-BC) who has been treating eating disorders for a little over two years. She conducts primarily individual and group art therapy sessions, although will occasionally conduct family art therapy sessions as well. Vivian's work focuses on many of the same targets that are addressed in individual and group therapy, however, approaching these targets through nonverbal mechanisms. Some of Vivian's favorite things to work on with patients in her art therapy sessions include clarifying their values, separating their eating disorder voice from their authentic voice, exploring and expressing emotions, challenging perfectionism, and body image concerns. Vivian still feels new to eating disorders work and identifies her primary growth edge as learning to work more effectively with patients who present as "abrasive" or "shut down" during sessions.

Dietitian (Claire). Claire is a registered dietitian (RD) who is a recent graduate and new dietitian who is enjoying her first job treating eating disorders, although she's the first to admit some days are easier than others. She found herself eager to work with the population following her own experience with disordered eating in high school, but sometimes finds she's too connected to her work. She believes in ongoing supervision and has found it helpful to avoid disclosure around her experience, consistent with her program's policy. In her work with her patients, Claire provides group education on foundational nutrition-related knowledge and provides individual patient care where she assesses and addresses disordered food beliefs and helps to normalize her patients' intake, as well as develops a prescriptive meal plan to meet each of her patients' individualized nutritional needs. Claire could use more support on disconnecting from the emotional pull of the work and not taking her work home with her.

Psychiatric Provider (Ayesha). Ayesha is a psychiatric nurse practitioner (NP) who has an extensive history treating chronic suicidality in community mental health settings. Ayesha transitioned to eating disorders work a few years ago and has picked up on the nuances of the work quickly. Given her background working with patients with severe and complex mental health concerns, Ayesha is well-equipped to manage Megan's medication regimen, which includes an antipsychotic, multiple PRN anxiolytics, and an SSRI. She is also able to draw upon her previous experience to effectively manage Megan's self-injurious behavior and suicidal ideation. Given her previous background treating chronically suicidal individuals, Ayesha is tolerant of a slow pace of change with patients. Ayesha's primary growth edge is around exposure-based procedures. While many of Megan's multidisciplinary team members find value in implementing exposure-based interventions as soon as feasible in treatment, Ayesha is at times reluctant to fully support these interventions because of the distress they cause patients and because of fears that the exposures will result in increases in suicidality and self-injurious behaviors. Some members of the team worry that the PRN anxiolytics that Ayesha prescribes may be impeding the effectiveness of exposures they plan with their patients, while also recognizing the value of their use in anxiety management outside of these contexts.

Medical Provider (Carlos). Carlos is a Family Nurse Practitioner (FNP) who is new at treating eating disorders. He most often finds himself managing medications for bowel regularity, which helps patients physically tolerate the early stages of the refeeding process. He monitors labs, weights, and vitals, and works in conjunction with the rest of the multidisciplinary team on providing psychoeducation on the refeeding process. Because he is so new at the work, he is finding his interventions, such as prescribing laps around the unit following a meal to facilitate digestion or discussing weights openly with patients, are often at odds with the philosophical approach of the treatment program.

Case Manager (Terri). Terri is a Licensed Clinical Social Worker (LCSW) who has been in the field for nearly twenty years and working in the eating disorders field for the past five years. Prior to working with eating disorders, Terri worked as a case manager in a psychiatric unit embedded within a major regional medical center. Terri is responsible for conducting a comprehensive assessment of each patient's needs upon admission. Areas that Terri asks about include medical, psychiatric, and dental needs, the patient's current living situation, transportation needs, employment-related and school-related concerns, financial needs, and legal concerns. Terri is responsible for ensuring that patients transition in a smooth and planful way through levels of care and that they eventually discharge from higher levels of care into an outpatient level of care with a full treatment team in place and with any barriers to recovery sufficiently addressed. Terri also plays a critical role in situations in which a patient may need emergent transfer for medical or psychiatric needs that cannot be effectively managed at the facility where she works. While Terri is detail-oriented and focused on her work, she's recently been feeling "burnt out" on the work and admits she doesn't really understand the complexities of eating disorders. The feedback she's received from patients and colleagues is that she can seem irritated and dismissive at times.

Sous Chef (Emmanuel, goes by the nickname "Manny"). Manny has a Bachelor's Degree in the Culinary Arts and has been involved in cooking and food preparation since he was a teen. Manny came across working with eating disorders when he was looking for a culinary position a couple of years ago after relocating. He saw the job posting for a Sous Chef and decided that it could be an interesting experience to try something new. Manny's passion for this line of work continues to deepen with each passing day. He loves being able to impact the lives of patients so profoundly through the work that he does. Manny fulfills multiple roles, including cooking meals, running culinary groups, and facilitating individual culinary sessions with patients. Manny's direct work with patients focuses on helping them to overcome skill deficits specific to food preparation while also helping them address negative emotions they associate with the kitchen in an experiential way. Manny is incredibly invested in seeing his patients succeed, although this desire sometimes leads him to make choices that aren't always in his patient's long-term best interests. For example, he has been known to occasionally swap out a challenging portion of a meal for an easier one if he believes the swap will make it more likely the patient is able to complete their full meal.

Nurse (Kurt). Kurt is a Registered Nurse who specializes in working with psychiatric patients. He has been working with eating disorder patients for five years. Kurt is responsible for a variety of tasks, including assessing patients for medical and psychiatric stability, taking patient's weights and vitals, distributing and administering medications, placing nasogastric (NG) tubes, implementing in-the-moment coaching and meal support, and providing education to patients one-on-one and in the context of nursing-led groups. Kurt considers himself an expert at meal support and willingly volunteers to lead training on this topic for his peers. Kurt is known for his tough-love approach and finds himself getting frustrated at times with patients who aren't ready to commit to recovery. He is starting to warm up to the idea of examining the balance of acceptance versus change within his work with patients, although has difficulty imagining actually making changes in his approach to interacting with patients.

Mental Health Technician (Omkaar). Omkaar has a Bachelor's Degree in Psychology and is currently a first year student in a MSW program, where he is studying to be a psychotherapist. Omkaar was drawn to the field of eating disorder treatment after supporting his sister through her own struggle with Anorexia Nervosa. Like Kurt, Omkaar is also responsible for a variety of critical tasks, including monitoring patient and unit safety, providing in-the-moment coaching and meal support, facilitating therapeutic activities, overseeing patient outings, and ensuring that day-to-day unit operations run smoothly. He is well-versed in DBT and is quick to suggest skills to patients in distress. Because Omkaar is training to become a therapist, he is having to learn to navigate effectively providing patient support without veering into content that would be more appropriate for a therapy session.

One issue that sometimes arises when providing multidisciplinary care is who is responsible for what. What is interesting about eating disorders care in particular is that there is often more overlap in responsibilities than there is siloing of responsibilities. For example, a psychotherapist will primarily provide therapy (via individual, family, couples', and group therapy) focused on the eating disorder and comorbid psychiatric disorders while sharing responsibility for body image work and food, movement, and body image exposures with a dietitian. A psychotherapist may also share the responsibility of determining the appropriate level of care, assessing function of the eating disorder, and assisting in normalizing nutritional intake with the entire multidisciplinary team. As another example, the medical provider may manage the medical sequelae and the bowel regimen for nutritional rehabilitation while also sharing the responsibility for determining degree of weight suppression, monitoring labs and vitals, and collaborating on enteral feeding interventions with the dietitian on the team.

Finally, it is important to note that the makeup of Megan's team is likely to shift over the course of time, typically becoming more simplified as she transitions to lower levels of care. For example, for some patients, their outpatient team may consist simply of a psychotherapist, dietitian, and medical and/or psychiatric provider, although for other patients, their outpatient team might include a group psychotherapist, an art therapist, a yoga therapist, a recovery coach and/or an eating disorders support group.

Provider Exercise – Reflecting on Your Role as a Multidisciplinary Team Member

Whether multidisciplinary eating disorders care is embedded in your day-to-day practice, as it might be if you work at higher levels of care or within a multidisciplinary outpatient practice, or you are functioning as a solo outpatient practitioner who coordinates care with other outpatient practitioners, it can be helpful to take a step back to examine how you are approaching this element of your work. Below are some questions you might consider in exploring this topic further!

1. What is going well in terms of your multidisciplinary coordination of care? Where do you see opportunities for growth in terms of how you collaborate with other providers?

2. What barriers have you encountered with regard to multidisciplinary collaboration in the treatment of patients with eating disorders? What thoughts do you have about strategies you could try to overcome these barriers?

3. What is one specific change you would like to make in terms of how you approach multidisciplinary collaboration in the treatment of your patients who are diagnosed with eating disorders? How do you plan to go about making this change? (NOTE: If you cannot think of any changes you would like to make at the present time, we encourage you to revisit this specific question after reading more about DBT principles and strategies that can be applied across disciplines, as you may find ideas come to you then!)

Chapter 6

The Structure of DBT

The Modes and Functions of DBT

A common misconception about DBT is that it is "just teaching patients skills," when in reality DBT skills training is only one of the four modes that make up treatment! The four modes of DBT are individual therapy, DBT skills training, in-the-moment coaching, and case consultation meetings, and each of these modes serves a specific function. The majority of the remainder of this text will be explaining each mode in detail, so the following few paragraphs are simply intended to provide a bird's eye view of an incredibly complex and nuanced treatment.

The first mode of DBT is individual therapy and in psychotherapeutic work, the primary function of this mode is to help our patients improve and sustain their motivation for change, although individual therapy may serve other functions as well. As we have discussed throughout this text, eating disorders are oftentimes disorders of ambivalence, so it is critical to intentionally program into treatment a mechanism through which ambivalence can be directly targeted on an ongoing basis. What has been left out of the discussion around the function of this mode of treatment is that all members of a patient's treatment team can and do play a significant role in helping patients to increase and sustain their motivation for change! We will discuss a number of strategies later in this text that providers can subtly weave into their work to address this critical treatment target.

The second mode of DBT is DBT skills training, which serves the purpose of enhancing our patients' capabilities. While we will provide an overview of the specific types of skills discussed in the context of DBT skills training, it is also important to remember that each member of a patient's treatment team has skills they can teach a patient that will help with eating disorder recovery. Some examples of skills that can be taught by non-therapist members of a patient's treatment team include meal and snack planning (dietitian), administering insulin to manage diabetes (medical provider and nursing), engaging in yoga as a method of self-care (movement therapist), or identifying and creating an

DOI: 10.4324/9781003495604-6

Table 6.1 Modes and Functions of DBT

Mode	Function
Individual Therapy	Improving Patient Motivation
DBT Skills Training	Enhancing the Patient's Capacities
In-The-Moment Coaching	Generalizing the Skills to the Inpatient Milieu and the Outpatient Environment
Case Consultation Meetings	Enhancing the Capabilities and Improving the Motivation of Staff

outpatient team (case manager in a higher level of care). A question that each provider can ask themselves when a patient enters treatment to understand how skills training applies to their discipline is, "What skills does my patient have currently and what skills will they need to have to recover from their eating disorder that fall within my scope of practice?"

The third mode of DBT is in-the-moment coaching, the primary function of which is helping our patients apply what they have learned in treatment to situations they encounter in their day-to-day lives, known in DBT as skills generalization. In-the-moment coaching can also serve the purpose of offering space in between sessions to repair damage to the therapeutic relationship that may have occurred, in addition to being a mode of treatment where patients can communicate "good news" outside of usual session times. Later in this text, we will discuss in-the-moment coaching more broadly, in addition to how in-the-moment coaching techniques can be applied in the context of eating a meal or a snack with a patient, as well as ways in which in-the-moment coaching may look different at higher levels of care versus outpatient settings.

The final mode of DBT is case consultation meetings, which serve the function of enhancing the capabilities and improving the motivation of staff. The closest parallel we have found to case consultation meetings outside of the DBT world are Balint groups for physicians, although these are still considerably different from case consultation meetings in DBT. The main thing to note with regard to case consultation meetings in DBT for now is that unlike staff meetings, morning rounds, or other type of clinical meetings, where the primary focus of discussion is likely updates and treatment planning, case consultation meetings focus specifically on what support a provider needs to provide optimal clinical care and to adhere to DBT principles in the context of providing that care.

DBT and the Treatment of Eating Disorders at Higher Levels of Care

Before we transition from discussion of the overall structure of DBT, we thought it was important to comment briefly on DBT and the treatment of eating disorders at higher levels of care. DBT as it was originally developed is a treatment that was designed to be conducted at an outpatient level of care and is a treatment that aims to avoid hospitalization whenever possible. For the individuals for whom this treatment was originally developed, this makes good sense, as it helps patients to learn to apply skills in the environments and situations in which they are most needed, in addition to preventing the inadvertent reinforcement of maladaptive behaviors for patients who find higher levels of care to be reinforcing (e.g. reinforcing expressions of suicidal ideation vis a vis admission to a hospital).

The nature of the treatment of eating disorders, of which medical and nutritional rehabilitation is often a critical component, as well as the nature of eating disorders themselves (e.g. brain-based, ego-syntonic disorders) suggest that more flexibility is warranted when considering levels of care in the use of DBT in the treatment of eating disorders. Wisniewski and Ben-Porath (2015) suggest an alternative approach for considering the level of care at which a patient diagnosed with an eating disorder might be treated, as well as the criteria that would suggest a step-up or step-down in level of care might be appropriate. They encourage the consideration of multiple angles, including American Psychiatric Association (APA) levels of care criteria, insurance criteria, case conceptualization, learning history, and the patient's own wise mind. When provider and patient don't see eye-to-eye, continued discussion until a synthesis can be reached or until patient or provider can offer a compelling enough argument from a wise-minded place to convince the other party to shift their perspective is encouraged.

Chapter 7

The Biosocial Theories of the Development of Eating Disorders

As part of setting the stage for using DBT principles and strategies in your work with patients diagnosed with eating disorders, it can be helpful to understand a DBT-based perspective on how eating disorders come to develop. There are a number of reasons why understanding the development of eating disorders through a DBT framework can be beneficial. First, as you review each of the biosocial theories, you will find that these theories are absent of blame toward patients and their families as it pertains to the development of the patient's eating disorder. In embracing these theories as a lens through which we can understand the experience of our patients, we are better able to maintain compassionate and nonjudgmental stances toward our patients and their families. Relatedly, many of our patients and their families long for an explanation as to why the eating disorder developed. Having something you can share with them that provides an explanation can help shift the focus on understanding the why to figuring out how to move forward. Finally, the biosocial theories help to provide context as to why certain strategies and skill sets are emphasized in DBT. In other words, the biosocial theories provide a rationale for the treatment components that make up DBT.

The Biosocial Theory of the Development of Borderline Personality Disorder

It is first important to understand the biosocial theory of the development of Borderline Personality Disorder (originally described in Linehan, 1993, pp. 42–62), as this biosocial theory served as a starting point of sorts for the development of the biosocial theories associated with specific eating disorders. The biosocial theory of the development of Borderline Personality Disorder hypothesizes that this disorder evolves out of a transaction between a biological dysfunction in the emotion regulation system and an invalidating environment, which in turn results in pervasive emotion dysregulation. As individuals attempt to regulate their emotions through maladaptive coping mechanisms, the risk for further

DOI: 10.4324/9781003495604-7

emotion dysregulation is increased and behaviors begin to develop that characterize the Borderline Personality Disorder diagnosis. To get a better understanding of the biosocial theory, let's take a look at each individual component.

The biological dysfunction in the emotion regulation system component refers to elements of our patients' biology that make them prone to emotional vulnerability. There are four characteristics that define emotional vulnerability. First, patients who are emotionally vulnerable tend to have a high negative affect at baseline. Second, they have a higher sensitivity to emotional stimuli, meaning that the threshold for a stimulus or situation to evoke an emotional response is lower than it is for most individuals. Third, they tend to have more intense responses to emotional stimuli. Finally, once they have had an emotional response, their return to a baseline emotional state tends to be a slower process.

Temperament is also a factor when it comes to biological dysfunctions in the emotion regulation system. Children who are at risk for emotional vulnerability tend to have a temperament that is characterized by high threat sensitivity, low effortful control, high reward sensitivity, and high negative affectivity. High threat sensitivity refers to increased full system (e.g. emotional, cognitive, behavioral, physiological) responses toward threatening stimuli, regardless of whether the threat is real or perceived. Low effortful control is characterized by difficulties engaging in self-regulation behaviors, like inhibiting maladaptive responses or planning and enacting adaptive responses. High reward sensitivity refers to an increased tendency to detect, seek, and derive pleasure from positive stimuli. Finally, high negative affectivity is characterized by increased levels of discomfort, frustration, shyness, sadness, and inability to be soothed. It is perhaps worth noting that many of these temperamental traits overlap with temperamental traits of individuals with specific eating disorder diagnoses.

Finally, there are a few other biological differences that are common among individuals who have a biological dysfunction in their emotion regulation system. This subset of individuals tend to have increased activity in the limbic region of their brain coupled with decreased prefrontal brain activation, which would be expected for individuals who experience intense and enduring emotional reactivity while also indicating they experience difficulty in downregulating their emotions. Other biological factors believed to be related to emotional vulnerability include heredity, intrauterine factors, brain injury, and early learning experiences that affect brain development and brain functioning.

Before we discuss specific examples of invalidating environments, it is important to make a couple points about invalidating environments more broadly. First, what constitutes an invalidating environment falls on quite a broad spectrum, from an environment where mild, unintentional misunderstandings occur with some degree of regularity all the way to environments where significant forms of emotional, physical, or sexual abuse are occurring. Second, it is important not to confuse invalidating environments as being part of a transactional model with invalidating environments "causing" a disorder to develop.

There are three types of micro-level environments that commonly emerge as invalidating environments individuals with Borderline Personality Disorder and other psychiatric illnesses encounter. The first of these environments is the disorganized family, which is characterized by neglect or maltreatment. In this type of environment, displays of emotion are often ignored or punished. In some circumstances, this creates a dynamic in which emotional escalation is reinforced, as intense emotions may be the only ones attended to and taken seriously. The second type of invalidating environment is the "perfect" family. In this type of environment, displays of emotion are considered to be taboo and the ease of problem-solving and achieving goals is oversimplified. Finally, the last type of invalidating environment is the "normal" family. This type of environment is characterized by a poorness of fit between the individual and the individual's family members.

Invalidation can also occur at a macro-level, in the forms of stereotyping and discrimination. Racism, sexism, homophobia, transphobia, xenophobia, anti-fatness, and so forth are all forms of pervasive invalidation that minority communities experience. Furthermore, the impacts of these forms of invalidation may be further compounded when an individual is a member of multiple minority communities. The principle of interrelatedness and wholeness from the dialectical worldview suggests that in order to understand someone, understanding both these micro-level and macro-level factors and their transaction with the individual is critical in understanding that individual's experience.

Now let's take a look at what happens when an individual's biological predisposition to emotional vulnerability transacts with an environment that punishes, ignores, dismisses, or trivializes displays of emotion and difficulties that can accompany experiencing intense emotions regularly. Individuals whose emotional experiences are routinely invalidated tend to internalize the message that their emotions are indeed not valid and instead begin to look to others for how they should think and feel. They also fail to learn how to effectively respond to or manage their emotional experiencing, which can lead to a pattern of suppressing emotions and then expressing them intensely, since ongoing suppression of emotion is not a sustainable way to approach coping with intense emotions. As this transaction occurs over the course of time, pervasive emotion dysregulation develops.

The Biosocial Theory of the Development of Bulimia Nervosa and Binge Eating Disorder

The overall structure of the biosocial theory of the development of Bulimia Nervosa and Binge Eating Disorder is quite comparable to the biosocial theory of the development of Borderline Personality Disorder, with the exception of the addition of vulnerability to food cues and reward sensitivity as biological elements influencing the likelihood of the development of Bulimia Nervosa or Binge Eating Disorder. While the model is indeed quite similar, there are a few subtle differences originally outlined by Safer, Telch, and Chen (2009) that we will describe below.

As with the biosocial theory of the development of Borderline Personality Disorder, a biological dysfunction in the emotion regulation system is also a component of the model for the biosocial theory of the development of Bulimia Nervosa and Binge Eating Disorder. What is different about this component of the model when applied to Bulimia Nervosa and Binge Eating Disorder is that this specific model offers the possibility that the biological dysfunction was either present prior to the development of a person's eating disorder or that the biological dysfunction may occur as a consequence of eating disorder behaviors. In the case of the latter circumstance, as a person initiates using eating disorder behaviors as a method of modulating emotions, eating disorder behaviors are reinforced and the biological dysfunction in the emotion regulation system begins to develop. For example, if a patient engages in purging which results in a powerful reduction of anxiety, they are more likely to use this as a coping mechanism in the future. As they rely on purging over and over again as a method of anxiety reduction, this behavior becomes an automatic, overlearned response for how to manage intense anxiety when it is present.

What is unique to the biosocial model for Bulimia Nervosa and Binge Eating Disorder is that the biological dysfunction in the emotion regulation system is coupled with a vulnerability to food cues and reward sensitivity. Vulnerability to food cues and reward sensitivity can manifest in a number of different ways. Some individuals struggle with temporal discounting, which is a cognitive deficit that involves difficulty resisting short-term rewards, like binge foods, in favor of long-term rewards. Other individuals struggle with hedonic hunger, which refers to an increased appetitive drive or preoccupation with highly palatable foods when not physically hungry. Of note for these particular individuals, there is increased connectivity between emotion centers and reward centers, which manifests as the reward value of palatable foods being particularly high under states of negative affect. A third type of challenge that individuals with Bulimia Nervosa and Binge Eating Disorder may experience is reduced reward activation to the taste of food. These individuals anticipate a high reward in advance of eating a food, however they have a decreased neural response to the actual taste of the food. It is hypothesized for these individuals that binge eating might serve as an attempt to match their actual experience to the anticipated taste. The last type of difficulty individuals may experience has to do with deficits in inhibitory control processes within the cortex that appear to be specific to food rather than a broader class of stimuli.

The combination of the biological dysfunction in the emotion regulation system coupled with vulnerability to food cues and reward sensitivity then transacts with invalidating environments, resulting in pervasive emotional dysregulation. The previously described types of invalidating environments can, and often do, apply to individuals diagnosed with Bulimia Nervosa and Binge Eating Disorder. There are also other ways in which society's intense focus on body weight, shape, size, and appearance can create an invalidating environment for individuals with Bulimia Nervosa and Binge Eating Disorder. For example, mixed messages are often conveyed through media, where one moment the enjoyment of rich and savory foods is encouraged and celebrated, and the next moment whole categories of foods are moralized as "bad" and dieting is encouraged. Weight-related teasing and the impossible standards conveyed by Western cultural expectations for beauty also add additional layers to the invalidating environments that individuals with Bulimia Nervosa and Binge Eating Disorder experience.

The Biosocial Theory of the Development of Anorexia Nervosa

The biosocial theory of the development of Anorexia Nervosa, which is known more broadly as the biosocial theory for disorders of overcontrol, focuses on the bidirectional transactions between nature, nurture, and coping (Lynch, 2018). Although these components are comparable categories to the components present in the other biosocial theory models, you'll notice that the specifics of each component are quite different from the components of the other models we have reviewed.

The nature component of the biosocial theory of the development of Anorexia Nervosa refers to a variety of biologically predisposed characteristics that tend to describe individuals diagnosed with Anorexia Nervosa. First, individuals diagnosed with Anorexia Nervosa tend to have a low reward sensitivity, meaning that they have a higher threshold that has to be met for a stimulus to be rewarding. Individuals with low reward sensitivity tend to be less excitable and tend to experience less spontaneous pleasure. Second, individuals diagnosed with Anorexia Nervosa are predisposed to low novelty seeking as a trait, meaning they prefer familiar experiences and planfulness over novel experiences and spontaneity. Third, individuals diagnosed with Anorexia Nervosa also usually have high threat sensitivity, meaning that they are more prone to states of defensive arousal and anxiety and more likely to interpret stimuli in their environment as threatening. Fourth, individuals diagnosed with Anorexia Nervosa tend to have high inhibitory control, meaning they have a higher capacity for distress tolerance, delayed gratification, and self-control. Finally, individuals diagnosed with Anorexia Nervosa tend to be highly focused on details rather than global processing.

The nurture component of the biosocial theory of the development of Anorexia Nervosa focuses on sociobiographical variables that reinforce, maintain, or exacerbate the overcontrolled coping style that we will discuss shortly. This type of environment reinforces being accomplished, appearing competent, following rules, being persistent, and expressing emotions indirectly. In contrast, behaviors that are punished include making mistakes, seeking attention, displaying emotion, and showing vulnerability and weakness.

The interaction between the nature and nurture components of the biosocial theory of the development of Anorexia Nervosa ultimately results in an overcontrolled, maladaptive coping style characterized by excessive self-control, avoiding risks, masking emotions, and maintaining social distance. What is learned from the transaction between nature and nurture is that through engaging in overcontrolled coping, aversive consequences can be avoided. Furthermore, this style of coping is also likely to be intermittently reinforced by the environment, further strengthening this method of coping as an overarching way of approaching day-to-day living. While short-term consequences of this approach to day-to-day life can be reinforcing, overcontrolled coping has a number of negative long-term consequences, including social ostracism, increased negative affect, and decreased overall life satisfaction.

The Spectrum of Overcontrol to Undercontrol

Another lens through which eating disorders can be understood that directly relates to the biosocial theories of development of eating disorders is the spectrum of overcontrol to undercontrol. DBT is a treatment that was developed to target emotional, interpersonal, behavioral, and cognitive dysregulation, in addition to self dysfunction, all of which are ways in which undercontrol manifests. Both Bulimia Nervosa and Binge Eating Disorder are thought to be disorders of undercontrol, where goals of treatment include helping patients to regulate their emotions and behaviors. Examples of behaviors that would be considered to be undercontrolled include bingeing, purging, substance use, and self-injurious behaviors. In contrast, RO DBT is a treatment that was developed to treat disorders of overcontrol, like Anorexia Nervosa, Restricting Type. Goals of treatment when targeting overcontrol include increasing flexibility, receptivity, and emotional expressiveness. Examples of overcontrolled behaviors include perfectionistic behaviors, compulsive planning, masking emotional expression, making comparisons to others, and avoiding novel experiences.

So why might it be helpful to think about eating disorders along this spectrum? First, conceptualizing eating disorders in this way can help to inform specific treatment interventions. For example, a patient diagnosed with Anorexia Nervosa, Restricting Subtype with no comorbidities might benefit from interventions like wearing mismatched socks to challenge perfectionism and rigidity or practicing having "small talk" with someone to target aloofness in social interactions. For a patient with Bulimia Nervosa, these same treatment interventions might be perceived as enjoyable, as wearing mismatched socks could be perceived by an undercontrolled individual as fun or humorous. Or in the case of making "small talk," the goal for an undercontrolled individual might be to have them speak less and listen more, rather than to share more as might be the case with someone with Anorexia Nervosa, Restricting Subtype. Second, this spectrum can help to conceptualize patients who have a clinical presentation that reflects both ends of the spectrum, like a patient who is diagnosed with Anorexia Nervosa, Bingeing and Purging Subtype, which has both overcontrolled and undercontrolled features, as well as patients who are diagnosed with comorbidities that are common in individuals with eating disorders and that fall at ends of the overcontrolled-undercontrolled spectrum, like Obsessive-Compulsive Disorder, Substance Use Disorders, and various personality disorders, like Borderline Personality Disorder and Obsessive-Compulsive Personality Disorder. These patients require careful consideration of what aspects of their clinical presentation are overcontrolled and what aspects of their clinical presentation are undercontrolled, which in turn can inform more nuanced treatment interventions.

Bringing DBT to Life – Applying the Biosocial Theory and the Overcontrol-Undercontrol Spectrum to Megan

Let's take a moment to reflect on Megan and to see how the biosocial theories of the development of eating disorders and the spectrum of undercontrol-overcontrol might assist us in case conceptualization and treatment planning. You might be wondering where Megan fits within both the biosocial theories of the development of eating disorders, as well as the spectrum of undercontrol-overcontrol, given her diagnostic makeup. Anorexia Nervosa, Binge Eating and Purging subtype would seem to be a diagnosis that fits within both biosocial theories and one that has both undercontrolled and overcontrolled features, whereas Megan's comorbid Alcohol Use Disorder and features of Borderline Personality Disorder suggest a more undercontrolled presentation. The complexity of Megan's presentation was one of many reasons we selected her as our patient to follow throughout this book. When working with patients diagnosed with eating disorders, diagnostic complexity is more often the rule than it is the exception. Let's start by taking a look at how Megan fits within each of the biosocial theories of the development of eating disorders, and then review ways in which the spectrum of undercontrol-overcontrol is relevant to her presentation.

The Biosocial Theory of the Development of Bulimia Nervosa and Binge Eating Disorder. When we think about the biological dysfunction in the emotion dysregulation system, we can hypothesize that the use of eating disorder behaviors early in the development of Megan's eating disorder were attempts to manage weight, however these behaviors likely evolved to serve the function of affect regulation and now have become overlearned, automatic responses to unpleasant emotions. There is other information that we can glean from Megan's vignette that suggests she may be biologically predisposed to being more reactive to emotionally evocative stimuli, experiencing emotions more intensely, and having more difficulty returning to an emotional baseline. From a hereditary standpoint, there is mention that Megan's mother may be a more emotionally expressive individual, which might suggest this quality was passed on to Megan. Megan's later suicidality, self-injurious behavior, and substance use, while not definitive indicators, are suggestive of the presence of intense emotional experiencing and difficulties with effectively regulating negative affect.

When we examine the vulnerability to food cues and reward sensitivity, some interesting questions arise. Does Megan have difficulty resisting short-term rewards, leaning to an increased vulnerability to binge eating, or are the instances of binge eating that she engages in secondary to acute food restriction? Does the reward of binge eating increase when she is experiencing heightened negative affect? What are her experiences immediately prior to and during an instance of binge eating and do these experiences map on to what is suggested by the biosocial model of the development of Bulimia Nervosa and Binge Eating Disorder? All of these questions could be areas for exploration by Megan's providers to help determine the extent to which this aspect of the biosocial theory of the development of Bulimia Nervosa and Binge Eating Disorder captures Megan's experiences.

In looking at the invalidating environment component of the biosocial model of the development of Bulimia Nervosa and Binge Eating Disorder, Megan was raised within a chaotic family system where she was a witness of regular verbal and physical abuse of her mother by her father, which specifically included comments about weight, physical appearance, and emotional expression. With regard to emotional expression specifically, one can imagine that Megan's witnessing of emotional expression being punished likely encouraged inadvertent suppression of her own emotions, which in turn contributed to pervasive emotion dysregulation over the course of time. In addition to witnessing her father's negative comments toward her mother about her weight and physical appearance, Megan was also the target of bullying by her siblings specifically focused on her weight, as well as the recipient of problematic messages from her pediatrician about "watching her weight." As Megan begins to develop her eating disorder, her eating disorder behaviors are further reinforced by the reactions from her family, teachers, and peers. Weight stigma pervades every aspect of Megan's social fabric. Finally, Megan is a survivor of childhood sexual assault that was coupled by accusations that she was being dishonest about what she experienced. This is considered an extreme form of invalidation that has likely played a significant role in the intensification of Megan's mental health symptoms over the course of time.

The Biosocial Theory of the Development of Anorexia Nervosa. Now that we've seen ways in which Megan both fits and doesn't fit within the biosocial theory of the development of Bulimia Nervosa and Binge Eating Disorder, let's take a look at what she fits and doesn't fit within the biosocial theory of the development of Anorexia Nervosa. In terms of the nature component of the biosocial theory of the development of Anorexia Nervosa, some of the information in Megan's vignette suggests she may have some of the biologically predisposed characteristics that are common in individuals with Anorexia Nervosa. Megan does not come off as particularly excitable or sensitive to reward in the vignette describing her, although further information gathering is likely necessary to determine if this is indeed the case. Megan expresses a strong preference for planful experiences and describes surprises as being aversive, rather than neutral or positive. Finally, at times Megan appears to have high inhibitory control, specifically as it pertains to restrictive eating behaviors and scholastic achievement, yet at other times she demonstrates a high degree of impulsivity, demonstrating how this specific model doesn't quite fit patients like Megan.

When looking at the nurture component of the model, there are certain characteristics that appear to overlap with Megan's home environment growing up. Megan's parents expressed an appreciation for hard work and scholastic achievement, in addition to modeling hard work and persistence through pursuing overtime hours to provide for their family. Although not explicitly stated in Megan's vignette, one might hypothesize given Megan's father's volatility, particularly when under the influence of alcohol, that rule following was important to avoid aversive consequences. In the absence of concrete data however, this would be another area for a therapist or other treatment team members to explore as they get to know Megan further. Finally, it is clear in Megan's vignette that open emotional expression in the household was frowned upon and often met with aversive consequences. As with the nature elements of the biosocial theory of the development of Anorexia Nervosa, the nurture elements of Megan's environment do not neatly fit within the model, although many of the elements described in the model are present.

Finally, when we examine the coping aspect of the model, we can see how the transaction between nature, nurture, and coping would result in some of the symptoms and behaviors that Megan is displaying at present. Through displaying self-control with food and with school, through masking her emotional expressions, and through maintaining social distance, Megan learned she was able to avoid aversive consequences. And in the case of self-control around food and school, behaviors like restricting coupled with subsequent weight loss and scholastic achievement were reinforced, further strengthening self-control in these areas as a method of effectively coping.

Spectrum of Overcontrol to Undercontrol. As is common with patients diagnosed with Anorexia Nervosa (specifically, Anorexia Nervosa, Binge Eating and Purging Subtype), coupled with multiple comorbidities, you can see that Megan presents with both undercontrolled and overcontrolled behaviors. Bingeing, purging, substance use, and self-injurious behaviors are generally thought of as undercontrolled behaviors, whereas restriction of food and fluids are behaviors that would generally be considered to be overcontrolled behaviors.

Megan also demonstrates some overcontrolled personality traits, including:

a. Avoidance of uncertainty: Megan does well on a schedule and does not like surprises; she weighs herself compulsively and tracks her caloric intake to be as accurate as possible.
b. Hyperperfectionism: Megan believes that any grade less than perfect is considered failure; she engages in food tracking in her journal which she describes as "almost ritualistic" and compulsive.
c. Premeditation and planning: Megan reports her previous suicide attempts were the result of careful planning with high intentionality; her self-injury to inner thighs is always in the same place with the same implement.
d. Low social connectedness: Megan avoids close relationships due to "trust issues" and states she is a "hermit."

As with the biosocial theories of the development of eating disorders, Megan also has a mixed presentation of undercontrolled and overcontrolled behaviors. Given that Megan doesn't fit neatly within these models, you may be wondering why we have found them to be useful ways of thinking when it comes to patient care.

The Value of the Biosocial Theories. One benefit of using these ways of thinking about our patients is that they can help us to assume a more objective and non-judgmental stance. They give us a framework that can help us to understand how our patient's behaviors developed, the mechanisms by which these behaviors have been strengthened and maintained, and the current function or functions that these behaviors serve. With a patient like Megan, who might be dismissed as "treatment savvy" or a "professional patient," these models remind us that eating disorders are brain-based illnesses with an incredibly complex etiology where the majority of factors at play are outside of the scope of our patients' control. Eating disorders are not a choice and not a form of manipulation and these models can help us to reaffirm this, not only for ourselves as providers but for our patients as well. The other benefit from the biosocial theories is that they can help with case conceptualization, which in turn informs our treatment interventions. For example, if through further assessment, we come to find that Megan's bingeing behaviors are serving the function of regulating negative affect, this would suggest that one area of focus for treatment would be helping Megan to develop more adaptive skill sets for tolerating and regulating her emotional experiences.

The Value of the Spectrum of Overcontrol to Undercontrol. There are also two distinct benefits for thinking about our patients' behaviors on a spectrum of overcontrol to undercontrol. First, we will discuss the DBT Treatment Target Hierarchy a little bit later in this text, but in short, behaviors that fall at extreme ends of the overcontrol and undercontrol spectrum often make for helpful targets in treatment. Second, by identifying these as behaviors falling on the overcontrol to undercontrol spectrum, we can start to think about these behaviors almost like knobs on a music producer's mixing board. Which of these behaviors need to be dialed up and which ones need to be dialed down? Sticking with the music production metaphor, the answer is usually not to turn a knob from "10" to "0" or "0" to "10," but rather to appropriately calibrate each knob. For example, for a patient who is aloof and distant socially, the goal would not be for them to behave in a way that is overly connected to the point they routinely over-disclose personal information and lack appropriate boundaries. Rather, the aim might be to help them develop a small network of close friends with whom they are willing to share more personal information when appropriate. Similarly, the goal for a patient who engages in regular instances of binge eating is not to have them become overly rigid with when, what, and how much they are eating, but rather to help them become more mindful and connected in their food choices. So when we metaphorically think of our patients' behaviors as a mixing board of knobs, we are able to be thoughtful in calibrating these knobs through the treatment interventions we select.

Provider Exercise – Reflecting on the Biosocial Theories and Overcontrol-Undercontrol Spectrum

Think about a patient with whom you currently work and make some notes about how you see the biosocial theory related to their specific eating disorder and the spectrum of overcontrol-undercontrol applying to their clinical presentation. Does this lens help you to better understand their experience or conceptualize their case? Why or why not? How might you apply this information in the context of clinical care? After having a chance to reflect on this activity, consider sharing your thoughts (ensuring they are appropriately de-identified) with a trusted peer for their feedback.

Chapter 8

The Stages of DBT

Now that you have some frameworks that can help you to understand the etiology and maintenance of your patient's eating disorder, we want to shift to providing you with a high-level view of DBT as a whole, as this will help you to place the interventions we will spend most of this book discussing into a context. DBT is separated into five distinct stages: the pretreatment stage and stages one through four. It is worth mentioning here that if you are working with a patient with an active eating disorder diagnosis, your patient will almost always fall into either the pretreatment stage or stage one of treatment. With rare exceptions, only patients who are in full remission from their eating disorder would be considered ready to progress to the latter stages of DBT treatment. It is also important to note that progression through the stages is by no means linear, particularly when working with patients diagnosed with an eating disorder. We have both worked with many patients who have progressed from the pretreatment stage of treatment to stage one of treatment, only to return back to the pretreatment stage of treatment and then back to stage one of treatment again. We've also watched patients progress to later stages of treatment and return to stage one of treatment in the context of a relapse. Although not inevitable, this non-linear progression through stages of treatment is common, and patients with this type of path can still ultimately achieve sustained recovery. Let's take a look at each of the stages of DBT treatment.

The Pretreatment Stage

The focal points of the pretreatment stage are twofold: orientation and commitment. In order for a patient to commit to treatment, they must first understand what they are committing to. This is where orientation comes in. While orientation is an ongoing process throughout treatment, orientation at the beginning of treatment specifically may focus on a number of topics, including information about the background, roles, and responsibilities of the patient and treatment

DOI: 10.4324/9781003495604-8

providers, details about the specific type of treatment being provided, and what the patient can expect the progress through treatment to look like.

The other component of the pretreatment stage of treatment is obtaining commitment from your patient to participate in treatment focused on helping your patient make the changes they want to make in their life. This can be more of a challenge when working with patients diagnosed with eating disorders in comparison to other psychiatric diagnoses. Many of the child and adolescent patients with whom I (AHK) have worked have been brought to treatment by parents and caregivers, rather than of their own volition. The initial common ground I have found with these patients rarely has anything to do with their eating disorder directly. Rather, we are able to find shared goals like "returning to school" and "getting out of treatment." While the initial paths we see to achieving these goals are often quite different, we at least have a shared endgame toward which we can work. With adult patients, who often do have a choice in whether to seek treatment and to pursue recovery, finding common ground with a highly ambivalent patient is typically a more nuanced matter. There are a number of strategies we will be exploring shortly that can help to enhance motivation for treatment and motivation for change.

Stage One

Stage one of treatment has the overall goal of helping patients to move from a state of behavioral dyscontrol to one of behavioral control. This is done by focusing on directly addressing any behaviors that put a patient's life at risk, that get in the way of treatment, and that impede on their quality-of-life, in addition to addressing any behavioral skills deficits. Specific behaviors that fall into each of these categories will be discussed in extensive detail in Chapter 12, so for now it is sufficient to know that this is the stage in which your patient's eating disorder is directly targeted, with the aim of achieving a full remission in symptoms.

Stage Two

The overarching goal of stage two of treatment is to move patients from a state where they have behavioral control but may still be experiencing intense emotional suffering to having the ability to experience a wide range of emotions without intense anguish. Other comorbid diagnoses your patient may have that were targeted in stage one of treatment may continue to be areas of focus in stage two of treatment. Of note, symptoms related to posttraumatic stress specifically are only an area of focus in stage one of treatment from a symptom containment standpoint. Thus, stage two of DBT is when the focus on posttraumatic stress symptoms shifts from symptom containment to symptom resolution.

Untreated trauma-related symptoms can put individuals at risk for relapse, so stage two of treatment is critical for many of the patients with whom we work. Common goals for this stage of treatment associated with trauma specifically include helping the patient accept that the traumatic experience occurred, reducing self-invalidation and self-blame associated with the traumatic event, and decreasing emotional, behavioral, and cognitive symptoms resulting from the traumatic experience. Other areas of focus in stage two of treatment that are not necessarily directly related to comorbid diagnoses include addressing inhibited grieving, feelings of emptiness, and any real or perceived sense of being an "outsider."

Stage Three

Stage three of treatment is focused on helping your patient to increase respect for self and decrease individual problems in living, with the overarching goal of helping your patient come to a spot where they experience ordinary happiness and unhappiness. Respect for self refers to the ability to value, believe, and validate oneself, including one's thoughts, emotions, and behaviors. Because of the nature of eating disorders work, addressing targets that are the focus of stage three of treatment often begins in stage one of treatment, and for many individuals diagnosed with an eating disorder, respect for self is a treatment goal that can take considerable time to achieve. Stage three of treatment also focuses on decreasing individual problems in living. Individual problems in living refer to everyday challenges that many people face and can cover quite a broad array of targets, including time management, interpersonal difficulties, stress management, and so forth.

Stage Four

Stage four of treatment has the overarching goal of helping patients to move from a state of incompleteness to one of freedom. This stage focuses on searching for and finding meaning, connectedness, and more sustained positive affect. While stage four of treatment has not been written about extensively, it requires maintaining gains from the previous stages of treatment, coupled with an enhanced focus on the application of mindfulness in day-to-day living, and may include spiritual work as well.

Provider Exercise – Identifying Stages of Treatment for Patients on Your Caseload

Because patients who are being treated at higher levels of care (Inpatient, Residential, Partial Hospitalization, or Intensive Outpatient) will almost always be in either the pretreatment stage or stage one of treatment, those of you who are treating patients solely at these levels of care can bypass this provider exercise. For those of you who spend some or all of your time treating patients in an Outpatient setting, you may find this activity to be of interest. For each patient on your caseload, give consideration as to which stage of treatment they would fall under, if you were using a DBT framework to guide your care. Consider your rationale for placing each patient in their specific stage of treatment and whether what stage you placed them in might lead you to consider a different focus for treatment at the present time. If you want to expand upon this exercise further, consider sharing your reflections (ensuring they are appropriately de-identified) with a trusted peer, ideally someone who is familiar with DBT.

Chapter 9

Getting Your Patient's Buy-In

Eating Disorders and Motivation for Change

It is well-established that for many patients diagnosed with an eating disorder, ambivalence around eating disorder recovery is pervasive. While most of the literature in this area focuses on Anorexia Nervosa, ambivalence around the desire for treatment, change, and recovery is seen across the entire spectrum of eating disorders. Before we explore ways to enhance motivation for change, we thought it might be useful to examine factors that may at least partially account for ambivalence across each diagnosis, drawing from literature as well as our own experiences. What you will notice is that the ambivalence seen in eating disorders can often be explained by the remarkably complex interplay of various psychological and biological factors and there are likely many factors that have yet to be discovered.

Ambivalence in Anorexia Nervosa

Understanding ambivalence in Anorexia Nervosa must start with an understanding of what drives and maintains the behaviors observed with this diagnosis. It has been well understood that internal reinforcers (e.g. a sense of control or accomplishment) are often more important than external reinforcers (e.g. a compliment on weight loss or having self-control around energy intake) in maintaining the illness (Garner, et al., 1982). As one might imagine, such an ego-syntonic disorder leads to high treatment dropout rates or avoidance of treatment altogether. More often than not, we have seen our adult and adolescent patients being brought into treatment by family or friends, oftentimes against their will. Regardless of level of care, much of the work centers around ambivalence and enhancing motivation. Let's start by taking a look at ambivalence for a patient diagnosed with Anorexia Nervosa, Restricting Subtype.

Vignette #1: "Millie." Millie is a 14-year-old, White cisgender female diagnosed with Anorexia Nervosa, Restricting Subtype, that developed during her involvement in travel soccer around age 11. She recalls her coach discussing

DOI: 10.4324/9781003495604-9

her physique to her parents, stating, "I think the few extra pounds she's carrying is holding her back. She could be a better performer if she lost a bit of weight." By eliminating snacks and discarding her packed lunch daily, Millie was able to lose 15 pounds and saw her performance and speed improve, landing her a spot as the starting forward. After the season ended, Millie recalls it being difficult to "flip the switch" and eat normally again. Her parents grew increasingly concerned as her weight continued to decline and they noticed a pattern of avoidance and isolation from her peers. Furthermore, menarche was never achieved, despite other developmental indicators she was on track prior to weight loss. Her parents ultimately decided to seek outpatient treatment after witnessing Millie refuse to eat any of her lasagna, which she previously considered to be her favorite food, or her birthday cake on her twelfth birthday. Reluctantly, Millie agreed to meet with a therapist and dietitian but remained minimally engaged until we find her now at age 14. She states she only shows up to sessions because she "has to" and because her parents threatened to take her cell phone away if she declines to attend. She reports placing high value on her eating disorder and becomes defensive when her treatment team attempts to set goals around improving intake and gaining weight. She has made no measurable progress in outpatient care so far, and her team has started to recommend a step-up to partial hospitalization.

While the inclination of a newer provider might be to focus heavily on medical sequelae of maintaining low body weight (particularly through adolescence) along with the psychological consequences of social isolation, exploring the maintaining factors of her eating disorder will assist in understanding her resistance and ambivalence and get us further along in treatment. As an adolescent patient with minimal engagement in treatment, the more fruitful work would be around motivation enhancement and exploring her ambivalence to make change and ultimately to recover from her eating disorder.

A number of themes have emerged from qualitative research examining self-reported maintenance factors of eating disorders, although with a focus primarily on Anorexia Nervosa specifically. These themes include security and control, avoidance, mental strength and skill, communication, and confidence (Nordbø, et al., 2006; Serpell, et al., 1999). Prompting care from others has been identified as an additional maintaining factor, particularly for adolescents (Nordbø, et al., 2006).

As Millie's therapist gathers information to assist her in exploring factors that may be maintaining Millie's eating disorder, the following hypothesized functions emerge:

1. *Sense of accomplishment.* Both of Millie's parents have successful, high-powered careers. Her father is the owner of an engineering firm and her mother works as an emergency room physician. Additionally, Millie is the

youngest of three children. Her oldest sister currently attends an Ivy League college and is on track to follow in her mother's footsteps, with admissions offers from numerous prestigious medical schools that she is in the process of considering. Millie's other sister is also accomplished academically, in addition to excelling at playing the violin. While Millie also does well academically and has begun to excel at soccer, she does not feel as though she is as accomplished as her other family members and notes that her eating disorder is what sets her apart. With further exploration by her skilled therapist, Millie also acknowledges core beliefs that she is a failure and that she is unlovable.

2. *Attention and care-seeking.* With two parents working in intense jobs and parenting three children, Millie has sometimes felt invisible within her home. While her parents have always made efforts to spend quality time with each of their children, Millie has noticed that as her eating disorder has progressed, both her mother and father have been more attentive and caring. She's afraid recovery from her eating disorder would lead to less familial support.

3. *Sense of control.* Although Millie's household might not appear chaotic to others, she has experienced it as such and notes that her eating disorder gives her a sense of control and predictability.

4. *Management of body image distress.* Millie acknowledges that she currently experiences a great deal of body image distress, however she predicts that the body image distress she would experience once weight-restored would be unbearable.

Now let's take a look at ambivalence for a patient diagnosed with Anorexia Nervosa, Binge Eating and Purging Subtype.

Vignette #2: "Kyle." Kyle is a 37-year-old, Black trans male with a long standing history of Anorexia Nervosa, Binge Eating and Purging Subtype. He states his eating disorder "has always been there, in one form or another," noting that he has experienced body image distress since the age of three or four. Kyle's eating pathology emerged at twelve, as body changes associated with puberty began to heighten the incongruence he felt between his gender identity and his external appearance. He started restricting his intake at that time to prevent development of hips and breasts, with the secondary desired outcome of achieving amenorrhea at a lower weight. In high school, Kyle started binge eating, purging, and abusing laxatives, along with severe energy restriction. Kyle endorses a significant history of bullying throughout high school and also notes that while his parents have said that they love him no matter what, they have had difficulty accepting that he is a trans man. At the present time, Kyle states his intention is to achieve "net zero" with energy intake and some days finds he is successful with restriction of food and fluid alone. Other days he finds himself engaging in binge eating episodes that last several hours, always coupled with purging throughout his binges, as well as excessive laxative use. Of note, Kyle also engages in self-injurious behavior via cutting.

Kyle has been in and out of treatment facilities and has had difficulty complying with the recommendations made by his treating providers. Kyle states that he feels like his providers "don't get it" and are insensitive to his gender dysphoria, noting that his providers have been unwilling to allow him to pursue gender affirming medical care at the same time he is completing eating disorder treatment. At higher levels of care, Kyle has been frequently misgendered by staff who are dismissive when Kyle corrects them, only further contributing to the pervasive invalidation Kyle has experienced in treatment and in the world more broadly, not only as a trans man but also as a Black man. Kyle recognizes the significant and pervasive impact that his eating disorder and self-injurious behaviors have had on his life, while also acknowledging crippling ambivalence around recovery from his eating disorder.

Although the data are still limited on the prevalence rates of eating disorders in transgender individuals, one study utilizing a large sample of college students found that 15.82% of transgender study participants had met criteria for an eating disorder during the past year (Diemer, et al., 2015), which is a rate nearly four times greater than the rate of eating disorders in the general population. There are a number of factors that are thought to account for the increased prevalence rates of eating disorders in the transgender community. The most common factor that arises in the research literature is that eating disorder behaviors can serve the function of suppressing an individual's physical characteristics associated with the sex they were assigned at birth and/or accentuate physical features that align with their gender identity (Algars, et al., 2012; Diemer, et al., 2018). Another related although distinct factor is that visual conformity unfortunately plays a significant role in the safety and well-being of members of the trans community. Research suggests that trans individuals who are more visually gender nonconforming are at higher risk for violence, discrimination, and poorer health outcomes (Diemer, et al., 2018; Gordon, 2016). In other words, "passing" can be a matter of life or death for someone who is trans. Finally, the Minority Stress Model suggests that stress-induced responses to victimization, discrimination, and internalized stigma may put individuals who identify as trans at greater risk of development of an eating disorder (Diemer, et al., 2015; Diemer, et al., 2018; Gordon, 2016; Watson, et al., 2016).

Kyle's newest multidisciplinary team has received training in working with transgender and nonbinary individuals diagnosed with eating disorders and as such, are better equipped to assess factors that may be contributing to Kyle's ambivalence about treatment and recovery. The following is a list of the hypothesized factors Kyle's team has been able to identify thus far:

1. *Gender dysphoria.* Kyle has clearly stated that his eating disorder behaviors have served the function of minimizing the development of breasts and hips, as well as suppressing menstruation. Furthermore, Kyle has noted that his previous providers have been unwilling to allow him to pursue gender affirming medical interventions while receiving treatment for his eating disorder. However, there is evidence that suggests that pursuing gender affirming medical interventions when desired can reduce eating disorder symptoms in transgender individuals through reducing non affirmation and enhancing body satisfaction (Testa, et al., 2017). Given that Kyle has not been permitted to pursue these interventions, his ambivalence about making changes to eating disorder behaviors is entirely understandable.

2. *Security.* Kyle is unfortunately all too aware of the horrific violence perpetrated against transgender individuals and members of the Black community and believes that his eating disorder behaviors are a necessary part of staying alive, absent the option to seek gender affirming medical interventions. Kyle has difficulty imagining giving up his eating disorder when he feels it will put him at risk for increased physical and emotional harm.

3. *Control.* As a member of multiple marginalized communities, Kyle's eating disorder also gives him a sense of control when so many elements of his lived experience are outside the scope of what he can individually impact. Many aspects of Kyle's lived experience feel chaotic and painful, and he has difficulty imagining giving up one of few things that give him a sense of agency in his own life.

4. *Emotion regulation.* As an individual who has faced chronic invalidation and discrimination, Kyle's eating disorder behaviors and self-injurious behaviors appear in part to be serving the function of helping to regulate negative affect. Although Kyle has been through multiple episodes of treatment, he has not learned as part of his previous treatment episodes how to apply the skills he has acquired to some of the unique challenges that he faces as a Black trans man. His team imagines that it must be hard for Kyle to think of giving up methods that have been effective in regulating emotions in the absence of having knowledge of how to regulate his emotions more skillfully.

Ambivalence in Bulimia Nervosa

Next we'll consider a vignette of a patient with Bulimia Nervosa.

Vignette #3: "Paul." Paul is a 45-year-old cisgender male who works full-time as a civil litigation lawyer. Paul has a history of Alcohol Use Disorder, Severe, Borderline Personality Disorder, Major Depressive Disorder, Moderate, and Generalized Anxiety Disorder. Paul has recently started bingeing and purging following the separation from his wife of eleven years, Susan. Ten months ago, Susan left Paul and took their two young children with her, citing frustration with Paul's alcohol use as a main precipitating factor. While Paul has a history of receiving treatment for his alcohol use, a substance that he reports he would turn to in times of high stress and uncertainty, he admits he'd "fallen off the wagon big time" when Susan decided to leave. Paul vowed to stop drinking, and found himself quickly turning to new behaviors, including binge eating and purging. Paul started bingeing in the office on nights when the stress of work and loneliness of marital separation felt overwhelming, with extreme fullness leading to purging via self-induced vomiting. Paul has been bingeing and purging five nights a week, often for multiple hours in his office with a private bathroom. Paul hasn't touched alcohol in months. Although Paul's functioning appears to have substantially improved since returning to abstinence from alcohol use, those closest to Paul have the sense that something is amiss, although they attribute their feelings to Paul's recent separation from his wife.

Co-occurring eating disorders and substance use disorders are a common phenomenon. Fifty percent of patients diagnosed with an eating disorder will also abuse a substance, and 35% of individuals who abuse substances will also meet criteria for an eating disorder (CASA, 2003). Bulimia Nervosa tends to have the highest association with substance use, followed by Binge Eating Disorder (Calero-Elvira, A., Krug, I., Davis, K., Lopez, C., Fernandez-Aranda, F., & Treasure, J., 2009). Interestingly, there is emerging evidence that suggests that rather than specific eating disorder diagnosis being related to the likelihood of someone struggling with a comorbid Substance Use Disorder, purging behavior specifically has the greatest association with comorbid Substance Use Disorders (Root, et al., 2010). Lastly, Alcohol Use Disorder, with which Paul has been diagnosed, tends to be most common among individuals diagnosed with Bulimia Nervosa, Binge Eating Disorder, and Anorexia Nervosa, Bingeing and Purging Subtype (Gregorowski, Seedat, & Jordaan, 2013).

The comorbidity between Bulimia Nervosa and Substance Use Disorders can be explained at least in part by common genetic, biological, environmental, and personality-related factors. Abnormalities in reward-seeking neurotransmitters can result in the combination of reward-seeking behaviors and impulsivity, both of which are common in Bulimia Nervosa and Substance Use Disorder (Dawe and Loxton, 2004). Personality traits (including a lifetime history of Major Depressive Disorder and neuroticism) and the tendency to self-medicate have been hypothesized to be predisposing traits in women that lead to an increased risk of individuals with Bulimia Nervosa developing a Substance Use Disorder (Baker, et al., 2007).

Paul's primary therapist, who specializes in the treatment of Substance Use Disorders specifically, has encouraged Paul to seek specialized care for his eating disorder, however Paul has been highly resistant to this idea thus far. Paul's therapist hypothesizes that the following factors are keeping Paul from pursuing treatment for Bulimia Nervosa:

1. *Emotion regulation.* Paul gets immediate relief from his anxiety, depression, loneliness, and stress when he engages in bingeing and purging. He feels unable to tolerate these emotions without relief of bingeing and purging now that he is no longer drinking.

2. *Management of suicidality.* Related to managing affect, Paul reports an increase in suicidality on the few nights he does not binge and purge. He feels it is "all [he] has left" and becomes defensive when his therapist suggests pursuing treatment that will target his bingeing and purging behaviors more directly.

3. *"The lesser of two evils."* Paul has recommitted to cessation of alcohol use after the significant role it played in his recent separation from his wife, however he finds that he has "symptom-swapped" and binge eating and purging are now serving similar functions to his alcohol use, as described above. He is relieved that he is no longer turning to alcohol and even reports his urges to drink are a lot lower since he started bingeing and purging. Although on some level he wishes he could stop bingeing and purging, he does not feel these behaviors have the same detrimental effect on his life as his alcohol use did.

4. *Guilt and shame.* Guilt and shame have been emotions that have been more prevalent for Paul throughout his life and Paul has tended to take the approach of avoidance when faced with these emotions. Paul is deeply ashamed of his behavior, especially as a middle-aged man with a high-powered career. At the present time, avoidance feels more comfortable to Paul in the short-term, even though avoidance is playing a role in perpetuating his guilt and shame over time.

5. *Self-hatred.* Paul also struggles with deeply rooted self-hatred and a chronic sense of emptiness. Paul has engaged in a variety of maladaptive behaviors over the course of his life, like self-injurious behavior as a young adult and episodic alcohol use throughout his adult life. He believes he is deserving of punishment and is skeptical of the belief expressed by his therapist that he is deserving of a life worth living.

Ambivalence in Binge Eating Disorder

While less outwardly common than the strong ambivalence often seen with Anorexia Nervosa, ambivalence about change and recovery is often present for individuals diagnosed with Binge Eating Disorder. The initial motivation for many individuals seeking treatment for Binge Eating Disorder is the secondary outcome of expected weight loss as well as resolution for a behavior that is perceived as detrimental, time-consuming, and for some, expensive. However appealing recovery may be at the start of treatment, as treatment progresses we have seen many patients struggling with ambivalence around the therapeutic work that is necessary to make progress. Let's take a look at our final vignette.

Vignette #4: "Louise." Louise is a 52-year-old, White cisgender female who recalls a long history of overeating beginning at age six. Growing up, Louise was an only child living in a single parent household who had a contentious relationship with her mother, who felt Louise was "way too emotional" and "a burden." Her mother was also a chronic dieter who imposed the same strict dieting regimens she maintained for herself on Louise as well. There were no sweets, fatty meats, or dairy permitted in the household, and Louise was not allowed to eat after 6:00pm. Louise's mother was clear in the message that thinness equated to success, noting that this would be a crucial factor in Louise being "the marrying type" as she entered adulthood. Louise recalls memories of her mother verbally shaming her eating habits, both in the home and in public, and weekly weigh-ins determined her weekly monetary allowance. Many nights she went to bed hungry or craving something she was forbidden. She started stealing candy from the corner store and hiding it in her room, finding she would lose control whenever she had access to it. This secretive eating was what she looked forward to the most in her day and it served as her escape after numerous challenging interactions with her mother throughout the course of the evening. Louise lived at home throughout college and noted that her secretive eating continued throughout her undergraduate years. After graduating, Louise moved into a place of her own and her secretive eating escalated into frequent binge eating episodes, sometimes occurring multiple times in a day. She is now socially isolated and reports having little outside of her binge eating. She has been in outpatient treatment with a myriad of providers for over fifteen years. Louise presents as engaged in therapy sessions, citing a high level of motivation to recover and lose weight, despite weight loss not being a treatment target of her outpatient team. Louise has a pattern of experiencing marginal improvement in the frequency and intensity of her binge eating behaviors at the start of a new therapeutic relationship, however notes that she "quickly sinks back into old behaviors, especially when things get rough." When asked to explore her motivation for recovery, Louise has always reported she's highly motivated to lose weight and get her life back, but on some level remains ambivalent around recovery of her eating disorder.

Unlike with Anorexia Nervosa and Bulimia Nervosa, little has been written or researched about ambivalence in Binge Eating Disorder. One study examining an adapted motivational interviewing intervention for Binge Eating Disorder that demonstrated positive results hypothesized that one of the factors driving ambivalence in pursuing treatment and recovery is an extensive history of unsuccessful attempts to stop binge eating. These authors suggested that the primary reason that the adapted motivational interviewing intervention was effective was due to enhancing confidence for change and self-efficacy (Cassin, et al., 2008).

To begin to unpack the maintaining factors of Louise's Binge Eating Disorder and what may get in the way of her motivation for recovery, one must investigate both emotional and neurobiological factors at play.

1. *Affect regulation.* Louise's binge eating behaviors very likely serve the function of regulating negative affect. For Louise, this likely began as a young child when she would engage in binge eating to assist in managing the distress caused by the relationship with her mother. Considering the biosocial theory, we can assume there is a biological dysfunction in the emotion regulation system and she is ill-equipped to manage her emotions without reliance on a maladaptive behavior such as binge eating. This behavior, after years of overuse, has become an automatic way of reducing emotional distress. Given the pervasiveness of Louise's negative affect, it makes sense that it would be challenging for her to reduce bingeing behaviors, since these behaviors are so effective in achieving short-term relief.

2. *Vulnerability to food cues/hedonic hunger.* While Louise's initial turn to highly palatable foods as a young child was likely secondary to imposed restriction of these foods by her mother, it is also possible Louise also experiences hedonic hunger, which refers to an increased appetitive drive or preoccupation with highly palatable foods when not physically hungry. For individuals who experience hedonic hunger, these palatable foods are particularly more desirable under states of stress.

3. *Reward pathways.* Understanding the neurological underpinnings that make it difficult to abstain from binge eating are worth exploring with a client like Louise. There are known alterations in the reward processing part of the brain of someone with Binge Eating Disorder, affecting brain regions responsible for anticipation of eating, how the body responds physically to food, and decision-making around eating, including whether to continue eating or not. One common theme for many individuals with whom we have worked who are diagnosed with Binge Eating Disorder is that they are seeking the sensations they experience at the time of their very first bite of a binge episode.

4. *Lack of alignment between patient and provider goals.* We would be remiss to not mention patient-desired weight loss as an aspect of Binge Eating Disorder treatment that can result in diminished motivation. Many patients who seek treatment for Binge Eating Disorder do so with the primary intention of losing weight and many treatment providers do not hold the perspective that weight loss is a clinically sound goal for treatment. Unfortunately, lack of alignment in goals can impact a patient's willingness to continue engaging in care. With Louise, this is very likely one factor leading to her

history of frequently switching providers and the ambivalence she experiences around her recovery.

Bringing DBT to Life – Exploring Megan's Ambivalence

Now let's return to Megan and explore some of her ambivalence to committing to eating disorder recovery. Megan, like many of the patients we have treated, appears to have perhaps never fully embraced treatment and the opportunity to work towards eating disorder recovery. As you may remember, when we met Megan she stated only early in her eating disorder treatment did she have "full intention of actually recovering." As time went on, she reports engagement in treatment was more about appeasing friends and family than it being an effort to work towards her own recovery. If our intention as providers is to help Megan have a positive outcome from this treatment episode that helps to set her on the path toward sustained recovery, it is critical that we begin to develop hypotheses about factors driving her ambivalence and target these factors in the context of treatment. Based on the information we have about Megan so far, the following are functions that we hypothesize Megan's eating disorder behaviors may serve that are contributing to her ambivalence about treatment and recovery:

1. *Managing distress.* From an early age, Megan learned that both eating disorder behaviors, like bingeing, purging, and restricting, as well as other maladaptive behaviors, like alcohol use and self-harm, can serve the function of decreasing the intensity of the negative affect she experiences, helping her to "numb out" and escape. Although Megan has an arsenal of DBT skills that she can draw from, she acknowledges that the potent effectiveness of her maladaptive behaviors in reducing distress short-term is hard to give up. While she notes that DBT skills can be helpful, her experience thus far is that their effects on reducing negative affect and distress simply aren't as potent as the effects of her maladaptive behaviors.
2. *Feeling competent.* Megan has a strong drive for perfectionism. She recalls being a great student and was acknowledged for her academic performance in the depths of her restriction. Megan has previously noted, "I may not be good at much, but I'm really good at my eating disorder; I can lose weight quickly when I want to. And when I'm in my eating disorder, I get the outcomes I want in life, like in school and with my job. I do better all around." Megan experiences a sense of pride when she is able to restrict intake at the same time her peers are completing and has had periods of her previous treatment stays where she has silently competed with her peers to be the "sickest one in treatment." The ways in which "success" at her eating disorder can be easily quantified, for example, through weighing herself, measuring her body, and calorie counting, has only fueled her focus on becoming "better"

at her eating disorder. Seemingly paradoxically, Megan is also terrified that if she truly put forth the effort to enter into sustained recovery, she wouldn't recover "right" or "perfectly," so there is no sense in trying.

3. *Being in control.* Megan has noted that so many aspects of her life have often felt outside of her control and that her eating disorder gives her a sense of control when everything else feels chaotic. Megan has stated that at these times, she is able to channel her mental and emotional energy into "doing her eating disorder as well as possible," which pulls her attention away from other aspects of her life that feel less secure, stable, or predictable.

4. *Eliciting positive reinforcement and avoiding punishing responses in the context of interpersonal interactions.* Megan has a history of receiving positive reinforcement from her environment when she has lost weight and punishing responses from her environment when she has consumed foods that others consider to be "unhealthy" or when she has appeared to gain weight. Although her core support system has been educated about eating disorders and has since learned to refrain from comments about body weight, shape, and size, as well as comments that moralize different types of food, Megan acknowledges that this learning history has had a profound impact on her and that the pervasiveness of diet culture and fat stigma still results in her hearing many body-related and diet-related comments in day-to-day life. Megan also expresses skepticism that her family members' belief systems have actually changed, noting that they "know what to say and what not to say," while also acknowledging that she isn't sure that they are presenting authentically in their interactions with her.

5. *Quelling trauma-related fears.* Megan believes that if she were to weight restore, her secondary sex characteristics, like breasts and hips, would be more visible to others. Megan endorses fears that if these parts of her body were to be more prominent, she would be at increased risk of unwanted sexual attention and perhaps even sexual assault. Megan finds relief in the "invisibility" that comes along with her eating disorder.

In addition to the functions that Megan's eating disorder behaviors may serve, there are additional factors that we hypothesize are contributing to her ambivalence around treatment and recovery.

1. *Hopelessness.* Megan has a chronic sense of hopelessness and doesn't believe she can recover. Megan cites her multiple treatment episodes as evidence that she has "failed" before and will "fail" again. Megan acknowledges that there are times where she does experience a sense of hope, however it is often fleeting and she quickly finds herself deflated and hopeless again.

2. *Fear of the unknown.* As a patient who regularly vacillates between eating disorder behaviors, suicidal ideation, self-injurious behaviors, and substance use, Megan finds the prospect of giving up all of these ways of coping

to be daunting. Historically, when Megan's eating disorder behaviors have improved, she has experienced a worsening of her other comorbid mental health conditions, and vice versa. While Megan acknowledges that her life is painful as it is currently being lived, she is terrified of what a life without behaviors might be like. "Better the devil you know than the devil you don't," Megan has quipped previously.

3. *Poorly defined values.* As we will discuss shortly, Megan has a vague sense of her values, however they are not particularly well-defined, nor is it necessarily clear to Megan how to go about living into her values in day-to-day actions or through establishing and working toward long-term goals. In other words, at this point in treatment, Megan does not have a particularly compelling "why" for pursuing her recovery.

4. *Lack of interpersonal connectedness.* Related to the previous point about values, Megan also has a dearth of interpersonal connectedness in her life. Outside of her relationships with her mother and siblings, which are at times strained, her close interpersonal relationships are limited to a small number of middle school friends. Megan does have some more superficial relationships with individuals she has met in treatment, which have been a bit of a double-edged sword for her. While these friendships have been helpful when they have been recovery-focused, many of the friends she has met in treatment have struggled with their own ongoing behaviors or relapses. When her friends are struggling, Megan finds it hard to focus on her own treatment and at times, her friends' struggles increase her own desire to return to or increase the frequency of her own behaviors. As such, Megan has limited meaningful interpersonal connections, which can often be of help when it comes to motivation to work toward recovery.

Provider Exercise – Exploring Patient Ambivalence

Think of a patient with whom you are currently working who expresses significant ambivalence. How do you conceptualize their ambivalence? What factors seem to be at play? What feels missing in terms of your understanding of their ambivalence? Feel free to make notes in the space below. If you would like to take this exercise a step further, spend some time brainstorming interventions that you think could be useful in targeting your patient's ambivalence. We will be reviewing various interventions shortly and you may find having a list of your own ideas to be helpful before beginning the next section of this text. If you feel comfortable doing so, you may find it to be useful to share reflections from this exercise (ensuring information is appropriately de-identified) with a trusted peer, ideally someone who is familiar with DBT. Did their input give you any different perspectives or interventions to consider?

Building a Life Worth Living

Now that you have an understanding of how motivation is relevant across eating disorder diagnoses, including how it can impede with both willingness and ability to make change, we want to discuss strategies that specifically target motivation and help to set the stage for change-oriented work. As you saw in the examples we shared, our patients' eating disorder behaviors have very real and very compelling functions that they serve. Before we can even start to consider the "how" of beginning to make change, we have to help our patients identify and connect with a powerful "why." As we discussed in the DBT assumptions earlier, many of our patients experience their current lives as unbearable. Although not a polar opposite to unbearable, on the other side of the dialectic from unbearable is what results from taking action to build a life worth living. Building a life worth living involves helping our patients to create a life where they are regularly engaging in activities that cultivate positive emotions, like joy, contentment, and pride, are taking action steps toward achieving long-term goals, are doing activities that evoke a sense of mastery, and are living in increased alignment with their values. For many patients diagnosed with an eating disorder, as their symptoms intensify and their identity becomes increasingly more entwined with their eating disorder, they no longer have the time, energy, or desire to engage in activities that once brought them positive emotions, to focus on long-term goals they have, or to consider who they want to be as a person outside of their eating disorder. Setting the stage for making incredibly painful and anxiety-provoking changes means revisiting (or in some cases, visiting for the first time) and intensifying our patients' connection to their life worth living and helping our patients to know that working toward their life worth living is possible. Of note, it is worth mentioning that in RO DBT, "building a life worth living" is adapted slightly to be "building a life worth sharing," which is defined as "learning how to flexibly adapt one's behavior to ever-changing circumstances to achieve a goal or live according to one's values, in a manner that accounts for the needs of others" (Lynch, 2018). The emphasis on flexibility and interpersonal relationships highlights some of the unique challenges that overcontrolled individuals encounter with elements of this piece of therapeutic work.

Helping a patient take the first steps toward building a life worth living starts with getting as robust a picture as possible in terms of the qualities our patients want to define them, the values patients want to guide their life, short- and long-term goals they have, and activities that might bring them a sense of pleasure or mastery. Assessing values and goals can be accomplished through discussion, although many handouts and homework assignments exist that can facilitate this process as well. I've (AHK) used writing assignments, values-focused card sort activities, tools assessing the importance of various life domains, and so forth as additional tools in helping explore a patient's values. Like with values and goals, gathering information about what activities a patient believes might bring them pleasure or a sense of mastery can also be done through conversation and supplemented by lists of activities a patient might consider.

So when and how do you go about initiating this conversation with your patient? I (AHK) have found that it can be helpful to introduce the concept of "building a life worth living" and linking this to values and goals early in treatment, even within my initial assessment with a patient, and then treating "building a life worth living" as a thread that runs throughout treatment. One of my previous supervisors said that "all roads lead to values" and I believe there is wisdom in this statement. Whenever I find myself having trouble finding shared goals and targets with a patient, feeling "stuck" with a patient, or simply a bit lost in treatment, finding the thread of "building a life worth living" can help to keep treatment moving forward.

In terms of how to go about initiating the "building a life worth living" conversation, Charlie Swenson (2016) suggests that three tasks in this conversation must be considered. The first of these tasks is the dialectical task, which involves exploring and intervening in the patient's dialectic of wanting to build a life worth living while also wanting to maintain their eating disorder. Few patients walk through our doors fully committed to giving up their eating disorder and pursuing building a life worth living. As such, it is important as a provider to be able to explore the functions our patients' eating disorder behaviors serve for them and seek to genuinely understand why they may not want to give these behaviors up. At the same time, it is also important to begin discussing our patients' values, goals, hopes, and dreams, and how treatment can help them increase their alignment with their values and move closer to achieving their goals, hopes, and dreams.

The second of these tasks is the behavioral task, which focuses on helping our patients to vividly envision a life worth living and then translate their vision into realistic goals and associated treatment targets. Many patients with whom I (AHK) have worked are able to articulate a vague description of their life worth living (e.g. "I want to be a good friend," "I want to have a meaningful job") that lacks the vivid detail that is often needed in order to make pursuing a life worth living feel like a worthy goal. A wide range of physiological (e.g. cognitive impairment associated with malnourishment), emotional (e.g. hopelessness), and cognitive (e.g. the belief one is not worthy of a life worth living) factors may have interfered with your patient being able to articulate a more vivid picture of their life worth living to date. It is important to gain an understanding of these barriers and to target them accordingly as you work with your patient to add detail, depth, and nuance to the description of their life worth living. Once you have a more vivid picture of your patient's life worth living, you can then start to identify specific goals and treatment targets associated with those goals. For example, if being a reliable, dependable friend who follows through on commitments is part of your patient's life worth living, an associated goal might be for your patient to schedule a certain number of social obligations each month and to follow-through on them. Behaviors that impede your patient's ability to achieve this goal that could be potentially viable targets for treatment could be avoidance of social eating situations (e.g. your patient might have a tendency to cancel brunch plans with friends) or isolating behaviors associated with symptoms of depression.

The final task is the relational task, which refers to maintaining a focus on cultivating a strong therapeutic relationship in the context of initiating the "life worth living" discussion. This means bringing forward all of the qualities you would typically bring forth in establishing rapport, like authenticity, curiosity, and compassion, within the context of the "life worth living" discussion. Of note, it is also important to attend to your balance of acceptance versus change in the context of this discussion. Knowing when to sit with a patient's ambivalence about change and when to push for increased alignment with their life worth living is critical in maintaining good therapeutic rapport.

Before we share a bit about Megan's life worth living, we thought it could be helpful to comment on scope of practice in the context of life worth living discussions. While assessment of a patient's life worth living and designing and implementing assignments to assist in increased alignment with a life worth living are more within the wheelhouse of therapists and psychiatric providers, there are still ways in which other disciplines can be actively involved in discussions and interventions related to building a life worth living. First, any provider can encourage and reinforce comments made by a patient about topics related to their life worth living. For example, if a patient shares that they spent time with friends over the weekend even though they felt like isolating, you don't have to be a therapist or psychiatric provider to express pride in their choice to engage in adaptive behaviors in the face of having urges to do otherwise. Second, there are many discipline-specific activities that providers can suggest that also are likely to be consistent with a patient's life worth living. For example, a dietitian might help a patient to plan to go to brunch with a friend. While planning for exposures to challenging foods and challenging meal contexts is within the scope of practice of a dietitian, in this example this plan also helps to bring a patient closer to ultimate goals they may have around social connectedness. Finally, when providing meal coaching or in-the-moment coaching, it can be useful to weave reminders of their life worth living into the process. For all of our patients it is critical to make the connection between the challenging things we are asking them to do and the life they ultimately would like to lead.

Bringing DBT to Life – Megan's Life Worth Living

One of the assignments that Megan's therapist gives her for homework during her first week in treatment is to write about the type of person she would like to be in various life domains. Here is what Megan came up with:

Family

"My mom and I are close, although we could be closer. I want to be a good listener rather than her just listening to my problems all the time. I want her to be able to trust that I will be dependable and supportive, particularly as she gets older. My brothers and I are not close, and I'm okay with that – we're really different people. I do want to have good interactions with them when we are together in-person. I also want to feel like we can work together as a team as my mom gets older and may need our help more."

Intimate Relationships

"I want to be married one day, but not any time soon. As a partner, I want to be a good friend, a good listener, loving, and dependable. I want to participate in activities we both like – I know I'd love to be able to see live music and go to museums with my partner. I want my partner to feel like he or she is part of my family."

Parenting

"I don't think that I want to have kids, but I do want to have pets. I grew up with dogs, so I think I'd like to have at least one when I feel a bit more stable in my home life."

Social Life

"I want to be a fun, dependable, trustworthy, supportive, and caring friend. I wish that I felt closer to the friends I have currently. I also want to meet some new people who share interests similar to mine, although the thought of meeting new people makes me nervous. Probably for the best that I find some friends who don't have eating disorders themselves."

Work

"I want to be seen as a diligent, responsible, and trustworthy employee. It's important for my work to feel meaningful to me. I enjoy helping others. I want to get my job back at the pharmacy when I'm in a more stable place."

Education and Training

"I want to go back to school to earn my PharmD so I can be a pharmacist. As a student, it's important for me to take my studies seriously and to get good grades. I also hope to be a lifelong learner."

Recreation

"I want to spend more time outdoors, maybe finding new trails to hike. I like books too, and I like reading about philosophy. When I'm at my sharpest I can read a couple books a week, so I would want to get back to that. I have a pile of books I've been meaning to read. I also like caring for animals and although I don't think I'm ready for it, I'd like to foster dogs some day."

Spirituality

"If I'm honest with myself, spirituality isn't really my thing. This isn't important to me."

Citizenship

"I like helping people, although it's also hard to be around people, so I don't really know what to do about that. I do want to volunteer at my local animal shelter once I'm out of treatment. I also think it's important to stay up-to-date on politics and to take action where I can, although I do not have any desire to be involved in things like canvassing or phone banks."

Physical Self-Care

"I want to be active and athletic. I need to have fewer bad habits and more good habits."

One observation you may have about Megan's completed homework assignment is that the writing is a bit more simplistic than what you might expect for someone of Megan's age. You also might notice that in some sections, Megan's description of her life worth living in those value domains is somewhat vague. It appears as though Megan's malnourished state has compromised her cognitive abilities at this point in treatment. When Megan's therapist reviews Megan's homework assignment with her during their next therapy session, she asks Megan if she can make some notes on her homework assignment where she would like Megan to elaborate more on her thoughts. Megan expresses openness to this and is able to expand upon the assignment to an extent, although it is apparent to her therapist that she is still struggling to envision and describe a more vivid life worth living. Megan's therapist makes a note to herself to continue to revisit Megan's vision for her life worth living to build upon over time and instead chooses to focus on identifying some specific and concrete steps that Megan can take each week to help her more closely align with her values. Megan's therapist also makes a note to revisit concrete action steps Megan can take to more closely align with her values around the time that Megan will transition to PHP, as returning to her home setting will create additional opportunities for actions Megan may decide she would like to take. Finally, Megan's therapist shares information about Megan's life worth living with the rest of Megan's treating providers, so they can use this information in their interactions with Megan, as appropriate.

Provider Exercise – Building a Life Worth Living

Reflect on the patient whom you wrote about in the "Exploring Patient Ambivalence" provider exercise and consider the following questions:

How do they define their life worth living? What qualities do they want to describe them as a person?

As you think about your patient's life worth living and qualities they want to describe them as a person, what feels vague or missing to you? What questions might you ask your patient in order to gather more information?

How do you plan to go about exploring your patient's life worth living further? Are there specific approaches or activities you would like to use during your sessions?

Commitment Strategies

Commitment strategies are a set of strategies that can be used to help increase and sustain a patient's motivation for change. In terms of timing of their use during a course of treatment, commitment strategies are particularly useful at the beginning of treatment and at times when a patient's motivation for change is waning. However, given the ambivalence many of our patients experience around making change, it is often helpful to weave at least one commitment strategy into most one-on-one sessions with clients. Let's take a look at each commitment strategy and how they apply in multidisciplinary eating disorders care (for a more in-depth discussion of the commitment strategies, readers are encouraged to review Linehan, 1993, pp. 284–291).

Evaluating the Pros and Cons. Evaluating the pros and cons involves looking at the benefits and downsides of one or more behaviors or courses of action. This strategy is helpful not only with patients who are ambivalent about making change, but also with patients who are more motivated to make changes, as this strategy can further strengthen their commitment to change. Some examples of pros and cons in eating disorder work include:

1. The pros and cons of engaging in a specific eating disorder behavior versus using skills to manage urges to engage in that specific eating disorder behavior.
2. The pros and cons of maintaining a vegetarian diet versus the pros and cons of incorporating meat into one's diet.
3. The pros and cons of returning to a competitive sport.
4. The pros and cons of discharging against medical advice from a treatment center versus the pros and cons of remaining in treatment.
5. The pros and cons of taking an anti-anxiety medication before meals.

Table 9.1 Pros and Cons of Binge Eating Versus Pros and Cons of Using Skills to Cope with Binge Urges

Pros of Binge Eating	Cons of Binge Eating
- Decreases my anxiety - Helps me "numb out" - Relieves stress - Feels good at the beginning - Excitement around planning to eat binge foods - Comfortable routine for me – one of the only things I look forward to - I get to eat what I really want	- Expensive - Creates stress because of credit card debt - Physical fullness afterward is unbearable - Time-consuming - Keeps me isolated from friends and family, the planning alone keeps me distracted when with others - Guilt associated with lying about binges - I don't always taste the food - Shame associated with the binges and related behaviors (eating food I have already put in the trash, stealing food) - Weight gain
Pros of Using Skills to Cope With Binge Urges	**Cons of Using Skills to Cope With Binge Urges**
- Helps me feel competent and in control - It is a step in the right direction toward having a healthier relationship with food - Don't have to deal with guilt, shame, or excessive fullness - Cheaper - Gives me more time to do other activities	- Don't get the "high" associated with binges – there is nothing else that feels the same - Have to deal with discomfort of sitting with urges - Takes effort - Have to deal with stress and anxiety

Table 9.2 Pros and Cons of Engaging in Food Exposure Versus Pros and Cons of Continuing to Avoid Certain Foods

Pros of Engaging in Food Exposure	Cons of Engaging in Food Exposure
- Feeling less fear over time (maybe?) - Adds more variety to my diet, which means I can eat with friends more easily - Eating different types of food will make me look less "weird" at meals - Less time spent reviewing menus and stressing out about restaurant choices - Makes it more likely I'll be able to eat in spontaneous social situations (parties, work events) - I might actually enjoy it?	- Potentially uncomfortable texture or feeling when I'm chewing and swallowing - Possibility I might vomit or choke - Having to deal with anxiety during exposure, I don't know how anxious I'll feel and how long the anxiety will last - Might smell gross and make me feel nauseous - Nervous feelings leading up to the exposure - Takes time to plan and do exposures

Pros of Continuing to Avoid Certain Foods	Cons of Continuing to Avoid Certain Foods
- Easier in the moment - Less fear about nausea, vomiting, or choking - Easier to plan and grocery shop for meals I eat alone	- Probably less healthy - Limits food-related activities I can do with friends and family - Continue to live in fear of bodily reactions to foods

In order to get a better sense as to how pros and cons can work, let's take a look at a couple of specific pros and cons lists.

There are a few important points to make about pros and cons. First, as you review pros and cons with your patient, be sure that you are paying attention to which of the pros and cons are short-term consequences versus which of the pros and cons are long-term consequences. What you'll often find is that the pros of maladaptive behaviors and cons of adaptive behaviors tend to be short-term consequences, which can sometimes help to shift how patients are thinking about their lists. If you look at the example of the pros and cons of binge eating above, you'll notice that binge eating for this particular patient both relieves stress and creates stress, with the stress that is created likely lasting longer than the stress relief associated with binge eating. Second, not every item in a pros and cons list will have the same value, so it can be helpful to have patients mark which items are most important to them. In the second example above, the patient notes that a pro of avoiding certain foods is that it is easier in the moment, however they note that a con is that it is likely unhealthy to have such a limited array of foods they are eating. In this case, they might rank their health as more important than the ease associated with continuing to make the same choices they have made about food previously. Related to these first two points, it is also important to note that the number of items in a pros or cons column should not necessarily determine someone's course of action. Just because there are more pros by number alone does not necessarily mean that specific course of action is in your patient's best interest. Finally, it can be helpful to think of the cons of an adaptive behavior as potential problems to be solved and the pros of a maladaptive behavior as outcomes your patient might be able to achieve through more skillful behaviors. For example, one of the pros identified for binge eating in the example above was that it relieves anxiety. If this is important to your patient, it can be helpful to explore whether there are other strategies the patient can use to achieve a similar outcome. Similarly, many of the cons identified for using skills to cope with urges to engage in binge eating can actually be targeted by skills as well!

Playing Devil's Advocate. Playing devil's advocate involves taking up the side against change, the side of the status quo, in the hopes the patient will take up the side for change. Let's take a look at an example:

Dietitian: "It still seems like the selections you're making with your food are still pretty rigid."

Patient: "I know you've tried to sell me on the importance of 'flexibility', but I know myself...if I start to relax around my portions, I'll lose all control and keep gaining weight, so I have to eat this way."

Dietitian: "So counting your almonds, weighing your food, and eating out of measuring cups is working out just fine for you then."

Patient: "No, it's not great. I am spending more time stressing about my food than just about anything else. And I can't eat unless I can measure or weigh my food, so I'm pretty limited."

Dietitian: "So, where would you like to go from here, and how can I support you?"

Patient: "Ugh, I don't know. I can try to eat more 'flexibly'. I'll start by getting rid of my food scale. But if I start to gain more weight, I'm going back to what I know works."

Foot-in-the-Door/Door-in-the-Face Techniques. Foot-in-the-door and door-in-the-face techniques got their start as sales tactics, however they have subsequently been used strategically in the context of behavioral healthcare. The foot-in-the-door technique involves making an easier request, followed by a slightly harder request, whereas the door-in-the-face technique involves making a larger request than what you think your patient will be willing to commit to, and then backing down to a smaller request that you think they will buy into. Here is an example of how this might look in the context of a dialogue with a patient:

Dietitian: "I know that you are still having difficulty believing that a dessert after dinner can be a part of normative eating, so I'd like to focus our work there this week. I'd like to set the goal of having you have dessert after dinner all seven days this week."

Patient: "There is absolutely no way I'm going to do that. I can do three days at most."

Dietitian: "I'm hearing that three days sounds doable, and I know you are capable of doing hard things. Could we shoot for four days?"

Patient: "That's asking a lot."

Dietitian: "I recognize that it is, and you've told me before that when you are in wise mind, you know this is an important next step for you. So what do you think?"

Patient: "Alright, alright. I'll give it a shot."

The above example shows how this technique might work for a patient who is more willing and able to make change. At times, use of this technique requires considerably smaller commitments as a starting point. Let's take a look at another example:

Dietitian: "In reviewing your meal logs, I noticed that you're regularly eating evening snack, which is a great improvement! Seems like it's generally fruit or a savory food...I see pretzels, cheese sticks and fruit. When's the last time you had a sweet dessert?"

Patient: "I don't like sweets."

Dietitian: "You don't like sweets or your eating disorder doesn't like sweets?"

Patient: "... I don't know. I can't remember the last time I had sweets."

Dietitian: "What if we set a goal around it? Every night this week I want you to incorporate a sweet snack."

Patient: "What! No. Not going to happen."

Dietitian: "Three days?"

Patient: "No. I'm not ready, and like I said, I don't even know if I like sweets..."

Dietitian: "How about we start small. Is there one sweet component of snack you can add, even one time this week?"

Patient: (sigh) "I can probably eat some chocolate chips with my pretzels and nuts."

Dietitian: "Sounds like a great place to start."

Connecting Present Commitments to Prior Commitments. Connecting present commitments to prior commitments is exactly as it sounds. If a patient has previously committed to a certain course of action and their commitment is fading or their behavior isn't aligning with this commitment, it can be helpful to revisit their original commitment. You can see a variation on this strategy in the previous example provided, where the dietitian reminds the patient that when they are in wise mind, they know that challenging themselves by incorporating desserts into the array of foods they consume is an important part of their recovery process.

Mental Health Technician:	"Hey, I noticed you've been isolating after meals recently. What's going on?"
Patient:	"Nothing, I'm fine, I just want to be left alone."
Mental Health Technician:	"I can't do that, I can tell your urges are high. I know that was a difficult meal."
Patient:	"I just need alone time, I have high urges right now; if I act on them, I'll feel better."
Mental Health Technician:	"I remember when we first met and you asked me directly if I could help engage you after meals and snacks because that's when you're most likely to engage in self-injury due to the shame you feel after eating. Do you remember that?"
Patient:	"Yeah. Forget it though...I just want to be left alone."
Mental Health Technician:	"I totally understand wanting to be left alone and I know that when you are in wise mind, you and I have the shared goal of helping you to decrease your self-harm behaviors. Am I right about that?"
Patient:	"Ugh, yeah.."
Mental Health Technician:	"Okay. I'm wondering if you and I could chat for a few minutes and come up with some ideas of other things you could try instead of self-harm to get through this difficult moment."
Patient:	(sighs) "Okay, I'm willing to give that a shot."

Highlighting the Freedom to Choose and Absence of Alternatives. Highlighting the freedom to choose and the absence of alternatives involves openly acknowledging all of the options a patient has available in a given situation, while simultaneously highlighting the limitations of those options. This strategy takes advantage of research that has shown that commitment to a course of action is increased when a person feels they have chosen that course of action freely and that commitment also increases when people believe there are no other viable alternatives to their selected course of action. Here are some examples of how this might play out:

Adolescent Patient: "You can't force me to eat. I'm not eating."
Outpatient Medical Provider: "You are one-hundred percent correct. I can't force you to eat."
Adolescent Patient: (sitting quietly, arms folded)
Outpatient Medical Provider: "Look, continuing to restrict is totally your choice, and when your parents brought you in for your appointment today, they shared with me that they think hospitalization is their only option if things don't change."

Adult Patient: "I don't know why I'm still here in treatment. In fact, I'd like to discharge today. I'm totally fine."
Patient's Husband: "You can't discharge today. I'm terrified. You're not coming home until you complete treatment."
Adult Patient: "Oh yes, I am. Come on, we're leaving."
Patient's Husband: "Oh no, we're not. You are not coming home, plain and simple. I'm not driving you."
Residential Therapist: "Mary, it's totally your choice whether you'd like to stay in treatment or not, and I'm hearing Cameron say that you can't come home with him if you leave. Am I understanding things correctly?"
Patient's Husband: "Absolutely."

Using Principles of Shaping. Using principles of shaping involves being willing to accept smaller commitments and associated actions with the goal of working on establishing larger commitments over the course of time. Just as our patients can get stuck in black-and-white, all-or-nothing thinking, so can we as providers! When we are speaking with our patients about making incredibly challenging changes in their lives, many of which are changes they feel ambivalent about or even directly opposed to making, it can be helpful to take a step back and explore whether there are steps in between where your patient is currently and where you hope to help your patient get. For almost any patient situation, there is probably a step in between where you and your patient can find common ground. Let's take a look at a couple of examples:

Patient: (sitting at table and staring at plate, while other people at the table have gotten started with their meals)

Nurse: "Alright, Melissa. Go ahead and pick up your fork and get started with dinner."

Patient: "There is no way I am completing this meal today. Are you kidding? This is seriously impossible."

Nurse: "Whoa, whoa, whoa…I didn't say anything about the whole meal. I just said let's focus on getting started. Let's take a look at your plate…between the broccoli, potatoes, and chicken, what looks most doable?"

Patient: "NOT the chicken."

Nurse: "Okay, well let's start with the potatoes then. I'll join you in eating them. Let's you and I both start with a bite."

Patient: "I told you that I'm fine with restoring some weight to avoid step-up to a higher level of care, but I'm not willing to give up being vegan."

Dietitian: "I hear what you're saying and I'm imagining how challenging weight restoration is going to be if we can't incorporate animal protein into your diet. Look, I gather that all meat is off the table right now, and I'm wondering about other animal by-products, like milk, butter, cheese…that sort of thing. Is there any wiggle room there to help us with this process?"

Patient: (deep sigh) "I'm willing to consider some of those things, maybe. But only if they are ethically and sustainably produced."

Dietitian: "I think that gives us a better place to start. Which of those items do you think would be easiest to obtain while also meeting your standards?"

Cheerleading. Cheerleading involves providing your patient with encouragement, highlighting the progress your patient is making, and expressing a genuine belief that your patient has the ability to overcome whatever brought them into treatment, in turn achieving and sustaining recovery and a life worth living. Cheerleading in the context of working with an individual diagnosed with an eating disorder is more nuanced than it might seem. Keeping in mind that many of our patients struggle with ambivalence around giving up their eating disorder in pursuit of recovery and a life worth living, they may not experience the same cheerleading statements to be reinforcing in the way that patients with other psychiatric illnesses might. For example, some patients might find the statement, "I'm so proud of you for completing 100% of your dinner today!" to be punishing rather than reinforcing. Statements like, "I can see you put in a lot of hard work today" can be a useful alternative to commenting specifically about completion and it is important to keep in mind that cheerleading is highly individualized. It can be helpful to ask your patient about statements that they find to be encouraging and statements that they find to be discouraging early on in the treatment process.

Agreeing on Homework. Agreeing on homework involves working collaboratively with your patient to identify at least one new solution or skill they are willing to practice in between sessions. In order to increase the likelihood of compliance, it is important that both you and your patient write down what was agreed upon and that you make a plan to ask your patient about the homework assignment as part of your next session. If you and your patient have agreed upon a particularly challenging assignment, you may want to make arrangements to check-in with them in between sessions to see how they are progressing and troubleshoot any barriers that have emerged. You may be wondering why agreeing on homework is one of the commitment strategies in DBT, since it doesn't necessarily seem directly tied into patient motivation. It could be argued that agreeing on homework ties in to using principles of shaping in that I have yet to meet a patient who wasn't willing to commit to doing a homework assignment in between therapy sessions, even if commitment hasn't always led to follow-through each and every time. If I can get a patient to make a commitment to trying something, that is a step in the right direction. If they not only commit to doing something, but also follow-through on their commitment, that is yet another step closer. And if they commit to doing something harder than I would have expected and follow-through, that is an even bigger stride toward recovery. Thinking about using principles of shaping as they relate to agreeing on homework, it is important to be thoughtful in selecting a homework activity with your patient, keeping in mind both their degree of ambivalence and their capacity to implement potential homework activities. Taking capacity out of the equation, here are some examples of assignments we might consider based on our patient's level of ambivalence:

Table 9.3

	Therapy-Related Homework	Nutrition-Related Homework	Med/Psych-Related Homework
Highly Ambivalent	- Track emotions and behaviors on a diary card - Complete a pros and cons list for a specific behavior and specific alternative behavior (e.g. bingeing vs. using skills to tolerate binge urges) - Do a homework assignment related to values and building a life worth living	- Track intake between sessions - Minimally commit to similar nutrition and fluid intake to avoid nutritional decompensation - Consider possible nutritional changes discussed in session - Consider reduction of compensatory behaviors - Commit to return to follow-up session	- Read about a medication their provider would like them to start taking but that they are reluctant to take
Moderately Ambivalent	- Conduct a chain analysis of a problem behavior and identify a new skill they are willing to try that targets a link in the chain analysis - Do a homework assignment that targets a secondary issue (e.g. depression), but that could have positive impacts on a primary issue (e.g. restricting)	- Complete a pros and cons list focused on nutritional change and/or compensatory behavior (e.g. reincorporating animal protein, adding a morning snack, decreasing caffeine intake, reducing time spent walking each week) - Work on a challenge food hierarchy - Engage in meal planning and grocery list creation - Commit to one to two agreed-upon nutritional challenges for the week (e.g. order in fast food for one meal this week; eat a meal in the dining hall instead of isolating in the dorm)	- Write a pros and cons list for taking a medication their provider would like them to start taking but that they are reluctant to take
Highly Committed to Change	- Engage in graduated exposures - Intentionally practice change-focused skills (e.g. Emotion Regulation, Interpersonal Effectiveness)	- Engage in graduated food-related exposures, with or without support of dietitian - Self-identify and engage in nutritional challenges without dietitian support	- Write out what skills they will use to help them follow-through on taking a medication they are reluctant to take and then fill the prescription

Bringing DBT to Life – Using Commitment Strategies With Megan

Megan:	"So, I just wanted to let you know…I've thought about it and decided to leave treatment tomorrow. I've gotten all I wanted out of treatment and it's time for me to go back to my life and job."
Claire (Registered Dietitian):	"Wait, what happened? You seemed to be very recovery-oriented on Tuesday when I last saw you and seemed open to the length of stay we discussed."
Megan:	"I just can't handle the weight gain and I honestly think I have the skills that I need to do this on my own. I'm not getting anything out of residential treatment right now."
Claire:	"I hear that and at the same time, you're still restricting portions of your meals on a daily basis, even with the support you have here."
Megan:	"I just need to leave and I'll be fine. I know myself."
Claire:	"Frankly, I'm really worried about you leaving care prematurely. You have done some really tremendous work in the time you've been here. You came in purging several times a day and at this point it's been over eight weeks since you've purged. I've seen huge leaps in your engagement, vulnerability, and willingness to try challenging foods. Your restriction has also really improved. I know you don't see it, but your progress is getting you closer to a life in recovery. *(Cheerleading)* I worry if you leave too soon and disengage from treatment, you will be taking some big steps backwards."
Megan:	"I won't take steps backwards, I really think I can do it on my own, and at a lower weight than you want me to be."
Claire:	"Sounds like the first step to eating disorder recovery is some weight loss. Am I understanding that correctly?" *(Playing Devil's Advocate)*
Megan:	*(quietly sulking)*

Claire: "Okay you're not going to like this, but I made you a promise the day you admitted. Do you remember? You told me when your eating disorder got loud, you'd want to leave early, and you asked me to help talk you into staying because you know you'd regret it if you left." *(Connecting Present Commitments to Past Commitments)*

Megan: "Did I say that? Well, I changed my mind. I still want to leave."

Claire: "My understanding was if you left care early, your mom would no longer help you with your rent, car insurance and cell phone bill. So… it's your decision to leave, but it might be pretty difficult to make ends meet without her help." *(Highlighting the Freedom to Choose and Absence of Alternatives)*

Megan: *(avoiding Claire's eye contact, visibly frustrated)*

Claire: "Look, I can see you're feeling frustrated. Can we slow it down a bit? How about we think through the pros and cons of you leaving." *(Evaluating Pros and Cons)*

Megan: "It's pointless. I know I want to leave. But… whatever. Pros: I don't have to weight restore anymore and get even fatter than I already am. In fact, I can lose ten or fifteen pounds, and I can return to my job and start making money again… I can use my own bathroom and get better sleep, since I'm not sleeping at all anymore. Cons: I might owe money to my insurance company if I leave, I might not get medical clearance to return to work, I'll have to let everyone know I didn't complete treatment, I'll have to figure out how to eat on my own, and I guess I might relapse. And I'll have to figure out my rent, car insurance, and cell phone situation."

Claire: "Sounds to me like you've got a lot to consider, and it sounds like there are some unknowns that could be helpful in decision-making. Look, I wonder if instead of just doing the whole cut-and-run thing tomorrow, if you'd be willing to discuss the medical clearance letter with your medical provider to at least get some more information to help you make the most wise mind decision you can? While you're at it, you could ask about your sleep medication regimen if it feels like poor sleep quality is contributing to your unhappiness here."

Megan: "Yeah, I guess I could do that."

Claire: "Are you okay with sleeping on this decision, then? I'm not asking you to commit to completing your treatment here, but will you at least commit to the next 48 hours?" *(Foot-in-the-Door/Door-in-the-Face Technique)*

Megan: "Ugh. Fine. You know me too well and if I really think about it, I'll likely just stick it out. Which is why I don't want to think about it and I want to just go! ...But yes, I'll think about it."

Claire: "Fantastic. In the meantime, I wonder if you're willing to revisit the pros and cons list we started together? I'd really like it if you were able to add additional pros and cons you might not have thought of in the moment, and maybe make a note for each pro and con whether it's something short-term or something long-term. I think that might help with accessing wise mind, too." *(Agreeing on Homework)*

Megan: "Yeah, I can do that."

Provider Exercise – Commitment Strategies

For this provider exercise, start by briefly reviewing the commitment strategies and then identify a patient who is struggling with motivation and/or ambivalence with whom you would like to try using commitment strategies during your next appointment. Once you have used one or more commitment strategies with your patient, use the prompts below to reflect on your experience. If you feel comfortable doing so, consider discussing your reflections with a trusted colleague for feedback.

Which of the commitment strategies did you use? How specifically did you use these strategies?

How did your patient respond in the moment? Did you notice any changes after the session in terms of your patient's thoughts, behaviors, or emotions?

What do you think went well in using the commitment strategies? What would you do differently in the future?

What other reflections do you have about your experience?

Chapter 10

The Therapeutic Relationship in DBT

We will be covering a lot of concrete strategies throughout this text, many of which we hope you will find useful in your work, and we would be remiss to not discuss the therapeutic relationship in the context of providing clinical care. Bruce Wampold has written extensively on this topic and in short, he has found that common factors like collaboration, empathy, alliance, and positive regard yield notable effect sizes when examining psychotherapy outcomes. We would not be writing this book if we didn't believe in the importance of and value of specific strategies and techniques and we want to spend some time discussing the therapeutic relationship because it has been found to be such a critical component of psychotherapy outcomes, yet is often not a topic of focus in discipline-specific training. For example, the dietitian-patient relationship is considered to be an important component of patient-centered care (Sladdin, et al., 2017), yet research suggests that exposure to the dietitian-patient relationship as part of the professional education of dietitians is variable (Nagy, et al., 2021) and that dietitians entering the eating disorder field often feel inadequately prepared, with communication being one area they identify where there are deficits in training (Heruc, et al., 2020). Given that communication skills are fundamental in establishing a therapeutic relationship, it can be reasonably deduced that dietitians do not feel adequately prepared for this task. Anecdotally, in conducting training on DBT with dietictians over the past number of years, many have alluded to the fact they did not feel they received exposure to material that prepared them for the nuanced aspects of navigating the therapeutic relationship and communication in the context of eating disorder work specifically. Furthermore, many of our (AHK, ETM) senior dietitian colleagues have mentioned that supervision and/or consultation, either from a therapist or psychiatric provider or from a senior dietitian with a history of multidisciplinary supervision and consultation, was necessary for them to develop their own skills in this area. We hope that the content of this chapter helps to establish a base of knowledge upon which providers who have not been trained on patient-provider therapeutic relationships can build.

DOI: 10.4324/9781003495604-10

Therapeutic Style in DBT

Therapeutic style in DBT refers to the interpersonal qualities we bring to bear in our interactions with our patients. Research that has been conducted on common factors in psychotherapy has found a number of elements of therapeutic style to be critical to psychotherapeutic outcomes, including collaboration, empathy, positive regard, and genuineness (Wampold, 2015). As we review more specifics about therapeutic style in DBT, you will notice that these elements are present. What perhaps separates DBT from many other psychotherapeutic interventions is the extent to which therapeutic style is discussed and utilized in a strategic manner and the ways in which more unconventional therapeutic styles are incorporated into treatment.

Validation

When we think about cultivating a positive therapeutic relationship within DBT, one the most valuable tools you have at your disposal is validation. Validation involves the combination of empathy, or an accurate understanding of our patients' lived experiences from their perspective, coupled with actively communicating to your patient that their perspective makes sense. Validation can manifest not only in our verbal responses to patients, but in our actions as well. For example, if a patient being treated in a residential level of care goes to the nursing station complaining of a headache, one way to validate the patient could be to verbally acknowledge their pain (e.g. "I hear you are in a lot of pain right now"), but perhaps a more powerful way to validate the patient is to provide an over-the-counter medication approved by their medical provider that can reduce the physical pain they are experiencing.

Why Validate? There are a number of reasons why validation is a critical treatment strategy. First, patients diagnosed with eating disorders are often ambivalent about change, yet treatment is ultimately a change-focused endeavor. Weaving validation throughout treatment provides a necessary counterbalance to an emphasis on problem-solving and behavioral change. I often think of "A Spoonful of Sugar," a song from the movie Mary Poppins, when I think about acceptance and change. Our patients are going to be more willing to accept treatment and an increased focus on change if they know that we understand just how painful and unpleasant change can be. Second, there is evidence that validation decreases emotional arousal, which in turn can help patients to emit more skillful responses. If you reflect on times when you've felt an intense emotion, like anger or anxiety, it can be considerably more difficult to respond skillfully than when your emotions feel less intense. Third, validation strengthens the therapeutic relationship and can help to repair relationship ruptures when they occur. If you reflect on conversations with your closest friends or family members, there is a good chance that you will find a healthy dose of validation woven throughout. Relatedly, if you think about a time you received a truly heartfelt apology from someone after an interpersonal conflict, most likely that apology included a significant amount of validation as well. Fourth, validation gives our patients feedback about their behavior, emotions, cognitions, and sensations. What you choose to validate provides our patients with important information. For example, if I have a patient who gets in an argument with a friend over the phone, some elements of their experience may have significant validity, like feeling the emotion of anger, whereas other elements of their experience may lack validity, like cursing at their friend and hanging up on them in response. Through the process of selective validation, we are teaching our patients to sort their behavior, emotions, cognitions, and sensations into "valid" and "not valid" categories, which in turn helps them to be more effective in navigating their day-to-day lives. Fifth, validating our patients helps to reduce their self-invalidation and increases their ability to self-validate. When we validate our patients, we are modeling for them the very behavior we want them to learn and implement, just directed inward instead of toward other people. Patients diagnosed with eating disorders are often masters of self-invalidation, particularly when it comes to their emotional experiences and the difficulty that goes along with making behavioral change. Their self-invalidation often mimics invalidation from others in their environment. Through providing our patients with validation, they can begin to see the wisdom in their own responses. Finally, validation can help to strengthen clinical progress. Research has shown that most people find validation to be reinforcing and that many people will take actions necessary to elicit validation from others. When we provide validation around things like making measurable clinical progress, trying new skills, or engaging with difficult parts of treatment (e.g. doing food exposures), we increase the likelihood of these things occurring again in the future.

The Six Levels of Validation. Validation can sound relatively simple at a surface level, however there is an incredible amount of nuance with validation done well. In order to help providers to get a better understanding of this nuance, DBT takes the broader treatment strategy of validation and breaks it down into both levels and types. The six levels of validation are as follows:

Level One – Staying Awake. This level of validation involves removing as many potential distractors as possible and putting your full focus into actively listening to your patient and making a wholehearted attempt to understand what they are communicating. Level one validation also requires that you recognize and let go of your own theories and biases that could influence how you take in information about what your patient is saying, feeling, and doing and instead approach each conversation with genuine curiosity, even if the conversation feels similar to conversations you've had before. While level one validation may seem simple on the surface, it actually requires a good degree of intentionality and attentional focus.

Level Two – Accurate Reflection. Level two validation involves verbally communicating an accurate summary of a patient's emotions, thoughts, assumptions, and actions. This is most commonly known as a "reflective listening," in that you are taking your patient's language and succinctly reflecting what they have shared back to them. When using this level of validation, it is important to be cognizant of using similar language to that of your patient.

Level Three – Articulating Unverbalized Thoughts or Emotions. This level of validation involves communicating thoughts or emotions that your patient has not explicitly expressed. It entails listening closely to what your patient is communicating and based on this information, imagining what they might be thinking or feeling beyond what they have shared. This level of validation is a form of "mind reading," to an extent. One point that is critical with this level of validation is that if your patient indicates you have not made accurate conclusions about what they are thinking or feeling, that you acknowledge your misunderstanding and seek to gain clarification.

Level Four – Validating in Terms of the Patient's Past History or Biological Dysfunction. Level four validation involves taking knowledge you have of your patient's history and using it to make sense of something a patient is experiencing in the present moment. For example, if a patient has a history of purging routinely after eating ice cream and they decide with their dietitian to do an exposure involving ice cream, it would make sense that they might be experiencing a great deal of anxiety on the day of the exposure. Level four validation can also involve making sense of the present moment in the context of a patient's biology. Eating disorders lend themselves particularly well to this form of level four validation, in that we know that eating disorders are biologically-influenced, brain-based illnesses where differences in genetics, neurotransmitters, and brain structures have been found. As a more concrete example, there is evidence that suggests serotonin-related dysfunctions in individuals diagnosed with Anorexia Nervosa create conditions where restriction is experienced as reinforcing, whereas consuming regular meals and snacks results in an uncomfortable increase in serotonin levels that are associated with an increase in anxiety and other negatively-valenced emotions.

Level Five – Validating in Terms of the Present Context. This level of validation involves seeking relevant facts in the current environment that can help you to make sense of a patient's behavior. For example, if you are working with a patient who already has heightened urges to restrict and they are experiencing a migraine with associated nausea, it makes sense that a meal that was likely already going to be a challenge is experienced as even more difficult than usual. It is important to note that if a situation presents itself where there are opportunities to validate both in terms of past history and present context, you should opt to validate based on present context first. Focusing on relevant history instead of what you are witnessing directly may be experienced as invalidating by some patients.

Level Six – Radical Genuineness. Level six validation is radical genuineness, which put simply, is being authentic and treating your patient as an equal. When coming from a place of radical genuineness, you are striving to validate your patient in a way that has the same degree of authenticity that you bring with your closest friends and family. We've heard many patients express how much they dislike being "therapized," which we have interpreted as providers using "cookie cutter" language in response to their patients, rather than approaching their patient as they would other people in their lives. Radical genuineness is freeing for both patients and providers. For patients, they know they are being seen and respected, just as they are in that moment. For providers, radical genuineness allows us to simply be ourselves in being wholly present with another person, quirks and foibles and all. Radical genuineness does not mean ignoring boundaries and professionalism, but rather allows us to access the best part of our genuine selves while remaining in a framework that puts the well-being of our patients first.

Examples of Types of Validation. There are four types of validation strategies that are both related to and independent from the six levels of validation: emotional validation strategies, behavioral validation strategies, cognitive validation strategies, and cheerleading. For a more extensive discussion of the types of validation, readers are encouraged to review Linehan, 1993, pp. 226–249.

Emotional Validation Strategies. Emotional validation strategies focus primarily on being aware of patients' emotional experiencing, accurately observing and describing the emotions we notice, and communicating the validity of our patients' emotional experiences. When we think about our patients on the spectrum of overcontrol to undercontrol, how emotional validation strategies are used varies for individuals who fall toward either of the ends of this spectrum. For patients who are more overcontrolled in nature, as we discussed earlier, they tend to mask their emotions, making it more difficult to read what they are experiencing and respond effectively. This same subset of patients is also more likely to struggle with alexithymia, meaning they may also be experiencing difficulty accurately observing and describing their emotional experiences. For these patients, emotional validation strategies focus on accurately identifying the emotion the patient is experiencing and helping them to develop the skills necessary to observe and describe their emotions as well. On the other end of the overcontrol-undercontrol spectrum, for patients who are more undercontrolled in terms of emotional expression, emotional validation strategies focus on giving ample space for emotional expression, while also being mindful to avoid approaches that amplify the intensity of the emotions the patient is experiencing. When working with patients who are more undercontrolled in terms of emotional expression, there can be a fear on the part of providers that by acknowledging their patient's emotional experience, there is the associated risk that the interaction will be derailed. When emotional validation strategies are applied thoughtfully, the opposite outcome often occurs. By focusing on the emotion the patient is experiencing, rather than the specifics of the situation that evoked the emotion, the intensity of the emotion is often reduced, and the interaction can be shifted to other important topics at hand. Conversely, avoidance of discussing the patient's emotion can not only result in the patient being "stuck" on the situation that evoked the emotion and the emotion itself, but also leave the patient feeling invalidated by their experience not being acknowledged and discussed.

Behavioral Validation Strategies. Instead of focusing on the validity of emotions, as was the area of focus with emotional validation strategies, behavioral validation strategies focus on the validity of our patients' behaviors. A subset of our patients can be self-critical and may take a punitive or invalidating approach in response to their behavior patterns. Other patients with whom we work may have been accused of consciously using their eating disorder behaviors or symptoms of other comorbid mental health conditions to achieve specific outcomes, like getting a loved one's attention and support. Behavioral validation strategies provide a sharp contrast to these perspectives and approaches to our patients' behavior. Behavioral validation strategies assume that all behavior is caused, and with this assumption in mind, that all behavior is therefore understandable. This does not mean that all behavior is effective when we consider our patients' goals and values, however when we consider what preceded the behavior, we can make sense of it. Eating disorder behaviors are an excellent example of behaviors that can both make sense and be inconsistent with goals and values. For example, when you consider the immediate relief that a patient experiences when they restrict, a relief that is driven at a biological level, you can understand why they would engage in this behavior when they are feeling intense anxiety. Behavioral validation strategies start with seeking to find a way that our patients' behaviors can make sense to us. Actively refraining from assuming our patients have conscious motives behind their behavior and challenging our patients when they assume these types of motives for their own behavior is another critical aspect of behavioral validation strategies. Finally, behavioral validation strategies move away from a focus on what our patients "should" have done when it comes to their behavior and instead focus on helping patients learn from their experience to prevent a similar situation in the future. Our patients may feel legitimately disappointed in their behavior and an emphasis on dwelling on the "should" may actually push our patients further away from developing the necessary skills to avoid a similar outcome in the future.

Cognitive Validation Strategies. Cognitive validation strategies are arguably the most difficult type of validation strategy to apply when working with patients diagnosed with eating disorders. Cognitive validation strategies focus on refraining from making our own assumptions and instead eliciting and searching for the truth in our patients' thoughts, beliefs, expectations, and assumptions. The challenge with eating disorders is that our patients' thoughts specific to topics related to food, physical activity, and body image are often quite distorted from reality, even to the point of sounding almost psychotic in nature in particularly severe eating disorder presentations. In situations where thinking is distorted such that a kernel of truth cannot be found, opting for emotional validation strategies can be a helpful approach. For example, if a patient expresses that they are afraid that their bones will liquify into fat if they eat ground beef, rather than searching for truth in a belief that is not grounded in reality, a statement like, "I can understand why it would be incredibly anxiety-provoking to plan a taco night this week if that is the message your eating disorder is giving you" might be helpful instead. There are also many situations in which our patients' thoughts will align more closely with reality and helping them to discriminate facts from interpretations and find the kernel of truth in their thinking can be a beneficial approach. For example, for a patient for whom significant weight restoration was a part of their treatment process, it is a common experience for friends and loved ones to have noticeable reactions upon seeing the patient for the first time after weight restoration has occurred. Trying to deny or refute that their friends or loved ones did indeed have a reaction to their weight would not actually map on to reality and is likely to be perceived as invalidating. Situations like these are where the sorting of facts (e.g., "I noticed that my friends had a visible reaction to seeing me for the first time after treatment") from interpretations (e.g., "They think I'm fat") is important. It is also important to acknowledge that the fat phobic, diet culture oriented society within which we live may influence the environment such that our patients' interpretations are indeed grounded within reality. Using the previous example, it is possible that there could be situations in which other interpretations have more validity (e.g. "My friends were worried about how thin I was previously and they now think I look healthy in a positive way."), however there also could be situations in which a patient's friends do indeed believe they are fat now that they have fully weight restored. In situations such as this one, there is indeed validity in the patient's initial interpretation, however not in additional thoughts that may follow (e.g. "If my friends think I'm fat, it means I need to lose some weight."). A final important element of cognitive validation strategies involves being able to honor situations in which a patient may arrive at a conclusion through intuition and situations in which a patient may hold different beliefs and values than our own. It is important not to assume that by virtue of your role as a professional, your perspectives and opinions are more valid than those of your patients.

Cheerleading. The final type of validation strategy is cheerleading. Cheerleading involves making statements that convey that you believe that the patient has the ability to engage in adaptive behaviors now and that they have the capacity to expand their abilities over time, moving them in the direction of recovery and a life worth living. Cheerleading is not taking an unreasonably optimistic view with regard to current and future possibilities for our patients. For example, it may not be reasonable to expect that a patient who has struggled for decades with chronic Anorexia Nervosa will be able to enter into full recovery and pursue their dream of becoming a world-class neurosurgeon, however it is reasonable to hold the belief that recovery and some form of personally meaningful employment is possible for even the most chronically ill of our patients. While cheerleading is a strategy that you should try to weave into each individual appointment with a patient, it's also important to note that cheerleading can actually contradict the other validation strategies we reviewed, so it is important to keep balance in mind when using cheerleading. In other words, expressing belief in your patient's ability to implement positive changes should also be accompanied with recognition that making change is often incredibly hard. There are also a couple of points specific to using cheerleading with patients diagnosed with eating disorders that are worth mentioning. First, because of factors like patient ambivalence, slow or inconsistent progress, pressures on providers to demonstrate rapid change, and so forth, it can be challenging for providers to remember to utilize cheerleading, particularly in a realistic and genuine fashion. It can be helpful to reflect on the DBT assumptions here, remembering that our patients are doing the best they can in any given moment, and that they need to do better, try harder, and be more motivated to change, all things that, as providers, we are equipped to help them with. Secondly, perhaps more so than with other psychiatric illnesses, with eating disorders, cheerleading must be thoughtfully individualized. For some patients, noting how proud you are that they were able to complete a meal can be experienced as reinforcing, whereas other patients may find the same statement to be aversive. We have found that in lieu of comments around meal completion, statements like, "I can see how hard you worked today" are generally experienced as positive and it is still important to get a sense as to the personal preferences of your patients.

Putting Validation in Context. Now that we've looked at validation in a more granular way, we want to take a higher level view to help you place validation within the broader context of DBT as a whole. If you remember our discussion earlier of the balance of acceptance and change in terms of a DBT provider's approach to treatment, this maps onto commonly used interventions within DBT. Validation is perhaps the most obvious acceptance-focused grouping of interventions and problem-solving is perhaps the most obvious change-focused set of interventions, which we will discuss in greater detail later. Mapping this onto eating disorder behaviors on the part of our patients, where we as providers may look at these behaviors as problems to be solved, our patients often have the perspective that these behaviors are actually the solution to the problem at hand. Helping our patients to begin to make change often first starts with being able to deeply acknowledge the kernels of truth in our patients' experiences (e.g. it makes perfect sense that one would want to find a way to decrease the experience of unrelenting and intense shame or anxiety and that absent knowledge of or the ability to utilize other methods of coping, one might turn to eating disorder behaviors) before introducing change-focused interventions.

Bringing DBT to Life – Using Validation With Megan

To demonstrate the value of the use of validation, particularly in the context of difficult discussions, let's return to Megan. To set the stage for this snippet of dialogue, Megan has recently stepped down to PHP and has been consistently denying any instances of bingeing and purging. Given Megan's extensive treatment history and history of periodic dishonesty with her treatment teams, Megan's treatment team has been both cautiously optimistic and skeptical. During morning rounds, Megan's medical provider shares that she got the results of Megan's most recent labs, indicating elevated CO2 of 33 mmol/L with downtrending potassium, which together is strongly suggestive of repeated episodes of purging via vomiting. Here is how the conversation between Megan and her went:

Medical Provider: (puts "Do Not Disturb" sign on door and silences office phone) (level one validation) "You got your diary card on you?"

Megan: "Sure do."

Medical Provider: (reviews Megan's diary card) "Alright, let's see here…looks like Tuesday was really tough for you. I see you restricted your afternoon snack and it looks like there was a lot of sadness and shame that came up on that day. Do you mind if I give your therapist a heads-up about how hard that day was? I imagine she'll definitely want to chat with you further about it." (level two validation)

Megan: "Yeah, sure."

Medical Provider: "Okay, let's see…what else…it looks like no instances of bingeing and no instances of purging, although I see some urges are still there. Megan, can I share something that's been on my mind today?"

Megan: "…um, okay?"

Medical Provider: "I know that you've been adamant that you haven't engaged in bingeing and purging since you started PHP and you know that I'm someone who always wants to take what you are saying and reporting at face value. That said, we got your most recent labs back today and one of the lab findings

	that came back is a strong indicator of purging that is happening pretty regularly."
Megan:	(appears caught off guard, and perhaps slightly tearful)
Medical Provider:	"...look, I can imagine if I was in your shoes and my medical provider just implied that they didn't think I was being honest with them, it would bring up a lot of emotions for me...maybe some shame, or maybe some anger." (level three validation)
Megan:	(sits silently)
Medical Provider:	"I know you've shared with me that conversations like this haven't gone well before, so I imagine it's got to be hard to share what you're thinking at the moment." (level four validation)
Megan:	"Yeah, the last time I had a conversation like this, I got kicked out of the program I was in."
Medical Provider:	"...so I bet you're worried that might be the endgame of our conversation today, too." (level three validation)
Megan:	"Yup."
Medical Provider:	"Can I share with you what I hope to get out of today's conversation?"
Megan:	"Sure."
Medical Provider:	"My goal is to figure out what's going on with this lab finding and if you're struggling, how the team and I can help you to get back on track. So talk to me...is there something going on that you've felt you couldn't be forthcoming about since you stepped down to PHP?"
Megan:	"Okay, I've been bingeing and purging again. And not just a little bit. A lot. And I feel awful about it. And I feel awful about lying."
Medical Provider:	"I can imagine it was really hard to share that with me right now, given all the emotions I'm hearing both the behavior and the lying are bringing up for you. Thank you for being honest with me." (level three validation)

In this particular situation, Megan's medical provider effectively navigated insistent, recurrent denial that a target behavior is occurring. The medical provider's nonjudgmental and skillful approach, specifically through the application of the six levels of validation, created a safe space for Megan to be forthcoming about her behaviors. One thing I (ETM) would like to highlight here is how easily and naturally the use of the six levels of validation can flow, even if the provider implementing validation is not a therapist with extensive DBT training. When a multidisciplinary team is working closely together, the effective use of validation strategies by one provider can open many doors for another provider. For example, you might expect Megan would now be comfortable enough to track this behavior on her diary card for the rest of her team to address and target in their own work with her.

Balancing Communication in DBT – Reciprocal Communication Strategies

In addition to validation, there are two groups of stylistic strategies within DBT that directly relate to the therapeutic relationship. Stylistic strategies refer to the ways in which a provider communicates with a patient, rather than what the provider is communicating or what treatment intervention they are applying. The first set of these strategies are the reciprocal communication strategies (for a more extensive discussion of these strategies, readers are encouraged to review Linehan, 1993, pp. 372–392), many of which have a substantial amount of overlap with the six levels of validation. What you may notice with the reciprocal communication strategies is that they align well with any training you may have received around the therapeutic relationship as part of your studies or post-graduate continuing education.

Responsiveness. Responsiveness refers to the extent to which you are attending to what your patient is communicating, both verbally and nonverbally and adjusting your verbal and nonverbal responses in a way that communicates that you are listening and that you are taking what your patient is communicating seriously. You can demonstrate responsiveness through a variety of nonverbal methods, including an attentive body posture, gestures like head nods or smiles, and appropriate eye contact. Responsiveness also requires verbal communication and can include things like reflecting back to your patient what you have heard, asking them to expand upon what they are saying, or answering a question they have posed to you directly. What you may have noticed about responsiveness as a strategy is that it can include employing all six of the levels of validation we reviewed previously.

Self-Disclosure. Self-disclosure is an admittedly complicated subject and one that requires consideration of a number of areas before applying it as a therapeutic strategy. For your specific discipline, it is important to know what ethical and legal limits or guidelines exist around self-disclosure, in addition to having a sense as to typical practices around self-disclosure within your discipline. If you work within a company or organization, your employer may also have explicit policies or guidelines or implicit workplace norms that can help to guide your decision-making around the use of self-disclosure. The purpose of self-disclosure is another area that has to be considered before using self-disclosure as a therapeutic strategy. Self-disclosure should always be in the best interest of the patient and relevant to the topic at hand. Finally, we will elaborate much further on your personal limits as a provider later in this text, however it is worth mentioning now that these must also be taken into consideration around the use of self-disclosure. While we hope to demonstrate that self-disclosure can have strategic clinical utility, it is also important not to force self-disclosure beyond your own limits.

Within DBT, there are two types of self-disclosure, the first of which is self-involving self-disclosure. Self-involving self-disclosure involves sharing your reactions to the patient and your interactions in the moment, as those interactions are happening. In some cases, self-involving self-disclosure might involve sharing your experience of what is happening from a process standpoint within a therapeutic session. Here is an example of how an interaction might look between a patient diagnosed with Bulimia Nervosa who engages in frequent restriction as a compensatory behavior:

Patient: "I honestly don't understand why we need to talk about me skipping dinner last night. It really wasn't a big deal. Pretty much everyone I know skips meals from time to time."

Therapist: "I know you don't see it as a big deal, but I do."

Patient: "I know the right things that I'm supposed to say here…that I believe all bodies deserve nutrition and that all bodies are good bodies…and I believe that for other people, I really do. I just don't believe it for myself."

Therapist: "I can understand why it would be hard to feel like those statements apply to you, given where you are in your overall treatment and recovery process. I think for a lot of people, behaviors have to shift before their thinking begins to. But I want to pause for a minute and go back to dinner last night. Why do you think I see missing dinner as a big deal?"

Patient: "Well, because I do think you think nutrition is important and because skipping my dinner wasn't following my meal plan."

Therapist: "Absolutely to both of those things. I'll also share that we have a number of examples since you've entered treatment where instances of restriction have resulted in instances of bingeing and purging and I know you've mentioned those are behaviors that you are motivated to stop."

Patient: "That's true. But I'm bingeing and purging much less now, and restriction has gotten so much easier. It seems like I could just keep restricting and everything would be fine."

Therapist: "Can I share something I'm observing in this moment?"

Patient: "Sure."

Therapist: "I'm feeling like we're at a bit of an impasse here. I think you and I have the shared goals of helping you to decrease and ultimately refrain from bingeing and purging. But it feels like we have fundamentally opposed goals when it comes to restricting. I'm curious what your perspective is?"

Patient: "I think that's it. I really don't want to binge and purge. But I really don't see what the problem is with restricting."

Therapist: "Well, I think one challenge is that restricting directly ties into bingeing and purging, so I'm having difficulty seeing a way to target those two things without targeting restricting as well. I know you've also mentioned wanting to work on your body image distress and I would imagine that would be hard for us to do when you're engaging in a behavior that directly conveys to yourself that your body is not okay as it is."

Patient: "I do know that when I've lost weight, even though I thought it would make me happier, it never does."

Therapist: "You've shared that with me before, and I think that observation is an important one. So where do we go from here? I can't force you to work on anything you don't want to work on, so I think it's important for us to figure out how to get on the same page with each other. What are your thoughts?"

In this example, the therapist is noting that from a process standpoint, she feels as though she and the patient are not aligned in terms of shared goals for treatment, opening up space for discussion about how to proceed. Other types of self-involving self-disclosure involve sharing how a patient's behavior is impacting you. Most patients are curious about their providers' reactions to them, so sharing your reaction can sometimes help in shifting behavior. It also provides an opportunity for patients to learn more about how their behavior impacts others, which in turn may be helpful in the context of other interpersonal relationships they may have. To provide some context for this next example, in this particular situation, a therapist who only provides treatment at higher levels of care is working with a patient who is in IOP. Although the patient has just recently transitioned from PHP to IOP, the therapist has been encouraging them to start looking for an outpatient team, since the therapist believes it may take some time for them to find multidisciplinary team members who they like and are willing to work with. This is the second week in a row that the patient has not taken any steps toward identifying an outpatient team. Let's take a look at how this conversation plays out:

Therapist: "So how's the search for an outpatient team going?"

Patient: "Um, I got the links you sent but I really haven't had time to look into them much."

Therapist: "So I totally know that it feels like the end of IOP is a long way away and I have to say that I'm starting to feel pretty worried that you haven't taken any steps toward finding a team just yet."

Patient: "There's just a lot that has been going on and I don't feel like I have to do it, like, right this second."

Therapist: "Here's the deal…I care a lot about you and based on the conversations we've had before, I know it hasn't always been easy to find a therapist who you connect with. I worry that it may take longer than you might think to find someone who would be a good fit. Also, I'm not going to lie…I really don't want to spend our last few weeks working together scrambling to try to find someone! What feels like a reasonable step you could take this upcoming week to get things moving?"

Patient: "I could at least take a look at the links you sent and pick at least five people who I'm willing to call to see if they'd be a good fit."

Therapist: "I think that sounds good, and can you do me one better? Would you at least call one of them to get the process a little further down the road? That would help me feel a bit better about where the process stands."

Patient: "That seems doable."

What you'll notice with this example is that it is a more subtle example of self-involving self-disclosure. The therapist in this example still shares the emotional impact the patient's behavior is having on them, as well as fears they have about what might come next if the patient doesn't begin taking action on identifying a team. The point here is that if self-involving self-disclosure as you imagined it feels like it goes beyond your own personal limits of what you are comfortable sharing, however you are someone who thinks this approach could be helpful, there are more subtle ways to weave this into the work you are doing.

The second type of self-disclosure in DBT is personal self-disclosure, which refers to sharing information about oneself, which can include both professional and personal information. Personal self-disclosure exists on a spectrum from benign (e.g. sharing information about favorite movies or music, disclosing information about your pets or favorite hobbies), to potentially influencing self-disclosure (e.g. your political viewpoints, religious beliefs, personal values), to highly personal self-disclosure (e.g. sharing your personal experience with a mental health diagnosis or significant medical condition).

The use of personal self-disclosure in treatment is a complex issue. Strategic self-disclosure is a form of radical genuineness that can enhance the therapeutic relationship and humanize you as a provider. For example, Henretty, et al. (2014) found that self-disclosures that reveal similarities between therapists and their patients are associated with a stronger therapeutic alliance. Strategic personal self-disclosure can also provide the patient with helpful feedback. For a patient coming from an environment where opinions expressed may directly contradict what would be helpful for a person diagnosed with an eating disorder to hear, open disclosure about your thoughts and opinions can be helpful. For example, many patients with eating disorders come from environments that reinforce a diet culture mentality and it can be helpful for patients to hear you express different perspectives without reservation. Finally, strategic self-disclosure can normalize skill use and give your patients stories they can reflect upon when they are attempting to apply skills. For example, I (AHK) always have relatively benign examples of both times I have applied skills to good success and times where my efforts at skill usage have not gone well. These stories help patients to realize that skills are for everyone and that even individuals who they perceive as skillful can struggle to apply skills in their own life on occasion. Furthermore, if the examples have memorable qualities to them (I tend to try to weave in humor or an element of suspense), they become stories patients can carry with them and remind themselves of.

On the other hand, personal self-disclosure can erode professional boundaries or shift the focus from the patient to the provider in a counterproductive way. This is where the use of case consultation teams and individual supervision as venues for exploring self-disclosure can be particularly beneficial.

More specific to eating disorders, a substantial percentage (24–47%) of eating disorder providers have experienced an eating disorder at some point in their life (Barbarich, 2002) and the question of self-disclosure around one's own experience of having an eating disorder has been a topic of debate. It is common for treatment programs to have either written policies or unwritten cultural "rules" about self-disclosure of an eating disorder history, although not all programs provide guidance on this matter and for individuals practicing independently, this becomes more a matter of one's own personal limits. For situations in which there are not explicit expectations with regard to self-disclosure of one's eating disorder history, there are a few things to consider that can be helpful in exploring appropriateness of disclosing more personal information:

1. *Your motivation for self-disclosure.* Be sure to check in with yourself about your rationale for disclosing the information you are sharing. While spontaneous disclosure of benign information about your life is not likely to be problematic, the sharing of more personal details should be well thought out with a focus on whether and how you believe the disclosure will benefit your patient.

2. *Whether your disclosure is about a resolved versus ongoing issue.* Perhaps with the very rarest of situations, disclosure about an ongoing issue shifts the focus from the patient to the therapist and runs the risk of substantially eroding appropriate therapeutic boundaries. Relatedly, if you choose to disclose

information about shared history with regard to an eating disorder, it is critical that you have been stable within your recovery for a significant period of time.

3. *The nature of the content disclosed.* Careful consideration should not only be given to what should be disclosed, but also in disclosing, what content you choose to share versus what content you choose to withhold. For example, if you choose to disclose information about a shared history with regard to an eating disorder, sharing information about specific skills you found to be helpful or providing words of encouragement that recovery is possible from the vantage point of your own lived experience may be helpful. Sharing details about your disorder (e.g. specifics about behaviors or numbers) is not likely to be beneficial to your patient and may actually be harmful in certain circumstances.

Warm Engagement. Warm engagement refers to a combination of responding positively to your patient coupled with demonstrating interest in your patient. Not only have a variety of common factors closely related to warm engagement been shown to contribute to positive treatment outcomes (Wampold, 2015), the use of warm engagement is also an opportunity for us as providers to model the very same interpersonal behaviors we want our patients to cultivate.

Not all providers find that what they imagine to be stereotypical warm engagement comes easily to them. If you are someone who relates to this sentiment, it is important to remember that all that is necessary for warm engagement is to demonstrate responding positively to your patient and showing interest in your patient. A few tips can be helpful here. First, make every effort to understand your patient and their behaviors, particularly those behaviors that may evoke negative affect on the part of you as a provider. Seeking to understand your patient demonstrates genuine interest and is likely to generate empathy, which in turn can help you to respond in a positive fashion toward your patient. Second, make a conscious effort to monitor your own emotional reactions to patients who are doing poorly and seek to find and highlight successes they are demonstrating. Finally, make intentional efforts to learn about and recall details patients share with you about their lives. Asking about how a pet or family member is doing, checking in about an event your patient was excited to attend, or asking what they thought of a book they read are all examples of showing genuine interest in your patient.

Genuineness. Genuineness refers to showing up as your authentic self in your interactions with your patients. Research suggests that genuineness is one of a number of common factors that contributes to positive treatment outcomes (Wampold, 2015). This certainly makes intuitive sense, in that both patient and provider are likely to find interacting in a genuine way to be preferable to interacting in a performative fashion. There are also additional benefits to genuineness beyond it being a factor in enhancing the therapeutic relationship. Many patients diagnosed with eating disorders struggle with interpersonal relationships in various ways. When providers interact with patients in a genuine way, this more closely mimics relationships a patient has with others in their life outside of treatment. This gives the patient a safe yet authentic space to work on enhancing their interpersonal effectiveness skills in a way that is likely to better translate to life outside of treatment than would be possible if the patients' providers were interacting with them in a more inauthentic fashion.

Balancing Communication in DBT – Irreverent Communication Strategies

Irreverent communication strategies assume the other side of the dialectic of the reciprocal communication strategies we just reviewed. Irreverent communication strategies are probably best grouped into two types of responses that are most often utilized when a patient is behaving or thinking in a way that lacks validity or when the provider finds themselves at an impasse in a session with a patient. Some irreverent communication strategies could be described as matter of fact, blunt, or confrontational responses to a patient's verbalizations or behavior, whereas other types of irreverent communication strategies would be described as quirky, unorthodox, or offbeat in nature. The main purpose that irreverent communication strategies serve is to maintain positive movement within an interaction with a patient, particularly if you are finding yourself in a "therapeutic rut" of sorts. We review irreverent communication strategies briefly below and readers are encouraged to review Linehan, 1993, pp. 393–397 for more in-depth coverage of these techniques.

Reframing in an Unorthodox Manner. Reframing in an unorthodox manner involves responding to what your patient is saying in a way that they aren't expecting. Let's take a peek at an example:

Psychiatric Provider: "I was hoping we could check-in about how your Zyprexa is working out for you?"

Patient: "Yeah, about that…I stopped taking it."

Psychiatric Provider: "Huh…well, it's your choice what medications you take, but you had mentioned you found it remarkably helpful the last time we checked in. I'm curious why you changed your mind?"

Patient: "I've already gained too much weight and I know that contributed. Also, I've decided this whole 'recovery' thing is not for me, so I'm giving up."

Psychiatric Provider: "So I should cancel our next appointment and pencil you in for three months from now when you'll need a higher level of care again?"

What a patient might be expecting in this situation is for the psychiatric provider to try to convince them to take the Zyprexa or to try to convince them that recovery is worth pursuing, however what you see here is not an opposite response, but rather a response that neither pushes for change or aligns with the patient's stated words. It is a response that lands oddly and in a way that begs for more conversation without forcing it.

Plunging in Where Angels Fear to Tread. Many patients are quite adept at detecting situations in which providers are avoiding being forthcoming with them. I (AHK) distinctly remember a time when I was working with an adolescent patient who was prone to becoming angry and I was trying to give her feedback about her behavior during groups. Worried about how she might react, I found myself taking an indirect and rather bumbling approach in trying to get to the point when my patient finally just said something to the effect of, "If you have something to say about how I behaved in group, just say it!" I share this story to communicate that many of our patients prefer a transparent, straightforward, concrete, and clear method of communication over an interaction such as this one. Plunging in where angels fear to tread honors that preference for authentic and non-avoidant conversation. Let's take a look at how this strategy might be used in a session:

Therapist: "So let's talk about the plan you and your dietitian made to try fast food this weekend. She mentioned that you're not thrilled about the idea."

Patient: "Because it's stupid. I'm not doing it. She can't make me, and you can't make me."

Therapist: "You're right, I can't make you. But I'm also going to call B.S. on this whole "it's stupid" business. If I remember correctly, last time you tried to eat a burger and fries, you ended up bingeing and purging. If that's not important to work on, I'm not sure what in the world is!"

Patient: "I don't even like burgers, I'm not wasting my money on ordering a meal that I'm not going to eat."

Therapist: "Here's the deal. Liking or no liking, I'd be a pretty crappy therapist to let you talk me out of this being the plan over the weekend. Rather than dismissing the plan outright, I'm wondering if we could start by talking about exactly what you're imagining will happen this weekend when you're doing this exposure?"

Patient: "Fine. This isn't me saying I'm doing it, though."

Using a Confrontational Tone. Using a confrontational tone is exactly how it sounds. When a patient begins to talk about responding to a situation in a dysfunctional manner or goes on a tangent that is distracting from a more important topic of discussion, the provider addresses this directly and firmly. Let's take a look at an example:

Dietitian: "Okay, I'm looking at your meal log entry for dinner last night, and it looks like you had a large garden salad with no protein, no dressing, and no accompanying sides. Am I seeing that correctly?"

Patient: "Yep, I thought that was close enough to meeting my exchanges."

Dietitian: (pauses and cocks head for a minute) *"Really?"*

Patient: "What?"

Dietitian: "Did you actually think a garden salad with just vegetables and nothing else going along with it is anywhere near adequate in terms of meeting your nutritional needs? It's not even in the ballpark."

Patient: "I mean, no...but the restaurant was out of what I had planned on getting and literally everything else on the menu looked impossible. I figured something was better than nothing."

Dietitian: "You're right, something certainly is better than nothing, and we've got to figure out how that something could actually meet your nutritional needs next time. Can we look at what some other options might have been?"

Patient: "Sure."

The example above is a gentler variation on using a confrontational tone. As an example of a more intense variation of this strategy, you could replace the dietitian's exclamation of, "really?" with a question like, "Are you freakin' kidding me?" to ramp up the intensity. The keys with using this specific strategy are that you have to have a strong therapeutic relationship with your patient and that this strategy fits within your overall therapeutic style. If either of these conditions are absent, it is likely that this approach will fall flat at best, or could cause a therapeutic rupture at worst.

Calling the Patient's Bluff. Calling a patient's bluff often involves taking an extreme statement by a patient at face value and responding to the statement as such. This is what this strategy might look like in a therapy session:

Therapist: "I see on your diary card that you've noted no urges to restrict all week... wow! What a change from last week!"

Patient: "Yeah! You know, I think everything just clicked, I'm feeling much better and I think I'm ready to discharge."

Therapist: "Wonderful! What a miraculous turnaround. Hey, since you're reporting such low urges to restrict with feeling ready for less support, let's celebrate with a donut! I saw some in the lobby and will pick up one for each of us."

Patient: *looks paralyzed*

Therapist: "...am I picking up on something here?"

Patient: *still looking paralyzed*

Therapist: "Look, as much as I wouldn't mind a donut right now, I'm not going to grab one for us. But what I do think I'm noticing is that even the prospect of eating that donut seems pretty terrifying to you. Can we chat about what was going through your mind just now?"

What you'll notice with this example is that the therapist takes the patient's self-report of a complete absence of eating disorder symptoms at face value, yet also gives the patient an "out" when it becomes clear that her bluff has been called. In other words, once the therapist has figured out that the patient is indeed likely experiencing more symptoms than she is reporting, she doesn't then expect the patient to go through with what would now be a spontaneous exposure to a fear food.

Oscillating Intensity and Using Silence. Oscillating intensity involves being strategic in adjusting your emotional expressions, voice tone, and body language in such a way that it doesn't align with the sentiment of what your patient is communicating. As a trainee a number of years ago, I (AHK) worked with a patient who had lots of active suicidal ideation and a very passive approach to problem-solving and our therapy sessions more broadly. I was struggling to make progress with her, so I took a videotape of one of our sessions to supervision with one of my supervisors at the time. No more than two minutes into reviewing the video, one of the reasons I had been having difficulty helping my patient to make progress became readily apparent. The more that my patient verbalized feeling suicidal coupled with a passive problem-solving style, the more that I became verbally and non-verbally activated. As a result of what I had seen, which was typical of our recent sessions, I decided to experiment with oscillating intensity and using silence during our next session. Instead of doing things like leaning forward and talking more when my patient verbalized suicidal ideation, I instead sat back in my chair and spoke far less than usual. To my surprise and relief, this approach led to my patient speaking more and being more willing to explore potential solutions to help decrease her suicidal ideation and take actions to make her environment more safe. Whenever I find myself feeling "stuck" with a patient in a specific session or over the course of multiple sessions, I often consider this specific strategy as a potential solution to get "unstuck."

Expressing Omnipotence and Impotence. Expressing omnipotence refers to implying that your expertise is necessary for a patient to make progress toward their goals and building a life worth living. In contrast to expressing omnipotence, expressing impotence means directly acknowledging your limitations as a provider or the limitations of your discipline-specific treatment strategies or treatment as a whole. The following are a couple of examples of expressing omnipotence:

Patient: "But how do you know it's possible for me to recover? I think I could get better for a little while, but I'm never going to be able to hold on to it, so what's the point in doing all of this hard work?"

Medical Provider: "Look, I don't know everything, but there are lots of things I do know. And I know you have the ability to recover. You're just going to have to trust me on this one."

Patient: "How do you know I need to eat this much? This meal plan is absurd and WAY more than my body needs."

Dietitian: "Look, I think we can both agree if you were in charge of determining what your body needs, you'd be losing weight, and rather quickly at that. And that can't happen if you want to return to school in the fall. I've taken into account everything I know from a nutrition science standpoint, in addition to considering individual factors in terms of your specific body. This meal plan is nutritionally adequate and what your body needs."

Now let's take a look at a couple of examples of expressing impotence:

Patient: "What are you going to do about it? It's not like you can force me to eat."

Therapist: "You're right. As much as I wish there was a way I could magically make sure you met all of your nutritional needs, day-in and day-out, I can't force you to eat."

Patient: "Can't you just go into my brain and fix it? Or give me a new brain altogether? Even taking all of the medication you've prescribed over the years, the anxiety around food is still there, and I still hate my body."

Psychiatric Provider: "If I could magically resolve your fear of weight gain and anxiety around food and your body, I would. But that's not how it works, even with the best medications I can offer. The most fruitful work we can do together right now is learning to tolerate all of that 'noise' in your head, so you can still eat and maintain an adequate weight."

Balancing Reciprocal and Irreverent Communication

Ongoing calibration to find the appropriate balance between reciprocal and irreverent communication in any given point in treatment as well as in the context of treatment over time is critical in maintaining our therapeutic rapport with patients while also helping them to move forward. Too much of an emphasis on irreverent communication can become a treatment-interfering behavior on the part of the provider. Utilizing excessive irreverent communication can also increase the likelihood of treatment-interfering behaviors on the part of your patient, like becoming withdrawn in session, refusing to engage in change-focused work, or discontinuing treatment altogether. Too much of an emphasis on reciprocal communication can also be a treatment-interfering behavior on the part of a provider and can result in stalled therapeutic change or patients feeling as though you don't take their problems seriously.

So how do you find a balance between these two approaches? From a big picture standpoint, it can be helpful to lean toward reciprocal communication earlier in treatment in order to facilitate the development of the therapeutic relationship. However as treatment progresses, any given session is usually a dance between reciprocal and irreverent communication. There is no prescriptive way to outline precisely when each set of strategies should be employed, rather it can be helpful to attune yourself to the flow within the session and consider switching approaches if you start to feel "stuck" within the session. What you will likely notice is that as you pay more conscious attention to your use of reciprocal and irreverent communication strategies, you will begin to develop more of an intuitive sense of how to go about weaving these throughout your sessions.

Playful Irreverence and Compassionate Gravity –
A Variation From RO-DBT

Playful irreverence and compassionate gravity are two critical therapeutic stances from RO DBT that have particular utility in working with overcontrolled patients (Lynch, 2018). Playful irreverence involves therapeutic teasing, which serves the dual purpose of signaling safety while simultaneously challenging your patient. In the context of our closest relationships, teasing can be a kind way to point out each other's flaws, while at the same time enhancing our interpersonal connectedness. Playful irreverence allows us to target maladaptive social signaling by our patients, but in a way that is kind. Furthermore, the use of playful irreverence models the very behaviors we want patients to utilize in their interpersonal interactions.

On the other side of the dialectic, compassionate gravity involves conveying to our patient through both verbal and nonverbal cues that we are taking their concerns and their experience seriously. By slowing the pace of our conversation, using a quieter tone, and assuming a more relaxed body posture, compassionate gravity also signals safety. While playful irreverence should generally be applied in situations where maladaptive social signaling is occurring, compassionate gravity should generally be applied in situations where a patient is engaged and genuine in their interaction.

The interplay between within this dialectic highlights that we both need to demonstrate to our patients that we understand them and take them seriously, while also challenging them and providing them with corrective feedback in a kind way.

Bringing DBT to Life – Balancing Reciprocal and Irreverent Communication With Megan

Megan:	"...this past weekend was hard. I tried to stay on track, but PHP is kicking my butt!"
Claire (Dietitian):	*[Nods warmly]* "Partial hospitalization certainly brings with it a new set of challenges. I'm sure you did better with intake than you think you did. Let's take a look." (warm engagement)
Megan:	"Saturday was my first full day out of programming. I ended up oversleeping and missing breakfast. I think it's my new medication…it makes me feel really drowsy all the time."
Claire:	"Gotcha. I imagine that drowsiness adds a whole additional layer on to the challenges that go along with transitioning to PHP. Be sure you mention the drowsiness during your next appointment with your psych provider. So, were you able to move your meal plan around to still meet your needs? It looks like the first time you ate was around noon." (warm engagement)
Megan:	"Yeah, I ate a bowl of oatmeal around that time."
Claire:	"I get that you were tired, but there's no way that met your nutritional needs. What else could you have selected that would've been more balanced and adequate?" (using a confrontational tone)
Megan:	"I dunno. Well, okay…I was staying with a couple of my friends for the weekend and they ordered pizza and wings to celebrate my first day out of programming, but there was no way that was happening."
Claire:	"Wait, so you had the option of eating fresh, delicious pizza and you opted for a sad bowl of soggy oatmeal? I'd like for you to do pizza tonight. What do you think?" (oscillating intensity, plunging in where angels fear to tread)
Megan:	[laughs] "Yeah, there's no way I'm doing pizza. I've been in recovery before without eating pizza. In fact, I can't think of the last time I actually ate a slice of pizza."

Claire: "I guess you make a point. Why start now? Sounds like a great idea to keep avoiding pizza. I hear bowls of instant oats are all the rage for social gatherings these days." (calling the patient's bluff, using a confrontational tone)

Megan: [shocked] "Woah woah woah! Okay, fine. I can try it tonight. Can I start with regular cheese pizza? I'm not ready for pepperoni."

Claire: [smiles warmly] "Yes, absolutely. I know this is a big leap for you, and I'm really proud of you for being open to this challenge. Cheese pizza is a great place to start. Now let's get back to reviewing the rest of the weekend…" (warm engagement, responsiveness)

Claire's ability to transition from a reciprocal to irreverent communication style and back quickly and seamlessly helps give this dialogue punch. Some of the features that make this approach effective can be difficult to capture in words, such as a shift in tone, volume, or intensity of one's voice or nonverbals such as sustained eye contact, head nods, or positioning in a chair, and these difficult to capture process elements can really help shape the conversation. I (ETM) also feel like this technique of dropping an irreverent bomb, so to speak, in the middle of a conversation can help quickly pivot the conversation into goal setting and make the session more efficient overall. However, it is also important to note that this technique can also come across as invalidating without careful balance of reciprocal communication.

Provider Exercise – Exploring Reciprocal and Irreverent Communication

For this provider exercise, start by considering where you tend to fall in terms of your balance between reciprocal and irreverent communication when you think about your patient interactions taken as a whole.

I--I
Reciprocal   Irreverent

Now consider the following questions:

Why did you select this particular location on the dialectic?

Does the balance between reciprocal and irreverent communication change across patients or across clinical scenarios? If yes, what do you make of this?

When you think about your patient interactions as a whole, are there any shifts you would like to make in terms of your balance between reciprocal and irreverent communication or how you apply these particular styles of inter-action? If yes, what specific things would you like to change?

The Therapeutic Relationship and Modeling Behaviors

The therapeutic relationship also provides a unique space in which we can model the very behaviors that we want our patients to develop. For patients who present as being more overcontrolled, we can model everything from being more casual to engaging in playful banter to demonstrating flexibility. For patients who present as being more undercontrolled, we can model things like being structured and organized, regulating our emotions and physiological responses skillfully, and navigating interpersonal interactions thoughtfully. For patients for whom these behaviors are challenging or even outside of their existing skill set, it can be helpful for them to see examples of the skills we hope they will develop and hone, particularly being demonstrated by someone whom they trust.

Another way in which the therapeutic relationship can be used as a tool for modeling behaviors has to do with how providers navigate alliance ruptures. When we consider Anorexia Nervosa specifically, some of the consequences that arise from the transactions that occur as part of the biosocial model of the development of Anorexia Nervosa are that patients learn to avoid conflict and open expression of emotion, both of which might be reinforced in the short-term but that are likely to cause interpersonal difficulties in the long-term. It is important for patients to have an opportunity to participate in interpersonal interactions where open expression of emotions and inner feelings, including those related to conflicts or disagreements, not only do not result in negative consequences but in fact enhance the intimacy of those interpersonal relationships over time. The therapeutic relationship between patient and provider offers a context in which these types of interactions can occur.

RO DBT offers a set of steps to follow in the event of an alliance rupture with a patient diagnosed with Anorexia Nervosa that models an effective approach to addressing conflicts and disagreements. In the event that a provider believes an alliance rupture may have occurred, the first step in repairing the rupture involves pausing whatever topic is being discussed in the session. It is important to note here that repairing alliance ruptures is not intended to take an excessive amount of time, so you can think of this first step as putting a bookmark in your session that you are likely to come back to shortly. Occurring concurrently with a pause in session contact, the second step of addressing an alliance rupture involves briefly disengaging direct eye contact. Temperamentally, patients diagnosed with Anorexia Nervosa are wired in such a way that they often find the experience of being the center of attention to be an uncomfortable one, so briefly disengaging eye contact can help them to feel more at ease. The third step of addressing an alliance rupture is also focused on body language and involves leaning back, taking a deep breath, relaxing one's facial expression, and doing an eyebrow wag. These changes in body posture send a message to the patient that they are safe. The fourth step of targeting an alliance rupture involves acknowledging that something has changed in the session, sharing your observations of what changed, and then actively soliciting your patient's observations as well. The fifth step in addressing an alliance rupture involves slowing down the pace of the conversation and giving your patient space to respond, as well as utilizing reflective listening strategies to facilitate continued dialogue and to ensure that you have a good understanding of your patient's experience. The sixth step in targeting an alliance rupture involves responding to your patient's self-disclosure in a way that increases the likelihood of self-disclosure in the future. This can be something as simple as sharing that you appreciated their willingness to be honest with you. The final step in addressing an alliance rupture involves checking-in with the patient to ensure that the alliance rupture has been adequately addressed from their perspective and that they are ready to return to the topic of discussion that was being explored prior to the alliance rupture (Lynch, Hempel, & Dunkley, 2018).

Alliance ruptures can and do occur with individuals diagnosed with Bulimia Nervosa and Binge Eating Disorder, although standard DBT is less prescriptive with regard to how to approach these alliance ruptures when they happen. However, research on alliance ruptures in general does provide some guidance on effectively navigating them when they do occur and this guidance aligns well with the "spirit" of DBT, as well as with more specific DBT principles and strategies.

In order to effectively address alliance ruptures, being able to identify when an alliance rupture has occurred is a critical first step. Alliance ruptures are generally thought of as falling in one of two categories: withdrawal ruptures and confrontation ruptures. Withdrawal ruptures are characterized by avoidance and withdrawal behaviors. Examples of withdrawal ruptures we have experienced in working with patients with eating disorders include shutting down in session (e.g. providing only minimal verbal responses, avoiding eye contact), disengaging from treatment (e.g. declaring an intention to leave treatment but refusing to discuss why, missing sessions), or avoiding discussion of certain topics. On the other hand, confrontation ruptures involve patients directly expressing negative feelings toward a provider or treatment in general. Examples of confrontation ruptures we have experienced in working with patients diagnosed with eating disorders include visible increases in negative affect and emotional expression coupled with confrontational comments (e.g. "If you really cared about me, you'd meet with me more than twice per week," "You don't understand me," "Treatment with you isn't working; I want to work with a different dietitian") or threats to "fire" a provider or to engage in maladaptive behaviors specifically in response to the alliance rupture.

Once it has been identified that an alliance rupture has occurred, guidance on how to proceed is less prescriptive and more dependent on the factor(s) driving the alliance rupture. Safran, Muran, and Eubanks-Carter (2011) outlined a number of common interventions providers use to address alliance ruptures, including repeating the therapeutic rationale for the intervention that may have prompted the alliance rupture, changing task or goals to better align with the patient's needs or goals in the moment, clarifying misunderstandings at a surface level and validating the patient's experience, exploring relational themes associated with the rupture, linking the alliance rupture to common patterns in a patient's life, and creating a new relational experience as a corrective contrast to previous relational experiences. Subsequent research focused on optimal responses to alliance ruptures based on the clinical consensus of experts suggested that validation of the patient's experience and exploration of the alliance rupture during the session in which it occurred were considered to be the two most appropriate immediate interventions, although experts also noted that change-oriented interventions focused on things like highlighting and altering patterns of behavior, thought, or emotion in the context of interpersonal interactions may be helpful interventions for future sessions (Eubanks, Burckell, & Goldfried, 2018). The take-home point here is that it is critical to be attuned to alliance ruptures and to address them promptly when they occur.

Bringing DBT to Life – Resolving an Alliance Rupture With Megan

In this patient vignette scenario, Megan has transitioned to PHP and is in an individual session with her dietitian, Claire. Claire has noticed that Megan's weight has started to trend upward since her transition to PHP despite being on a maintenance meal plan that Megan reports she is following. Although Megan is denying both episodes of bingeing and urges to binge on her diary card, Claire is having difficulty imagining what else might account for the trend she is observing. Megan and Claire are in the midst of an easygoing back-and-forth exchange about Megan's week when Claire decides to bring up her observations. Here is what transpires:

Claire: "Megan, I know that on your diary card you've been reporting no instances of bingeing or even urges to binge since you've transitioned to PHP. On one hand, I totally want to take what you are reporting at face value. On the other hand, I'm noticing some trends in your weight that make me wonder if there is more going on."

Megan: (curtly) "Oh, so you're saying I'm getting fat."

Claire: "No, that's not what I'm saying at all…"

Megan: (curtly) "Well, you're saying I'm a liar then."

Claire: "No, not that either…"

Megan: (mumbling almost inaudibly as she curls up tightly in a ball and turns away from Claire) "I don't want to talk about this."

Claire: "I'm sorry Megan, I couldn't hear what you said…"

Megan: (in a raised voice) "I *said* I. Don't. Want. To. Talk. About. This." (turns completely away from Claire; the sound of muffled sniffling can be heard a bit)

Claire: (takes a deep breath, ensures her body posture is relaxed) "Okay, we can pause for a minute." (Claire allows a few minutes to pass by quietly and she attends to her own physiological, emotional, and cognitive reactions) "Look, Megan…I get the sense that I really struck a nerve here. Can you help me understand what's going on?"

Megan: "I honestly haven't been bingeing but you bringing this up makes me feel like I must be getting fat and I was already having so much body image distress lately and this just makes it worse. And it makes me feel like I can't trust you or this meal plan you have me on."

Claire: "I get it. It must be incredibly difficult to keep pushing forward and meeting your nutritional needs when your body image distress is so loud. I know you're physically uncomfortable and that some days it feels intolerable. On top of that, I know you've had moments in our work together where you've had difficulty trusting me. It feels like right now, all of those pieces are colliding for you *and* what I'm asking is bringing up some strong emotions."

Megan: "… yeah. Not sure what else you want me to say. Can we wrap this up?"

Claire: "Sure, we can, but before we do…can I ask you something?"

Megan: (allows a few moments to go by without making eye contact) "Sure. What?"

Claire: "I would love for us to work on our relationship so you feel comfortable engaging in conversations about bingeing and purging. I know you'd rather not talk about it, but I wouldn't be doing my job if I ignored those behaviors. So tell me, how could I have gone about this in a different way? I clearly took a misstep somewhere, because you shut down pretty quickly."

Megan: "I don't know. I hate talking about those behaviors in general, but I really didn't like the tone you took. It felt too… accusatory. You should know better than to make a comment about my weight climbing. How did you think I would react?"

Claire: "I hear you. So it sounds like I could work on my tone next time we have a conversation like this?"

Megan: "Not just the tone. In the past, you've taken more of an open-ended approach that felt more inquisitive. That works better for me. I'm less likely to spin-out about my weight or shut down that way."

Claire: "That's really, really helpful. I appreciate you taking the time to share with me your experience and coach me a little on how best to work with you. How do you feel about me sharing this with the rest of your treatment team? We'd like to be as helpful as possible and want to collaborate with you around addressing behaviors that may bring up more shame."

Megan: "Yeah, I guess that could be helpful. Thanks for hearing me out, and for pushing me to talk about the things I don't want to. I know it's for the best, it just makes me uncomfortable."

Provider Exercise – Exploring Alliance Ruptures

For this provider exercise, think about one or more patients with whom you have had an alliance rupture and respond to the questions below. Once you have had a chance to reflect on these questions, consider discussing your reflections with a trusted peer.

1. What signs have you noticed previously that have suggested that an alliance rupture has occurred with a patient?

2. What approaches or strategies have you found helpful in addressing alliance ruptures?

3. What might you want to do differently in addressing alliance ruptures in the future?

Chapter 11

Dialectical Strategies

Dialectical strategies focus on effectively navigating the dialectical tensions that emerge in the context of treatment. Some of these dialectical tensions are at the core of DBT as a treatment, like the tension between acceptance and change or the tension between flexibility and stability. Other tensions are more specific to eating disorder treatment, like the desire to recover and the desire to maintain one's eating disorder or with an adolescent patient, the desire for autonomy and the pursuit of adulthood coupled with the fear of maturation. Dialectical strategies aim to bring out opposites, alternative points of view, and missing information, with the goal of creating a synthesis and balance, moving away from polarized extremes. Dialectical strategies can be exceptionally helpful in helping you get "unstuck" when you find you and your patient are at an impasse. Consider the dialectical tensions that might be present in the room and how you might have to shift to achieve balance. Is this a moment for more acceptance or more change? Is reciprocal communication needed or is irreverent communication more appropriate? Will validation or problem-solving be more well received? Do you need to hold firm or is it a time for compassionate flexibility? The frequently used metaphor of an effective session feeling like a dance between you and your patient is an accurate one, with specific dialectical strategies helping to direct the rhythm and the tensions within the room in an artful and nuanced fashion.

Now that you understand some of the broader aims of dialectical strategies, let's take a look at specific strategies that fall under the category of dialectical strategies. These include entering the paradox, the use of metaphor, the devil's advocate technique, extending, activating "wise mind," making lemonade out of lemons, allowing natural change, and dialectical assessment. Each of these strategies is discussed in further detail below and readers are encouraged to review Linehan, 1993, pp. 205–219 for a more comprehensive coverage of each of these strategies.

Entering the Paradox. Entering the paradox involves allowing your patient to sit with seemingly irreconcilable contradictions or dilemmas, rather than rescuing

DOI: 10.4324/9781003495604-11

your patient from the discomfort often associated with a situation for which there is no singular "right" answer. Perhaps the most common paradox that exists within eating disorder work is a patient's desire to recover coexisting with their desire to remain entangled in their eating disorder, however there are other paradoxes that exist as well. We will discuss exposure-based procedures more extensively in Chapter 16, however within exposure-based procedures exists the paradox that the actions that cause the most immediate emotional and physiological pain are the very same actions that ultimately alleviate suffering. For many patients with eating disorders, entering the paradox is particularly challenging and particularly beneficial. Entering the paradox is directly contrary to the rigid, black-and-white thinking with which many patients diagnosed with eating disorders struggle. Through encouraging our patients to enter the paradox, we are helping them to develop the ability to think and behave more dialectically.

The Use of Metaphor. The use of metaphor involves utilizing anecdotes, stories, and analogies strategically. There are a number of reasons why using metaphor can be more effective than simply stating a point or teaching something in a more didactic fashion. First, anecdotes, stories, and analogies are often more likely to grab our patients' attention than more didactic ways of conveying information. Second, the use of metaphor can help our patients to think more flexibly and creatively about a topic at hand. Finally, in presenting information in a more indirect than direct manner, we reduce the likelihood of our patients either rejecting or becoming argumentative about the points we are trying to convey. Although not a form of the use of metaphor, a strategy drawn from RO DBT called smuggling also has a similar aim. With smuggling, a provider plants a seed or a small part of a new idea without being overly enthusiastic or going into excessive detail. This gives the patient space to reflect on what the provider shared without feeling the need to react and take action in the moment. Finding ways to slow-play a point or make a point indirectly can help increase the likelihood that our patients will be more willing to consider the information we are sharing in certain circumstances.

To show an example of how the use of metaphor can work, I (AHK) want to share a story that I have often shared with patients with whom I have worked as a way of teaching the "effectively" skill, which you will learn about in Chapter 18. The essence of this skill is focusing on doing just what is needed in a situation, without getting caught up in emotions, the thought of whether something is "fair" or "unfair," and so forth. The story goes a little something like this:

When I was growing up, my parents always let me know that education was an important priority, one that was often expected to be at the top or near the top of my priorities list. The unintentional byproduct of this was that I had a play area in the basement of our house that would get quite messy during the school year while I spent my time focused on academics. On the very first day of summer break after my sixth grade year, all of the kids in our neighborhood headed outside to play. As I reached for the handle of our front door to join them, my parents stopped me and let me know that I wouldn't be going outside until the basement was tidied up. I immediately began to protest, telling my parents that it wasn't fair and that no other kids in the neighborhood had this expectation, however my parents remained firm. So how did I spend the first few weeks of my summer vacation? Sitting nearby a pile of toys and listening to the radio in the basement, stewing about how life wasn't fair and waiting for my parents to change their minds. At a point I began to realize that fair or unfair, the only way to get what I most wanted, which was to spend time with my friends, was to acknowledge the boundary set by my parents and clean up the basement. With that recognition, I was able to (admittedly begrudgingly) move from willfulness to willingness and utilize the effectively skill to jumpstart cleaning up my play area and enjoying the rest of the summer with my friends.

This example touches on all three benefits of the use of metaphor. First, most patients with whom I shared this story found it to be at least somewhat interesting and funny and some patients would periodically make reference to it throughout their time in treatment. Second, if I wanted to use this story to encourage flexible and creative thinking, before sharing what I actually did, I could ask patients to generate as many solutions as possible. What is likely to arise from this brainstorming session are solutions that are likely to be ineffective (e.g. do nothing and stay miserable, try to convince my parents to change their minds), solutions that might be temporarily effective but against my values (e.g. hide all of my toys rather than actually putting them away, sneak out of the house when my parents aren't looking), and solutions that might be possible, effective, and consistent with my values (e.g. clean the basement myself, ask my friends for help in cleaning up the basement, use my allowance money to pay for someone to clean the basement). Finally, this story normalizes that everyone struggles to use their skills at times, shows that using skills can be difficult, and demonstrates how we can take a compassionate and nonjudgmental stance toward willfulness.

The Devil's Advocate Technique. You may be seeing this and wondering, "Haven't we already covered this technique?" and the answer to your question is indeed, "Yes!" You may recall that playing devil's advocate was covered in the commitment strategies section, where the purpose in using this strategy was to cultivate and enhance your patient's motivation for change. When thinking about the devil's advocate technique as a dialectical strategy specifically, the targets of this strategy become our patients' extreme and rigid beliefs and rules, with the goal of them arriving at more dialectical thoughts and guidelines for their lives. To understand how this works with a target other than motivation in mind, it can be helpful to look at a couple of examples:

> I (ETM) was working with a patient at a residential level of care who struggled with extremely poor dietary variety coupled with lack of willingness to work on this specific target. She limited herself to a handful of foods, including almonds. I tried to target increased dietary variety from many angles, including through discussing the biological and physiological benefits of dietary variety and the importance of dietary variety from a practical perspective, as well as sharing various psychological and exposure-based interventions that could be used to improve dietary variety. None of these approaches were effective. When we would plan menus with variety, she would only eat the almonds. The client continued to express strong ambivalence around dietary variety specifically and recovery more broadly, making statements like, "There's no way I'm eating pizza and everything else you want me to eat when I leave here. I'm going to eat what I want." Many weeks into our work together and stuck in a dead-end conversation around her over-reliance on almonds, I dropped my resistance and stated, "I think you're right about the almonds, they're all your body needs. Let's go ahead and plan for approximately 450 almonds a day for the rest of your admission." The patient was astonished and responded, "What? No! I'm going to want different foods… eventually. I'm just afraid of the weight gain."

In another example, I had a client who was regularly engaging in slippery-slope exercise, which was the kind of movement that was deeply entrenched with her eating disorder, despite my recommendations to explore more enjoyable movement, such as hiking and dancing. I was making no inroads with her until I stated, "I actually think you should get a gym membership. You'll have access to a treadmill, machines that will do the math for you and tell you how many calories you've burned, high intensity cardio work-out classes…the whole she-bang!" The client immediately knew what I was doing with her and laughed, agreeing her exercise regimen was beginning to feel increasingly disordered. With both of these examples, you see ways in which the use of devil's advocate technique as a dialectical strategy helped to shift rigid behaviors and beliefs for both patients.

Extending. Extending is a strategy that involves taking extreme communications made by our patients at face value, often in a way where we are taking the patient more seriously than they take themselves. Having been a person who once practiced aikido, I (AHK) think that Linehan's description of extending being borrowed from this art of self-defense is an accurate one. One of my favorite moves in aikido was one where I started directly facing toward my practicing partner, who would then throw a punch toward me. As a first move,

I would sidestep and move with the flow of the punch while guiding my hand toward the wrist of my practice partner's punching hand. After grabbing their wrist, I would pull just a bit further, moving with the natural momentum of their punch and beyond a point of stability. In throwing them off balance a bit, it made subsequent movements focused on shifting them the exact opposite direction and eventually into a position of being pinned considerably easier. How does this translate to dialogue between a patient and a provider? Many of the situations I (AHK) have found extending to be useful involve situations in which the patient is making an extreme "if-then" statement.

One example that has come up for me (ETM) many times in the clinical setting is with working with the ambivalent patient who stumbles in their recovery. For example, one patient with whom I worked purged between sessions following a substantial period of time where he had been able to refrain from engaging in purging behaviors. The following session, he presented as somber and defeated, and stated something to the effect of, "I knew recovery wasn't for me. I just knew I couldn't do it. I've been sick for ten years already, so what's another ten more?" He then indicated that he planned to quit treatment for now, hinting he might seek help in the future. Previously with this patient I had taken a gentler approach, reminding him that recovery does not require perfection and that we can learn from slips and get back on track. However, at this moment, I leaned into the extending technique and replied, "That makes sense to me, I'll pencil you in for ten years out," while proceeding to show him my computer's calendar for the year 2028. The patient was surprised by my response, and this helped to shift the mood from defeated to playful and enhanced the patient's willingness to continue working on his recovery.

Activating "Wise Mind." We will expand upon wise mind at various points throughout this text, however in short, wise mind is a state of mind that takes into account all forms of knowing, including logic, emotions, body sensations, intuition, and so forth. Activating "wise mind" is considered to be a dialectical strategy because it is focused on helping patients refrain from only relying on a single way of knowing as the "be-all, end-all" way of knowing and using this limited perspective to guide their behaviors. For example, many patients with whom we have worked have used the bodily sensation of fullness as a rationale for restriction, operating under the assumption that the sensation of fullness is a sufficient indicator that their nutritional needs have been met. Contributing an additional challenge in this situation, a patient might also perceive their emotional reactions, like anxiety or disgust, as aligning with this conclusion. However, considering additional ways of knowing adds complexity to the picture. The patient may have received psychoeducation about their specific meal plan, ways in which hunger and fullness cues are distorted at the time a patient is receiving treatment and in early recovery, and that eating disorders are a brain-based illness with predictable emotional responses that also do not align with facts. If a patient is able to access logic, this information adds some counter-points to what they thought they knew to be true. Perhaps they might add on another layer of knowing, accessing their intuition that their multidisciplinary treatment team truly cares for them, and wouldn't recommend anything that was harmful or painful and unnecessary. Through accessing "wise mind," the patient faced with the decision of whether to follow their meal plan in the presence of sensations of fullness is likely to arrive at a different decision than simply relying on one way of knowing alone.

Making Lemonade Out of Lemons. Making lemonade out of lemons involves framing a situation that a patient finds to be undesirable as something that is positive in some way. This strategy is a bit irreverent in nature, so it is important that you both have good therapeutic rapport established with your patient and that you have a good understanding of why your patient finds the situation to be undesirable and have validated your patient's perspective. In eating disorders work, unplanned but natural exposures to feared stimuli are probably the most common situations where making lemonade out of lemons can be a helpful strategy. For example, if a patient who is receiving treatment at a residential level care has a situation in which they are plated an extra portion or has to eat something different than what they were expecting due to the kitchen running out of a certain item, they are not likely to perceive this type of situation as preferable and may be inclined to complain about the situation to you as their provider. Yet these types of unplanned exposures are exactly the types of situations your patient will need to be able to navigate successfully as they transition to lower levels of care. Framing these situations as a great opportunity to practice flexibility rather than an egregious error on behalf of the staff involved in the meal both highlights the clinical utility of the experience as well as prevents unhelpful dynamics from emerging between staff members.

Allowing Natural Change. For many of our patients, change is incredibly hard. This holds true even when the change seems to be a relatively minor one (e.g. change in a unit schedule or rule) or even one that is positive (e.g. discharging to a lower level of care, returning to school in the fall). It can be tempting to create an artificial degree of predictability and stability in order to avoid the possibility of evoking patient distress, however this approach fails to prepare our patients for life outside of treatment, where unpredictable events and lack of consistency are commonplace. Allowing for natural change is the middle ground between introducing change simply for the sake of introducing change and taking deliberate action to avoid introducing change whenever possible. It is important to note that increasing our patients' ability to tolerate and respond effectively to unpredictability and change are often relevant treatment targets that need to be addressed. One strategy for addressing these treatment targets are exposure-based procedures, which will be discussed more extensively in Chapter 16. When using these procedures, unpredictability and change are deliberately and thoughtfully introduced, however only once a patient has been properly oriented to these procedures and have agreed to their use as part of their treatment.

Dialectical Assessment. Marsha Linehan has previously noted that most errors of intervention are errors of assessment rather than errors of intervention and this observation highlights the significant value that dialectical assessment offers as a strategy. Returning to the dialectical worldview, it is important to remember that this worldview is both systemic and transactional. When we think about the cause of eating disorders, the reality is that there is no single cause, but rather complex transactions between a multitude of factors, including genetics, neurobiology, temperament, hormonal changes, cultural pressure for thinness, dieting, portion size escalation, food insecurity, and so forth (Schaumberg, et al., 2017). I (AHK) would argue complex, multifaceted causes do not lend themselves to a simple conceptualization of a patient's illness, nor to a generic, "one size fits most" approach to treatment interventions. Complex causes require thoughtful and robust conceptualizations that lend themselves to targeted and nuanced interventions. The spirit of dialectical assessment is captured nicely by the question, "What is being left out?" With dialectical assessment, one is constantly striving to achieve a deeper understanding of the multitude of factors that are influencing a patient's thoughts, emotions, and behaviors, and the ways in which the patient is transacting with and influencing their environment, and then using this information to further refine one's approach to treatment. This can open up new avenues for intervention that not only focus on helping the patient to make change, but also that consider ways in which the patient may be able to influence change in their immediate environment or even within broader systems. Tying dialectical assessment back to the therapeutic relationship, it can not only help with more effective treatment interventions, it can also improve the richness of validation that we use with our patients. The more we are curious about what drives our patient's thoughts, emotions, and behaviors and seek to learn more, the more the depth of understanding is enhanced and the more we are able to accurately convey that our patient's thoughts, emotions, and behaviors make sense.

Provider Activity – Exploring Dialectical Assessment

We (AHK, ETM) have found dialectical assessment to be one of the most helpful strategies out of all those that exist within DBT. To demonstrate the value of this specific strategy, we wanted to show an example of how case conceptualization of a patient can evolve drastically through continuing to search for what is being left out.

For this example, we will show how your case conceptualization for a patient diagnosed with Bulimia Nervosa might evolve with further information. The following is what you know about your patient after a few sessions with them:

Your patient has consistently been restricting some or all of breakfast. They report feeling paralyzing fear about plating and they often don't even enter the kitchen to attempt to plate. When they do enter the kitchen and attempt to plate, they report being overwhelmed by trying to select foods to meet their exchanges. Your patient also reports significant body image distress, noting that they find themself to be "disgusting" and "gross" and that they feel they "don't even deserve to be here because I'm in such a horrific body." In the space below, reflect on how you might be conceptualizing their restricting behaviors thus far:

In your next session with your patient, you are discussing another instance in which they have restricted breakfast and your patient notes that one specific fear that comes up for them is that they won't be able to find foods that meet their protein exchanges for breakfast. You learn that your patient's parents do not keep food items that could meet your patient's protein exchanges that they enjoy (e.g. peanut butter) around in large quantities because they have the belief your patient will binge on them, even though there is no history of these items being binge foods for your patient. As such, your patient usually has more limited protein options. Furthermore, you learn that your patient has a history of food insecurity where they were often faced with situations in which they had to eat various forms of meat that were "on the line" in terms of expiring. Meat is typically one of the protein options that is available. In the space below, reflect on how your conceptualization of your patient's restricting behaviors may have evolved with this additional information:

With your updated conceptualization of your patient's restricting behaviors in mind, you have been able to help them in making some progress with regard to decreasing their frequency of restriction, however they are still reporting high anxiety around breakfast in particular and they are continuing to struggle with intermittent restriction. In reviewing their meals and snacks from the past week, you notice that whenever the patient is successfully completing breakfast, it's always cold foods, such as cereal with milk or yogurt with fruit. When you reflect this back to the patient, you learn the patient avoids any food preparation that requires using any heating element, such as the stove, toaster, or toaster oven. What types of questions would you need to ask in order to use this information to assist with case conceptualization? Consider a couple of responses you think your patient might have to those questions and how this would further refine your case conceptualization.

Our hope is that with this exercise, you have been able to see the value of asking a question like, "What is being left out?" Assessment should always be a process rather than an event and furthermore, dialectical assessment suggests that there is no point at which one truly has the full picture.

Bringing DBT to Life – Dialectical Strategies With Megan

At the start of her seventh week of Residential care, Megan met with her medical provider (Carlos) for a session, where conversation promptly turned to the patient's desire to leave care Against Medical Advice (AMA). Carlos has grown accustomed to this conversation, as Megan often finds his visits aversive, particularly when he is sharing positive indicators of Megan's medical status. Megan, like many individuals struggling with an eating disorder, often finds herself making comparisons to peers, noting she "likes to be the sickest one." Megan's treatment team had successfully managed conversations around leaving AMA in the past through utilizing commitment strategies, like highlighting the freedom to choose and absence of alternatives and connecting present commitments to prior commitments. In this conversation, we see Carlos lean in through the use of the extending strategy.

Carlos: "Hi Megan, how are you feeling? Has your constipation improved? It looks like your intake has improved and I see your weight is trending up, vitals are improving, labs look great…great job!"

Megan: "Wow, okay…yeah…it's time for me to go."

Carlos: "What? Go where?"

Megan: "How do I sign an AMA form? I need to leave today."

Carlos: "Slow it down for a moment if you can…did something happen that makes you want to leave treatment?"

Megan: "I am the biggest one here. I'm obviously not sick enough to be here. I need to go."

Carlos: (brief pause, nodding) "Sure, okay…well, I can have the frontline team work on packing your bags and I can pull up the bus schedule for you since I know you don't have a car here. I think there's a bus early this evening. I should probably call over to nursing now, though, since it will take them a minute to get everything ready." (reaches for phone) (extending technique)

Megan: (appearing perplexed) "I... well...I might need more time than that."

Carlos: "First thing tomorrow then?" (extending technique, continued)

Megan: "I don't know, I don't know if my mom will let me leave, and I have to figure things out with my job..."

Carlos: "Look, forgive me if I'm mistaken, but I don't think you *actually* feel ready to leave treatment. If I had to take a guess, your eating disorder got pretty activated when I said you are more stable than you were and medically are on the right path."

Megan: (brief pause) "...yeah, I mean, I know you have to say that, it just really pisses me off to no longer be the sickest one here. It makes me want to pull back and start restricting again."

Carlos: "That totally makes sense to me, and I'd encourage you to bring this up with Serena. Can we agree it's not time to discharge and get you on your way to lunch after a quick physical exam?"

Megan: "Sure, yeah."

When Carlos pivots quickly in the conversation and engages in the extending technique, he throws Megan off balance for a moment, as she likely expected Carlos to talk her out of wanting to leave or to highlight the risks associated with leaving treatment prematurely. When he turns to extending, he takes her word at face value and calls Megan's bluff. It is important to note that in this situation, Carlos needs to feel confident Megan doesn't actually want to leave treatment or he will be helping her pack her bags shortly. This interaction opened up the possibility for Megan to consider her actual desires (e.g. to remain in care) and allowed her to be open with Carlos about the impact information he shares has on her (e.g. when you say x, it makes me feel y), which then allowed Megan to recommit to treatment for the time being. I (ETM) find this technique works exceptionally well when you have good rapport with a client and feel reasonably confident in your predictions of how extending might work. In working with eating disorders, which are often characterized by ambivalence, it is also important to have a plan to shift your approach in the event that extending does not work as intended.

Another dialectical strategy we'd like to provide an example of is making lemonade out of lemons. For this example, we're going to explore the use of this strategy in the context of Megan's avoidance of red meat (in the absence of an allergy, intolerance, religious or cultural belief). Megan reports she avoids beef and pork and has "since middle school," when she recalls seeing a documentary on farming practices. She states that ever since then, she finds the idea of eating beef and pork aversive and has no willingness to consume these products. On multiple occasions during her admission, Claire and Serena have attempted to explore this with Megan to try and untangle the eating disorder from her self-imposed dietary restriction. Although Megan has been adamant that her unwillingness to eat beef and pork is not related to her eating disorder, in exploring various hypothetical scenarios, it becomes clear that Megan's rigidity around red meat is likely to interfere with her ability to enter into a more sustained recovery. For example, during one session, Claire asks, "What if you were to cook out at a friend's house and they only had hot dogs and hamburgers?" to which Megan replied, "Well, then I wouldn't eat anything. I would eat when I got home." Claire attempted to work with Megan on exposures to beef and pork throughout her stay at a Residential level of care, however Megan refused to engage with this aspect of treatment. However, after transitioning to a Partial Hospitalization level of care, Claire and Serena took Megan to the local burger restaurant for a challenge lunch and Megan encountered an unexpected surprise.

Megan:	"Um, what is this?" (holding up the top bun of her burger, revealing several slices of bacon)
Claire (Dietitian):	"Oh would you look at that – I heard you order a turkey burger with no bacon, but I guess they misunderstood your order."
Megan:	"Yeah, no way. You know I don't do pork. I'm not eating this." (pushes the bacon cheeseburger away)
Serena (Therapist):	"What an incredible opportunity to push past some old beliefs about foods you can and can't eat! You've avoided targeting beef and pork this entire admission, and now here we are!" (making lemonade out of lemons)
Megan:	"I don't think I can. Maybe I can take the bacon off?"
Claire:	"You could…but what if you didn't? What if you just ate the bacon on the burger exactly as it came out?"
Megan:	(appearing overwhelmed) "No. I've been avoiding this since I was in middle school. I did *not* sign up for this. I mean…ugh. Even if I take the bacon off it's still going to *taste* like bacon. I'm not eating anything except maybe some fries."

Serena:	"Here it is again…that narrative you continue to carry that says you can't eat a full range of foods, in this case beef and pork. And here it is again, getting in the way of your recovery. What if you took a bite? That will also challenge your all-or-nothing, black-and-white thinking that we've been targeting for a while now."
Megan:	"You two are killing me (nervous laughter). Okay fine. ONE BITE."
Claire:	"That's the spirit, Megan!"
Megan:	(closes eyes and takes a bite of the bacon turkey burger) "… okay I did it. Will you two get off my back now?"
Serena (post-processing the meal):	"I have to reflect on something, Megan… you did something really incredible today. If the same scenario happened even a month ago, I really think it would've ended differently. Don't you?"
Megan:	"Yeah, I think you're probably right. I would've had a meltdown and restricted the entire meal. And probably would've been in a terrible mood the rest of the day."
Claire:	"And you didn't! You actually completed the whole meal. You really managed that situation beautifully, Megan. And we promise…we didn't plan for the restaurant to toss bacon on your burger!"

This is a great example of taking an unplanned, anxiety-provoking situation and turning it into a positive step towards a patient's recovery. A likely outcome of this naturalistic exposure could be increased self-efficacy (and perhaps a willingness to integrate beef and pork in the future) secondary to the success of this unplanned exposure. As mentioned above, part of the success of this intervention hinged on the patient's progress in treatment, as well as the rapport and support of the treating providers, who take this opportunity to encourage engagement with the food instead of having it replated without bacon. Other examples of making lemonade out of lemons include a client transforming an unexpected, uncomfortable conversation with an acquaintance about dieting into something recovery-oriented by asserting their needs and boundaries or a client seeing their weight at a PCP's office and reframing that information to support their recovery and progress made.

Provider Exercise – Dialectical Strategies

For this provider exercise, start by briefly reviewing the dialectical strategies and identify a patient with whom you think using these strategies could be helpful. Patients who might particularly benefit are patients with whom you are currently feeling "stuck" and/or patients who struggle with rigid or polarized thinking. Once you have used one or more of the dialectical strategies with your patient, use the prompts below to reflect on your experience. If you feel comfortable doing so, consider discussing your reflections with a trusted colleague for feedback.

Which of the dialectical strategies did you use? How specifically did you use these strategies?

How did your patient respond in the moment? Did you notice any changes after the session in terms of your patient's thoughts, behaviors, or emotions?

What do you think went well in using the dialectical strategies? What would you do differently in the future?

What other reflections do you have about your experience?

Chapter 12

Creating a DBT Treatment Target Hierarchy

As you are beginning to make inroads with regard to establishing rapport and getting your patient's buy-in around treatment and recovery, it can be helpful to simultaneously begin to think through what targets your patient might need to address in treatment in order to help them make progress toward their life worth living. The DBT treatment target hierarchy is a concise, triaged summary of all the targets you would like to work on with your patient over their course of treatment, broken into primary targets, secondary targets, and where relevant due to the patient's age, adolescent dialectical dilemmas.

Before we discuss what each of these categories involves, we'd like to outline the reasons why taking the time to identify and triage targets can be helpful. First, when you have a comprehensive, triaged summary of all of a patient's potential treatment targets, you can more effectively identify what is most important to focus on during an individual provider appointment and structure your time accordingly. Second, having a bird's eye view of all the things your patient is struggling with can help with a more comprehensive, holistic case conceptualization. You can both see individual pieces of your patient's struggle, as well as ways in which each piece links to the larger whole. Third, with a list of all of a patient's treatment targets available to the patient's treatment team, each member of the treatment team can see where their time and attention is best allocated. While there are many targets that will be shared by the team as a whole, there will also be targets that are most relevant to certain discipline-specific team members. Finally, the DBT treatment target hierarchy provides a comprehensive snapshot of your patient at the beginning of treatment, which becomes a baseline against which progress in treatment can be measured.

Primary Targets

Primary targets in DBT are any behaviors, emotions, thoughts, and urges that should or must be addressed in the context of stage one of treatment in order to help the patient move closer to their goals and building a life worth living. What

DOI: 10.4324/9781003495604-12

is unique about primary targets in DBT is that the sole focus is not only on the patient when it comes to identifying and addressing targets. The behaviors, emotions, thoughts, and urges of the patient's family members and supports, as well as the behaviors, emotions, thoughts, and urges of the patient's treatment team members can also become targets for treatment. Many providers often experience this as a confusing paradigm shift, so if you are having that experience as you read this, know that you are not alone! This shift in thinking about patient care becomes easier to understand as you look at more specific examples, so let's take an in-depth look at each of the four levels of primary targets within DBT.

Level One Target Behaviors

Patient Life-Threatening Behaviors. There has yet to be any evidence that has emerged in the treatment literature demonstrating that eating disorder treatment for a patient who is no longer living is effective. What you can logically conclude from this statement is that life-threatening behaviors of the patient must be targeted first and foremost in the context of treatment. Since this is a text that is focused on the treatment of eating disorders specifically, it is important to highlight that eating disorder behaviors can fall in any of the first three levels of target behaviors, depending on both their level of severity and the extent to which they put the patient at imminent risk of death. Some indicators that may suggest the patient is at imminent risk of death include severe bradycardia, significantly prolonged QTc intervals, and severe electrolyte imbalances. If you are not a medical provider, this underscores the importance of ongoing multidisciplinary collaboration that includes involvement of a medical provider, in order to help assess the severity of your patient's eating disorder behaviors.

There are also other behaviors that fall within the category of patient life-threatening behaviors. Suicidal behaviors are perhaps the most obvious grouping of behaviors that would be situated within this category. Suicidal behaviors include a wide range of behaviors, such as suicidal ideation, planning to commit suicide, communications about intent to commit suicide, obtaining lethal means, and fantasizing about suicide and/or expected consequences of suicide. The rates of completed suicides among individuals diagnosed with eating disorders are staggering, particularly in comparison to the general population. One study that examined suicide rates over an extended period of time among individuals diagnosed with eating disorders found that crude mortality rates were 4% for individuals diagnosed with Anorexia Nervosa, 3.9% for individuals diagnosed with Bulimia Nervosa, and 5.2% for individuals diagnosed with OSFED (Crow, et al., 2009). By comparison, the rates of death by suicide in the general population are 14.5 per 100,000 people (Kochanak, et al., 2019). The impact of suicide on individuals diagnosed with an eating disorder can also be examined through looking at the extent to which suicide accounts for deaths when a death has occurred. As an example, suicide is estimated to account for one in every five deaths of individuals diagnosed with Anorexia Nervosa (Papadopoulos, Ekbom, Brandt, & Ekselius, 2009).

The last major grouping of behaviors that fall within the patient life-threatening behaviors umbrella are self-injurious behaviors, which include behaviors such as cutting, scratching, burning, headbanging, punching, and so forth. One of the most common questions I (AHK) have been asked by supervisees is why self-injurious behaviors fall in the category of patient life-threatening behaviors, particularly in instances where the self-injurious behavior has a low risk of severe adverse medical consequences (e.g. scratching that results in only mild breaking of the skin). There are a number of reasons why self-injurious behaviors have been included as level one target behaviors. First, there is evidence that suggests self-injurious behavior is a strong predictor of future suicidal ideation and suicide attempts (e.g. Guan, Fox & Prinstine, 2012). Even though the risk of self-injurious behavior resulting in death may not be imminent, given it is a substantial risk factor for subsequent suicidal ideation and suicide attempts, it logically makes sense to target these behaviors aggressively in treatment. Second, self-injurious behavior may result in accidental death or medical consequences (e.g. severe infection, head injuries) that put a person at risk of death or severe, long-term medical consequences. Third, self-injurious behavior is fundamentally incompatible with the overall stated goal of treatment, which is to build a life worth living. There is simply no way to achieve a life worth living while actively and intentionally inflicting harm to one's body. Finally, as we will touch on further throughout this text, self-injurious behaviors may serve a similar function to a patient's eating disorder behaviors. In situations where this is the case, failing to address self-injurious behaviors creates a situation in which the core issues driving the patient's eating disorder are likely never adequately addressed. For those of you who have worked with individuals diagnosed with an eating disorder and who also engage in self-injurious behavior, it is a common phenomena to observe a worsening of self-injurious behaviors as eating disorder symptoms improve, and vice-versa. Successful treatment requires targeting both concurrently. As with suicide-related behaviors, self-injurious behaviors are also more common in individuals diagnosed with eating disorders than the general population. Estimates of the twelve-month prevalence rates of NSSI among US adolescents, young adults, and adults are 7.3%, 17%, and 5% respectively. In contrast, up to 72% of individuals diagnosed with eating disorders also engage in NSSI, with notably higher rates of NSSI among individuals diagnosed with Bulimia Nervosa and Anorexia Nervosa, Anorexia Nervosa, Binge Eating and Purging Subtype (Claes & Muehlenkamp, 2014).

Before we move on from patient life-threatening behaviors, it is important to briefly discuss the responsibilities of individual multidisciplinary team members as it relates to this subject. Obviously, if there is an imminent risk of loss of life (e.g. a patient's labs or vitals indicate the need for an ambulance to transport them to the hospital immediately; a patient has conveyed they have intent to commit suicide imminently and they have a plan and means to enact this plan), all members of the patient's multidisciplinary team hold the responsibility for prompt emergency intervention. But what about situations in which a patient struggles with low-severity self-injurious behavior or mild suicidal ideation? It is helpful for all members of a patient's multidisciplinary team to be aware of the self-injurious behavior or suicidal ideation, in that these behaviors can impact things like case conceptualization and recommended level of care, however it is not the responsibility of a dietitian or medical provider to be attempting to intervene with these behaviors. Rather, it is critical that they communicate with the therapist and psychiatric provider working with the patient about any new information they may hear, such that these members of the multidisciplinary team can follow-up in the context of their work with the patient.

Parent/Caregiver/Partner/Family/Support Life-Threatening or Treatment-Destroying Behaviors. Parent, caregiver, partner, family, and/or support life-threatening or treatment-destroying behaviors refer to any behaviors on the part of these individuals that put a patient's life at risk or create a situation in which it is impossible for treatment to be effective. The most obvious example of behaviors that would fall in this category are ones that would trigger mandated reporting, like abuse or neglect. Other behaviors that might reach this threshold include behaviors that actively and intentionally go against recommendations made by the patient's multidisciplinary team, like strongly suggesting the patient to restrict their intake when weight restoration is necessary or encouraging the patient to engage in compulsive exercise for purposes of weight loss, perhaps even joining with the patient in engaging in compulsive exercise as a family activity. While behaviors on the part of families and supports that reach this threshold are rare, it is important to be vigilant in monitoring for these behaviors and to actively intervene when they do occur.

Milieu- or Treatment-Destroying Behavior. Milieu- or treatment-destroying behavior generally refers to any behaviors that a patient might engage in that threaten their ability to remain in treatment because of the impact the behaviors have on others. Behaviors that fall in this category are most typically seen in the context of outpatient groups or in the context of treatment milieus at higher levels of care. Examples include aggression toward other patients, bullying of other patients, or sexual behaviors toward other patients. Behaviors that are not directed at patients themselves may also fall in this category. When I (AHK) was running DBT skills groups in an outpatient environment, I had a circumstance in which a few members of the group I was running witnessed another group member behaving aggressively toward his pet. The reactions that some of the group members had were intense; one group member immediately left the group with a stated plan to engage in self-harm and another group member stated that she felt a strong urge to leave group and use alcohol. Other group members indicated that they weren't sure they felt comfortable returning to group in the future if the group member they witnessed being aggressive toward his pet was going to be present. In a situation like this, the issue at hand must be addressed before group can proceed.

Provider Unethical, Severely Irresponsible, or Treatment-Destroying Behavior. One of the things that is both unique and powerful about DBT is that it is not just patient behavior that is taken into consideration in the context of treatment, but provider behavior as well. The last group of level one targets focuses on addressing unethical, severely irresponsible, or treatment-destroying behavior on the part of providers. Examples of behaviors that fall in this category include sexual behaviors toward patients, violation of state or federal laws pertaining to treatment, creating false documentation, and extreme interpersonal conflict among staff. Just as you cannot conduct effective treatment with a patient who is dead, you cannot conduct treatment if your license is suspended or revoked or if you are in jail for a crime. As such, as uncomfortable as it may be to acknowledge and discuss, provider behavior that runs the risk of these outcomes must be promptly targeted.

Level Two Target Behaviors

Patient Treatment-Interfering Behaviors. The first subcategory of level two target behaviors are patient treatment-interfering behaviors. This refers to any behaviors that the patient is engaging in that impede the effectiveness of treatment. While it might be considered rather obvious that one would need to address behaviors that are negatively impacting the effectiveness of treatment before forging ahead with further treatment interventions, the intentional focus on treatment-interfering behaviors is an aspect of DBT that is considered to be somewhat unique. While other therapeutic traditions certainly allow for space to address treatment-interfering behaviors, doing so is not necessarily systematically integrated into treatment protocols and procedures.

There are three general categories of behavior that fall under the broader category of patient treatment-interfering behaviors. The first category of behavior is made up of any behaviors that get in the way of the patient personally benefiting from treatment. There are three subcategories of behavior that fall within this overarching category. Nonattentive behaviors refer to any behaviors that result in a patient being either physically or mentally absent in terms of treatment and can include behaviors like missing or showing up late to appointments, using substances prior to appointments, or dissociating or having panic attacks during appointments. Specific to work with eating disorders, engaging in restriction to the point that cognitive abilities are impaired is another example of behavior that would fall in this subcategory. Non-collaborative behaviors refer to any behaviors that interfere with the therapeutic working relationship between patient and provider. Particularly when working with adult patients, where providers have little to no ability to influence patients' environments, active collaboration is essential for treatment to be effective. Examples of non-collaborative behaviors include lying, manipulating weights, arguing with provider suggestions, and withdrawing during sessions. Finally, noncompliant behaviors refer to situations in which the patient is not following-through in engaging in treatment interventions discussed, whether during appointments or outside of appointments. Examples of behaviors that fall in this category include refusal to follow a meal plan or recommendations around physical activity, not completing self-monitoring tools in between appointments, or refusing to get weights and vitals taken.

The second category of behavior is made up of any behaviors that may not personally negatively impact the patient, but that get in the way of other patients' treatment. In outpatient settings, behaviors in this category typically refer to open hostility, conflict, or judgment occurring in the context of DBT skills groups. In inpatient, residential, and partial hospitalization settings, the amount of time that patients are in each other's presence in a given day tends to create the opportunity for additional patient treatment-interfering behaviors to occur. These include engaging in behaviors that "trigger" other patients (e.g. engaging in eating disorder behaviors during mealtimes, detailed discussion around eating disorder symptoms or self-harm behaviors), conflict among patients in the milieu, and creating eating disorder "pacts."

The final category of behavior also consists of behaviors that may not personally negatively impact the patient, however that impact the patient's treatment providers in ways that increase their burnout or decrease their willingness to continue treatment with the patient. Behaviors that push the personal limits of providers are one subcategory of behaviors that fit within this overarching category. Examples of behaviors that fall within this subcategory include repeatedly asking for more frequent appointments or more frequent contact than the provider is willing and/or able to provide, interacting with a provider in a way that is overly friendly or sexually provocative, or making threats toward a provider or their family. This subcategory closely aligns with the concept of therapeutic boundaries. Another subcategory of behaviors that fall within this broader category are behaviors that push organizational limits. Rather than being limits that are set by an individual provider, these are limits set by the organization or company where the provider works. In general, behaviors that fall in this category are violations of unit or clinic rules, like bringing prohibited items on company premises or refusing to follow directions of staff responsible for managing a unit. The final subcategory of behaviors that fall within this category are behaviors that decrease provider motivation. Examples of behaviors that fall in this subcategory include noncompliance with treatment, judgmental comments toward the provider, and threatening to sue the provider or report the provider to their licensing board.

Patient Treatment-Enhancing Behaviors. DBT is a treatment that is not just focused on what behaviors patients and providers want patients to decrease, but also on behaviors that are helpful for our patients to increase and sustain as well. One category of behaviors that can be helpful for patients to increase and sustain are patient treatment-enhancing behaviors, which are defined as behaviors that make a provider want to continue working with a patient. Patient treatment-enhancing behaviors tend to be somewhat individualized from provider to provider, although one category of patient treatment-enhancing behaviors that is agreed upon by all providers is behaviors that demonstrate measurable progress toward treatment goals. Other behaviors that qualify as patient treatment-enhancing behaviors will vary from provider to provider or may even vary from patient to patient seen by a given provider. For example, I (AHK) have had situations in which I've simultaneously had patients on my caseload where for one patient, asking for help from staff was a treatment-enhancing behavior, whereas for another patient for whom a goal has been set to work on managing distress more independently, asking for help may actually fall in the category of a treatment-interfering behavior. We will discuss behavioral principles like reinforcement and shaping later in this text and for each of your patients, it can be helpful to have a sense of specific treatment-enhancing behaviors you want to shape or reinforce in order to help them emit these behaviors more frequently. Some behaviors that we have found to be reinforcing include completing diary cards in advance of individual sessions, following through on homework assigned in individual and group sessions, coming prepared to session with topics to discuss, expressing excitement when a skill or strategy learned in treatment has been helpful, actively participating in group and individual sessions, engaging in experiential activities, being honest, curious, and vulnerable, and expressing appreciation towards providers.

Parent/Caregiver/Partner/Family/Support Treatment-Interfering Behaviors. We are firm believers that the involvement of parents, caregivers, partners, family members, and other supports in eating disorder treatment when clinically indicated can have a powerful effect in helping to set and keep our patients on a path toward recovery and building a life worth living. While family members and supports can be some of our greatest assets in treatment, they can also interfere with treatment as well. For child, adolescent, and young adult patients, some common treatment-interfering behaviors on the part of families and supports include threats to remove the patient from treatment, failing to provide adequate supervision of the patient around meals and snacks, restroom use, and/or physical activity, and not adhering to provider recommendations. For family members and supports of patients across all age groups, some additional common treatment-interfering behaviors include missing, canceling, or arriving late to appointments, reinforcing ineffective behaviors, demonstrating high expressed criticism toward the patient, contacting providers excessively, and arguing with recommendations and information given by providers.

Alliance-Ruptures. The focus on alliance-ruptures as a treatment target is borne out of RO DBT, which prioritizes targeting alliance-ruptures over treatment-interfering behaviors when working with patients diagnosed with Anorexia Nervosa. Alliance-ruptures are defined as circumstances in which the patient feels misunderstood and/or situations in which the patient does not feel as though treatment is relevant to their problems. Unlike many of the other treatment targets within the DBT treatment target hierarchy, rather than viewing alliance-ruptures as problematic, they are viewed as opportunities for patients to practice navigating conflict in a way that enhances intimacy and connectedness (Lynch, Hempel, & Dunkley, 2015). Although alliance-ruptures were identified as a treatment target specifically in the context of working with patients diagnosed with Anorexia Nervosa, targeting alliance-ruptures has relevance in working with individuals diagnosed with Bulimia Nervosa and Binge Eating Disorder as well.

Provider Treatment-Interfering Behaviors. Something else that is unique about the focus on treatment-interfering behaviors in DBT is that this focus extends beyond patient behaviors to provider and team behaviors as well. There are four somewhat arbitrary categories into which provider treatment-interfering behaviors can fall that we review below.

Non-Adherent Behaviors. The first grouping of provider treatment-interfering behaviors are non-adherent behaviors. While your aim in reading this text may not be to work toward conducting DBT in such a way that it would meet the threshold to be considered adherent, it is important that when you've determined what principles and strategies you do want to apply in your work that you follow-through in utilizing these principles and strategies. For example, I have found that dietitians with whom I (AHK) have interacted with at conferences love the idea of incorporating DBT diary cards in their work. I will also add that many providers with whom I have worked forget to review diary cards routinely or fail to address patient diary card noncompliance when it occurs. This is an example of a non-adherent provider treatment-interfering behavior. Eating disorder work in general and DBT as applied to eating disorder work more specifically is a complex, nuanced, and ever-evolving subspecialty of clinical care that requires ongoing action on the part of providers through self-guided learning, attendance at conferences, and supervision and consultation in order to remain competent and stay current with best practices. Failing to stay abreast of new developments within the field and to adapt one's care accordingly is another example of non-adherent provider behavior.

Behaviors Creating a Therapeutic Imbalance. Behaviors that a create a therapeutic imbalance is another category of provider treatment-interfering behaviors. In DBT, as providers we seek not only to help our patients move toward more dialectical approaches with regard to thoughts, emotions, and behaviors, we also strive to embrace a dialectical philosophy ourselves and to model this philosophy in our clinical care. Yet work with eating disorders in particular is rife with possibilities for dialectical failures in our work as providers.

One common area of imbalance falls on the dialectic of acceptance versus change. We will engage in a much more extensive discussion about exposure-based procedures later and it can be helpful at this juncture to note that a subset of eating disorder providers tend to avoid exposure-based procedures, opting instead for distress tolerance oriented approaches to helping patients manage their distress around meals and snacks. While this approach may help them to meet their nutritional needs in the short-term, it does not help patients reduce the unpleasant emotional experiences that accompany eating or prepare patients to engage in social eating in a way that is socially normative. On the other side of this dialectic, providers can be focused on change to the point that it is experienced as invalidating. Because eating meals and snacks is such a relatively uneventful and routine part of everyday life for providers who have not experienced what it is like to have an eating disorder firsthand, it can be easy to forget to truly put ourselves in our patients' shoes to the best of our ability in the service of understanding the emotional anguish that our patients experience when faced with a meal or snack. A metaphor that was offered to me (AHK) early in my work with eating disorders is that for many of our patients, the fear they experience when tasked with completing a meal or snack is like the fear you would experience being faced with eating a plate of spiders. One time of doing this would be quite enough for the majority of people I know. Now imagine being faced with this task five or six times a day, with no end to that experience anywhere in sight. This offers a helpful reminder to be thoughtful about how much change may actually be possible for a patient at any given moment in time.

Another common area of therapeutic imbalance is the balance between flexibility and stability. When working with patients diagnosed with eating disorders, particularly patients who are more medically or psychiatrically compromised, there can be a pull to switch therapeutic approaches or to unilaterally transfer or refer a patient out when it appears progress is not being made. Helping our patients to make progress often requires both focus and patience, coupled with managing our own emotional reactions throughout the process. On the other side of this dialectic, there are certainly times where flexibility and creativity are called for. One thing that I (AHK) have found to be fascinating about eating disorders work is that for patients diagnosed with an eating disorder without additional psychiatric comorbidities, there is somewhat of a predictable course of treatment and treatment plan. However, for patients with a more complex psychiatric presentation or who have a more chronic eating disorder presentation, often one with many courses of treatment at higher levels of care, successful treatment outcomes may require deviation from "treatment as usual" in thoughtful ways if a more standard approach to treatment isn't leading to desired outcomes.

An additional area in which therapeutic imbalance may be present is the balance between nurturing versus demanding change. When operating from the extreme end of the nurturing side of the dialectic, a provider is assuming that their patient lacks the ability, whether due to skills deficits or motivational deficits, to make necessary changes independently. We often see this occur with meal support. Pushing our patients through excruciating challenges multiple times a day can be painful and the people providing patients with support can fall into the trap of ignoring eating disorder behaviors (e.g. permitting a patient to disassemble their turkey sandwich if it "gets them to eat it"), negotiating with the eating disorder (e.g. being willing to swap out challenging parts of a meal for easier food items), and/or loosening time constraints around meals in the hope that having extra time will allow the patient to complete. Another example of nurturing I (ETM) often see with newer dietitians is acceptance of a patient's dietary limitations without further probing. Patients will often present with an extensive list of foods not tolerated well, barring verified allergies and intolerances, or foods they ethically do not agree with. When examined, it becomes clear the restrictions are part of the eating disorder and should not be "honored" through modifications to meal planning. Excessive nurturing can also manifest in providing excessive support to patients, like having more frequent sessions with a patient than you typically would in the absence of a clear clinical rationale or providing a patient with significant support or coaching without them having made an effort to utilize skills more independently first. On the other side of the dialectic, demanding change when it is either beyond the patient's current ability or beyond what they have the willingness to do at the moment is an approach that is unlikely to be successful. Some common circumstances under which demanding change occurs are when providers are frustrated with a patient's slow pace of change or when a patient appears to be more skillful or willing than they actually are.

The last area in which therapeutic imbalance may be present is the balance between reciprocal and irreverent communication. A variety of factors can result in providers being overly vulnerable or friendly with their patients. For example, the accessibility of our patients when working at higher levels of care can be somewhat of a double-edged sword. On one hand, having the opportunity to work with patients more frequently and within the types of settings where they struggle the most can help providers with case conceptualization and treatment interventions and can help patients feel supported and to generalize skills in the situations where they are needed the most. On the other hand, providers being more frequently and readily accessible can result in therapeutic boundaries that might be overly flexible at times. Many treatment providers also have their own eating disorder histories, which also has both its own benefits and downsides. On one hand, lived experience can be incredibly helpful in providing authentic validation or in thinking through potential skills and strategies that might benefit a patient. On the other hand, there is the risk of sharing an unnecessary amount of information about one's own historical or current struggles with a patient without a clear clinical target for this degree of self-disclosure in mind. There are also pitfalls when providers fall too far on the other sides of these dialectics. Using the same examples as above, for a provider working at a higher level of care who is overly concerned about boundaries, having rigid rules around exactly when, where, and how patients can have contact can be experienced as cold and invalidating. Using the example of a provider who has their own history of an eating disorder, in attempts to avoid self-disclosure about their personal history, the provider might be experienced as being evasive or aloof. Thinking about irreverent communication more specifically, being overly blunt or confrontational without incorporating warmth and validation can have significant negative impacts on therapeutic rapport. Careful thought must be given to each side of the dialectic and how this polarity informs our responses to our patients.

Behaviors Showing Lack of Respect for the Patient. Behaviors showing lack of respect for the patient refers to a broad set of behaviors that fall under the umbrella of "professionalism." Behaviors in this category include being late to or missing appointments, appearing disinterested or watching the clock when interacting with a patient, allowing for interruptions during appointments, maintaining an unkempt office space, and so forth. These behaviors may be accidental, as in the case of lateness to an appointment in the context of a recent time change, or they may be indicative of burnout with a specific patient or professional burnout more broadly. While all professionals have likely engaged in behaviors showing lack of respect for patients on occasion, it is important to be vigilant about these behaviors, both to prevent them from becoming a pattern and as a sign of larger, underlying concerns that may need to be addressed.

Personal Factors That Can Impact Professional Effectiveness. The final subset of provider treatment-interfering behaviors refers to a subcategory of behaviors that require ongoing monitoring at minimum and that may need to be targeted if they begin to interfere with treatment. One set of personal factors that can impact professional effectiveness pertain to stressors at work and outside of work. In the workplace setting, time demands outside of patient care, like staff meetings and documentation requirements, can impact professional effectiveness by limiting the amount of time available for patient care. Outside of the workplace setting, required but not restorative tasks at home can limit the amount of time available for leisure and necessary self-care, like adequate time for physical activity and sleep. Another set of personal factors that can interfere with professional effectiveness has to do with provider reactions to their patients or to themselves. Working with patients diagnosed with serious psychiatric illnesses can evoke emotions like anger, fear, and sadness. These are common, natural, and understandable reactions that should not be pathologized, and it is important to monitor the impact these emotional reactions have on professional effectiveness. For example, if a provider is so afraid of being sued by the parents of an adolescent patient that it results in them making decisions that they don't believe are in the patient's best interest, this is likely a situation that needs to be addressed. Finally, diet culture, fat stigma, and food beliefs are pervasive within our society and providers are not immune to their impacts. In fact, individuals who have written about body image have noted that there is a certain degree of "normative discontent" around body image that is present and expected (Tiggemann, 2011). Furthermore, many providers who treat patients with eating disorders are in recovery themselves. With all of this in mind, it is critical that providers are mindful in an ongoing way of their relationships with food, physical activity, and their bodies, and proactively addressing issues that arise that have the possibility of negatively impacting patient care.

Team-Interfering Behaviors. The last category of level two targets is team-interfering behaviors. We will discuss the fourth mode of DBT, case consultation meetings, in much further detail in Chapter 20, including specifics about team-interfering behaviors. In short, team-interfering behaviors refer to any behaviors that interfere with the logistical functioning of case consultation meetings, like showing up late to meetings or failing to notify team members of upcoming absences, as well as behaviors that are inconsistent with the intended process of case consultation meetings, like fragilizing other team members or responding defensively to feedback.

The multidisciplinary nature of eating disorders work is also such that the scope of team-interfering behaviors could be expanded beyond the context of case consultation meetings to the functioning of a patient's multidisciplinary team as well. For example, if a dietitian puts a contingency in place with a patient that a therapist subsequently undermines, this lack of alignment between team members becomes an area that requires targeting in order for optimal treatment to be provided. Providing high-quality eating disorders treatment requires effective and timely communication, agreement upon a treatment plan with components of the plan delineated by discipline, and demonstrated professionalism among team members.

Level Three Target Behaviors

Level three target behaviors pertain to any behaviors that pose a significant impediment to our patients' quality of life. If you are working with patients diagnosed with a primary eating disorder, then the behaviors that are of most interest in this category are eating disorder behaviors that have not met the threshold of severity to be considered level one or level two behaviors. This might include low-frequency bingeing, purging, restricting, or compulsive exercise, as well as other disordered eating behaviors, like chewing and spitting, body checking, and calorie counting. Other behaviors that fall within this category are behaviors associated with comorbid psychiatric or medical conditions, severe interpersonal difficulties, financial problems, criminal behaviors, school-related or employment-related difficulties, and housing problems.

Level Four Target Behaviors

Level four target behaviors are the last of the stage one primary targets and these focus on increasing behavioral skills. Patients who enter into treatment for their eating disorder often have skills deficits in a number of areas. The DBT skills modules specifically focus on skills related to mindfulness, interpersonal effectiveness, emotion regulation, and distress tolerance. Additionally, there are another set of skills from RO DBT that focus specifically on targets relevant for overcontrolled patients. Finally, self-management skills are both woven into DBT skills modules and taught independent of them.

Unique to the treatment of eating disorders specifically, there are also skills a patient may need to develop around food-related topics. These skills may include following a meal plan, portioning, preparing food, grocery shopping, and so forth. We will elaborate upon these areas, as well as the DBT skills modules, in Chapters 16 and 18.

Secondary Targets

The secondary targets in DBT are captured by three dialectics, the poles of which represent extreme patterns of behavior in which our patients may engage. The value in identifying and addressing secondary targets is that they are often directly related to the primary targets with which our patients struggle and may even be a common thread across target behaviors of differing topographies. For example, a single secondary target may be functionally related to self-injurious behaviors, bingeing and purging, and substance use.

Emotional Vulnerability vs. Self-Invalidation. The first dialectic of secondary targets is emotional vulnerability versus self-invalidation. Emotional vulnerability refers to the experience of intense and pervasive emotional suffering. This emotional suffering is often characterized by feeling emotions both quickly and intensely, followed by difficulties returning to emotional baseline. Marsha Linehan describes individuals who struggle with emotional vulnerability as being the "psychological equivalent to a third-degree burn patient," where even the slightest of stimuli can result in an extreme emotional reaction. The treatment targets relevant to this side of the dialectic are increasing emotion modulation and decreasing emotional reactivity. The goal here is not to attempt to eliminate emotional experiencing, but rather to assist patients in increasing their ability to reduce the intensity of unpleasant emotions and to inhibit maladaptive actions taken in response to negative affect.

Emotional vulnerability is contrasted with self-invalidation, which involves taking on characteristics of the invalidating environments we reviewed when discussing the biosocial theories of the development of eating disorders. Self-invalidation can manifest in a number of ways, including invalidating one's emotional experiences coupled with attempting to suppress one's emotions, distrusting one's own perceptions and looking to others to define one's reality, responding to one's emotions with negative secondary emotions like shame, disgust, or anger, and oversimplifying the ease of solving one's problems. The treatment targets relevant to this side of the dialectic are increasing self-validation and decreasing self-invalidation. The goal here is to enhance your patient's ability to nonjudgmentally observe, describe, and experience their emotional states and counteract self-invalidating statements with self-validating ones.

While some patients for whom the secondary targets are relevant may only fall on one side of a given dialectic in terms of their patterns of behavior, often what you will observe with secondary targets is a vacillation between extreme ends of the dialectic. For example, I (AHK) have worked with patients who experience intense anxiety or shame in the context of trying to complete a meal or snack. However, instead of validating their emotional experiences and the challenges associated with completing a meal or snack, they engage in self-invalidation by saying things to themselves like, "This isn't hard. You just need to eat." Rather than reducing the intensity of their emotions or helping them to be more skillful in the context of meals and snacks, these messages often result in heightening the negative affect they are experiencing and a vicious cycle of emotional vulnerability and self-invalidation is set in motion.

Active Passivity vs. Apparent Competence. The second dialectic of secondary targets is active passivity versus apparent competence. Active passivity is defined as a coping style characterized by helplessness, coupled with actively working to get others to solve one's problems. Active passivity manifests in lots of different ways when working with patients diagnosed with eating disorders. I've worked with some patients who have held deeply seated beliefs that because eating disorders are brain-based illnesses, the only treatment interventions that could be effective must be in the form of medical interventions. When working with these patients, they have often been reluctant to try psychotherapeutic interventions and instead spend their energy focused on the belief that the solution to their problems lies in medication changes alone. Active passivity can also be displayed in behaviors that can appear like "splitting." For example, I have had many patients try to convince me (AHK) to talk to their dietitian on their behalf to request a decrease in their meal plan, rather than initiating these conversations themselves. Finally, active passivity can also manifest in patients expending a great deal of energy trying to get their environment to change to best meet their needs, rather than focusing on ways in which they could learn to respond more effectively to their environment. The treatment targets relevant to this side of the dialectic include increasing active problem-solving and decreasing active passivity. This is accomplished through both helping patients to develop the skills they need in order to be able to solve their own problems and through enhancing their willingness to implement these skills when needed.

The other side of this dialectic is apparent competence, which is defined as patients presenting themselves in such a way that leads others to inaccurately perceive them as being more competent, in control, and effective than they actually are. When I think of apparent competence in eating disorders work, I think of patients who have come to treatment in a significantly malnourished and medically compromised state, yet who immediately and consistently start meeting all of their nutritional needs once in treatment with no outward signs of distress. In some circumstances, their apparent competence has appeared to be driven by a strong desire to complete treatment as soon as possible, in the service of returning to something highly motivating outside of treatment, like going back to school or college. In other circumstances, patients with more of a "people pleasing" presentation have verbalized that they are completing simply because they don't want to be an inconvenience or disappointment to staff. The treatment targets relevant to this side of the dialectic include increasing accurate communication about one's abilities and decreasing the extent to which behavior is dependent on mood. As with active passivity, these treatment targets are also addressed through assisting patients in learning new skills, often with a specific emphasis on interpersonal effectiveness skills.

As with the first set of secondary targets we discussed, vacillation between active passivity and apparent competence is also common. I (AHK) have worked with patients diagnosed with severe and long standing eating disorders who have been able to complete 100% of their meals and snacks without engaging in compensatory behaviors immediately after being admitted to treatment with seemingly little signs of outward distress. I have also seen these very same patients struggle with other symptoms, like panic attacks or dissociation, with no outward evidence of attempts at skills use when these symptoms arise, instead relying heavily on staff to intervene in an attempt to address these symptoms.

Unrelenting Crises vs. Inhibited Grieving. The final dialectic of secondary targets is unrelenting crises versus inhibited grieving. Unrelenting crises refers to situations in which a precipitating event occurs that results in intense emotional pain, which the patient then attempts to escape by engaging in impulsive actions that perpetuate the state of crisis. An example of a series of unrelenting crises might look something like the following: A patient with a historical diagnosis of an alcohol use disorder, but who has been abstinent for years, gets unexpectedly dumped by their partner. In response to the intense sadness they feel, they find themselves at a bar later that day, drinking heavily. After a few drinks, they text a different ex-partner, with whom they "hook-up" with later that evening. In addition to an intense hangover, they experience a great deal of shame in response to both their relapse and their "hook-up," and begin engaging in cutting in an effort to decrease the shame they are feeling. What you see in this example is how quickly one crisis can lead into another when a patient lacks the necessary skills to tolerate or change their emotional experiences. The treatment targets relevant to this side of the dialectic include increasing realistic decision-making and judgment and decreasing crisis-generating behaviors. These treatment targets are addressed through a number of strategies, including helping patients to increase awareness of their emotional states and associated urges and act opposite to these urges, often coupled with the use of distress tolerance strategies.

The other side of this dialectic is inhibited grieving, which refers to the involuntary and automatic avoidance of cues associated with past losses and traumas, which prevents the individual from progressing through the normal stages of a grieving. As a result, the individual does not have the opportunity to habituate to the painful emotions associated with the losses and traumas they have experienced. Both histories of traumatic experiences and comorbid posttraumatic stress disorder diagnoses are common in individuals diagnosed with eating disorders. Prevalence rates for a history of traumatic events have ranged from 37% to 100% in individual studies, with a history of childhood sexual abuse being one specific type of trauma that increases the risk for development of an eating disorder (Tagay, et al., 2014). Of individuals who have experienced one or more traumatic events, individual studies of persons diagnosed with eating disorders have found that 4% to 52% meet criteria for a posttraumatic stress disorder diagnosis (Tagay, et al., 2014). There are also losses unique to eating disorders, specifically in the treatment and recovery process, that are worth mentioning here. For some patients, their identity itself is wrapped up in their eating disorder. For other patients, they experience their eating disorder as a close and trusted companion of sorts. The loss of the pursuit of a "perfect" body and the loss of reliably effective, albeit ultimately maladaptive, coping strategies are also often experienced during the treatment and recovery process. The treatment target for this side of the dialectic is to assist patients in being able to fully experience negative affect without turning to avoidance behaviors as a way to inhibit emotional experiencing.

As with the other two dialectics we have discussed in this section, you may also encounter situations where patients vacillate between unrelenting crises and inhibited grieving. Many of the strategies that patients turn to in order to inhibit their grief, while effective in the short-term, tend to create further crises. For example, if a patient who is struggling financially, but who finds relief in online shopping sprees ends up making multiple online purchases in an attempt to regulate their affect, they are likely to experience temporary relief while also worsening the crisis at hand. One can imagine that as the frequency and depth of crises at hand intensifies, that patients might also struggle to refrain from maladaptive behaviors that inhibit the grief they are experiencing, thus creating a vicious cycle of vacillating between extremes.

Dialectical Dilemmas Unique to Eating Disorders

As DBT has begun to be applied in the treatment of eating disorders specifically, individuals doing this work began to notice that unique dialectical dilemmas can emerge (Wisniewski & Ben-Porath, 2015; Wisniewski & Kelly, 2003).

Rigid, Overcontrolled Eating vs. Absence of an Eating Plan. The first of these two dialectical dilemmas is rigid, overcontrolled eating versus absence of an eating plan. Rigid, overcontrolled eating refers to clients focusing on every detail of their eating plan, including what they will eat, when they will eat it, how much they will eat, and so forth. Manifestations of rigid, overcontrolled eating include measuring, weighing or counting foods, refusing to eat any food beyond one's meal plan or beyond a caloric goal, difficulties deviating from a plan when needed (e.g. making a plan to go to a different restaurant if the restaurant where a meal was planned is closed), and so forth. On the other side of the dialectic, absence of an eating plan can result in inadequate intake (e.g. in the absence of understanding what one's body needs, underestimating those needs based on eating disorder thinking) or at the other extreme, binge eating.

Apparent Compliance vs. Active Defiance. The second of these dialectical dilemmas is apparent compliance versus active defiance. Wiśniewski and Ben-Porath (2015) define apparent compliance as, "Behavior in which the patient reports engaging in a sufficient amount of a behavior to demonstrate effort but does not engage in it enough to make appreciable change." For example, a treatment team might be working with a client who has a history of compulsive exercise via running who is trying to weight restore, yet isn't restoring weight at the pace that would be expected. The patient might say, "I haven't run one single time!" and while this may indeed be accurate, the team may discover through further assessment that the patient has replaced running with long, brisk walks multiple times per day. Although they are indeed following through with what was asked of them by their team, at least in terms of the very specific "letter of the law," this would be considered apparent compliance, as long, brisk walks are inconsistent with the intention of the team's treatment recommendation.

On the other side of the dialectic, active defiance is defined as willful behavior that is in direct opposition to treatment recommendations or provider or program limits. For example, a client who is eating 100% of their meal plan, yet is still failing to restore weight might be told by their dietitian that they need to increase their meal plan. Examples of active defiance in response could be restricting their next meal after this discussion or continuing to eat their previous meal plan rather than the revised meal plan created by their dietitian.

Adolescent Dialectical Dilemmas

The adolescent dialectical dilemmas are a set of dialectical dilemmas that apply specifically to the parents and guardians of adolescent patients and that can also apply to the adolescents themselves and even their treating providers (Miller, Rathus, & Linehan, 2007). It is also worth mentioning that when working with patients diagnosed with eating disorders specifically, patients who are chronologically young adults will often present as younger than their age. As such, we have found that these adolescent dialectical dilemmas are often relevant in the treatment of young adult patients as well.

Excessive Leniency vs. Authoritarian Control. The first of the adolescent dialectical dilemmas is excessive leniency versus authoritarian control. Excessive leniency refers to parents or guardians allowing for an inappropriate degree of self-directedness on the part of their adolescent child. This can manifest in a number of ways, including lacking appropriate rules in the household or refusing to hold the adolescent accountable around violations of existing rules, making too few developmentally-appropriate demands of their adolescent child, or giving into inappropriate demands made by their adolescent child. There are a number of ways in which excessive leniency manifests when it comes to eating disorders, including allowing the adolescent child to have inappropriate control over food choices (e.g. allowing the child to purchase fat free or diet products), allowing the adolescent child to engage in more physical activity than their treatment team has approved, or not holding the adolescent accountable to developmentally-appropriate tasks (e.g. household chores) out of fears that conflicts over these tasks could result in a return to eating disorder behaviors.

The other side of this dialectic is authoritarian control, which refers to placing extreme limits on freedom and autonomy. Authoritarian control can include setting extremely strict rules around social activities, curfews, schoolwork, and so forth, in addition to applying unnecessarily harsh punishments for violations of rules. When working with patients with eating disorders, the ways in which this side of the dialectic manifests are a bit more subtle and often well-intentioned. I (AHK) have worked with parents who were so blindsided and frightened by their adolescent's eating disorder that even once their child was on a solid path toward recovery, they were still reluctant to return freedoms that were reasonable and appropriate. For example, I have worked with parents who were initially unwilling to let their adolescent child go over to a friend's house for dinner, even though they would be appropriately supervised by adults who understood their eating disorder diagnosis and even though their child had a sustained period of abstinence from eating disorder behaviors.

The treatment targets for this dialectic are working toward increased authoritative discipline for parents who fall into either dialectical extreme and increasing adolescent self-determination for parents who fall on the authoritarian control side of the dialectic. What this looks like is ensuring there is appropriate and clear structure and rules within the home; that the rules have clearly delineated if-then consequences, both for compliance with the rules and for situations in which the rules are not followed; that the use of reinforcement is emphasized and the use of punishment and coercion are minimized; and that rules are balanced out with love, support, and opportunities for the adolescent to be heard. I (AHK) have found that for many adolescents transitioning from higher levels of care back into the home setting, it can be helpful to have a family therapy session where the proposed structure and rules of the home are discussed and the adolescent has an opportunity to provide input, although with all ultimate decision-making lying with the parent(s)/guardian(s) of the adolescent. Examples of relevant rules and structure that I have seen parent(s)/guardian(s) decide to put in place include expectations for meals and snacks (e.g. eating meals and snacks at set times with the family at the table and consisting of the same foods all family members are being served), participation in treatment (e.g. attending all scheduled sessions with providers, staying within a weight range), engagement in competitive sports (e.g. participation being contingent upon meal and snack completion), as well rules and structure for themes common across all adolescents (e.g. rules and structure around social media use). Having this conversation in the context of a family therapy session often helps parents and guardians to effectively navigate finding a balance between dialectical extremes.

Normalizing Pathological Behaviors vs. Pathologizing Normative Behaviors. The second of the adolescent dialectical dilemmas is normalizing pathological behaviors versus pathologizing normative behaviors. Normalizing pathological behaviors refers to parents and guardians failing to identify and/ or address behaviors that their adolescent child is engaging in that are extreme manifestations of normative adolescent behaviors that put their adolescent child's life and/or well-being at risk. There are a number of behaviors not directly related to eating disorders that fall in this category, including driving while intoxicated, engaging in unprotected sex, or initiating repeated physical altercations with peers. There are also certain behaviors specific to eating disorders that parents and guardians may have normalized prior to their adolescent child initiating treatment or that they may continue to normalize even after treatment has begun. Diet culture is pervasive throughout our culture and as a result, pathological behaviors associated with diet culture are oftentimes normalized or even rewarded. For example, I (AHK) have worked with adolescent patients whose parents initially complimented them on weight loss or new exercise habits, completely unaware that these were early indicators that their child had developed an eating disorder. I have also worked with parents of adolescent patients who have experienced difficulty letting go of the "good food"/"bad food" dichotomy who have wanted their adolescent child to be able to continue to avoid certain foods or food groups that they consider to be "bad foods." While there are certain individuals who can go through their lives avoiding certain foods or food groups and not develop an eating disorder, once someone has developed an eating disorder that has included avoidance of certain foods and food groups, returning to this approach is no longer a normative way to meet one's nutritional needs.

The other side of this dialectic is pathologizing normative behaviors. Behaviors like experimentation with substance use or sexuality, interpersonal conflicts with peers, identity exploration, and so forth are all normative adolescent behaviors. However, for many parents of adolescent children, there may be an intense desire to prevent these behaviors from occurring, even if doing so comes at a high cost to their adolescent child. For example, for an adolescent who has a distant history of significant bingeing and purging behaviors, a parent might find they are pathologizing the adolescent's choice to get "seconds" during a holiday meal out of fear that this was an indication they were returning to bingeing and purging behaviors.

The treatment targets for this dialectic are helping parents and guardians to accurately delineate which behaviors are normative adolescent behaviors and which behaviors are pathological adolescent behaviors. Psychoeducation about typical adolescent development can be helpful here, as well as supporting parents and guardians in developing their ability to access "wise mind" in discerning where a given behavior may fall. Some parents and guardians may benefit from discussion around the types of factors to consider in making such a determination, like whether the behavior was risky (and how much so), impulsive versus thoughtful, and/or related to the patient's individual treatment targets in some way. Determining whether a behavior is normative or pathological in the context of an adolescent struggling with an eating disorder can be incredibly tricky, given both the nature of the illness and the pervasiveness of diet culture messages throughout our society. For example, a parent might wonder if their adolescent who has a compulsive exercise history going on a slightly longer walk than usual is normative or an indication they may be moving in the direction of a slip or relapse. Alternatively, a parent who struggles with their own diet culture mentality may struggle to understand why it is not normative for their adolescent child to insist that they never be made to eat fast food. It is often hard enough for parents and guardians of adolescents to find their "wise mind" about what is normative versus not without a history of an eating disorder to be factored in as well, so parents and guardians of adolescent patients diagnosed with an eating disorder may need ongoing help in exploring this particular area.

Fostering Dependence vs. Forcing Autonomy. The final adolescent dialectical dilemma is fostering dependence versus forcing autonomy. Fostering dependence refers to behaviors on the part of parents or guardians that prevent their adolescent child from progressing towards increased autonomy in a gradual and developmentally-appropriate fashion. It is typical for adolescents to have increased ownership around completion of schoolwork and household chores and management of their time and money as they age. When parents and guardians are overly involved in these tasks, the adolescent child misses the opportunity to develop the skills needed to complete these tasks independently. Fostering dependence can also manifest in eating disorder specific ways. Thinking about the progression of an adolescent patient through treatment from a FBT-based lens, once a patient has weight restored, if this is a necessary treatment target, and has successfully remained abstinent from use of eating disorder behaviors, the next step in treatment involves a gradual return of control and choice around food to the adolescent. Parents and guardians who fall toward the fostering dependence side of this dialectic may struggle with allowing for this next step in treatment. Another way in which fostering dependence manifests in eating disorders treatment pertains to situations in which an adolescent patient may have fears around maturation. One common pattern of interaction I (AHK) have observed in these situations is the adolescent patient engaging in physical and emotional "clinginess" with one or both parents or guardians and the patient's parents or guardians responding through excessive caretaking in return. These patterns of interaction can be challenging to disrupt, in that the experience of these interactions is often reinforcing for both the adolescent patient and their parents or guardians and it can be hard for patients and their parents or guardians to imagine negative consequences associated with this pattern of interactions.

The other side of this dialectic is forcing autonomy, which refers to parents or guardians removing their support of their adolescent child and expecting a developmentally inappropriate degree of autonomy and self-sufficiency. Forcing autonomy can manifest in a number of different ways, including expecting the adolescent to assume adult responsibilities around the house, like parenting younger siblings or holding primary responsibility for all household chores, or expecting the adolescent to have greater personal and financial independence, like being solely responsible for taking care of their medical needs or paying for the majority of items needed for basic functioning. Forcing autonomy can also manifest in unique ways when working with adolescent patients diagnosed with an eating disorder. Parents or guardians may hold unreasonable expectations of an adolescent who is early in the treatment and recovery process to prepare and consume meals independently, while also refraining from engaging in eating disorder behaviors with little to no supervision. Even further toward this end of the dialectic, parents or guardians might even task the adolescent child with planning meals for the week and purchasing groceries on behalf of the family. Parents and guardians often struggle with recognizing that their adolescent child's eating disorder has altered the trajectory of expected autonomy given their chronological age and adjusting the expectations they hold of their adolescent child accordingly.

The treatment targets for this dialectic are striking a balance between promoting appropriate individuation while also encouraging reliance on others when appropriate. Promoting individuation involves parents and supports gradually moving from doing tasks on behalf of their adolescent to coaching their adolescent in doing these tasks to eventually expecting their adolescent to assume full ownership of these tasks. For example, for an adolescent who is early in recovery and about to head off to college, it is likely important that this adolescent begins to take ownership of tasks related to their recovery that they will need to be able to complete independently while at college, like planning meals and grocery shopping for these meals. Rather than expecting that their child will be able to do these tasks without any guidance, the parent and adolescent could begin to share in meal planning and grocery shopping each week, with the parent allowing the adolescent to do as much as they are able to independently, while also providing coaching around pieces they are still learning. On the other side of the dialectic, it is important for the parents of the adolescent to remain sufficiently engaged in their life to support them in their recovery process. Using the same example of a patient early in recovery who is headed off to college, it would likely still be beneficial for the patient to have releases of information in place so that their parents can communicate with their providers and that the patient's parents are regularly checking-in with them about how they are doing with their recovery as they transition to college.

The DBT-C Treatment Target Hierarchy

We have both worked in an eating disorder healthcare system that has treated patients who are as young as eight years of age and diagnosed with an eating disorder, and patients as young as five years of age have been diagnosed and treated for Anorexia Nervosa in other hospitals and healthcare systems. For those of you who have worked with children, adolescents, and adults, you have experienced how vastly different effective treatment can be for individuals who fall within these age groups. DBT-C is a treatment that was developed for pre-adolescent children, ranging in age from 6 to 13, who experience significant behavioral and emotional difficulties. Of note, DBT-C has not been utilized in clinical trials to determine its effectiveness in the treatment of eating disorders, however there are elements of DBT-C that make sense in the treatment of eating disorders in younger patients.

While many of the elements of standard DBT remain in DBT-C, there are some notable areas where modifications have been made, the DBT Target Hierarchy being one of those areas. The DBT-C target hierarchy if as follows (Perepletchikova, 2020):

Level One Targets: Decrease Risk of Psychopathology in the Future

1. Life-threatening behaviors of the child
2. Treatment-destroying behaviors of the child

3. Treatment-interfering behaviors of parents
4. Parental emotion regulation
5. Effective parenting techniques

Level Two Target Behaviors: Target Parent-Child Relationship

1. Improve parent-child relationship

Level Three Target Behaviors: Target Child's Presenting Problems

1. Risky, unsafe and aggressive behaviors
2. Quality-of-life interfering problems
3. Skills training
4. Treatment-interfering behaviors of the child

Secondary Targets: Three Core Senses DBT-C Aims to Help Parents Instill in Their Child

1. Sense of self-love
2. Sense of safety
3. Sense of belonging

   Take a minute to compare the target hierarchy above to the standard DBT treatment target hierarchy. One of the things you probably noticed is that there is a considerable amount of focus on the behaviors of the patient's parents, rather than the patient themselves. DBT-C operates under the assumption that behaviors of the patient's parents are key to achieving lasting changes in the patient's emotional and behavioral regulation, going as far as to say that the patient's behavior is irrelevant until their environment has the capacity to consistently and effectively promote progress. This means that the patient's parents must be committed to treatment, engaged in the treatment process, willing to follow through on agreed upon plans, and resolving their own skills deficits through acquiring and practicing new skills. In contrast, while the child's full involvement in treatment is certainly desirable, it is not necessary for treatment to be effective.

   Interestingly, this perspective is not entirely incompatible with how parents and guardians are viewed in the context of eating disorder treatment for adolescents and even young adults. Family-Based Therapy (FBT) is one of the most empirically-supported treatments for Anorexia Nervosa in child and adolescent populations, with emerging evidence that it is effective for children and adolescents with Bulimia Nervosa and young adults with Anorexia Nervosa as well. When taking an FBT-based approach, the patients' parents or guardians assume responsibility for the refeeding process and establish appropriate boundaries and structure, with the goal of eliminating the option for the patient to continue to engage in eating disorder behaviors. As we discussed earlier in this book, one of the challenges in working with patients diagnosed with an eating disorder is that there is often significant ambivalence and in some cases a nearly complete absence of willingness to work on abstinence from eating disorder behaviors. Rarely have we worked with a child or adolescent patient at a higher level of care who was entering into treatment on their own volition. Almost always they have felt as though they were forced into treatment by their parents or guardians after their eating disorder came to light and their stated main motivating factors for completing treatment are things like, "I want to go home" or "I want to go back to school." With this as the context in which a patient is entering into treatment (e.g. the patient's parents want them to get help; the patient has minimal to no internal motivation for treatment or recovery), the patient's parents or guardians become critical agents of change, particularly early on in the treatment process. This does not mean that simultaneous work is not being done with a focus on helping the patient to develop internal motivation to refrain from eating disorder behaviors in the pursuit of recovery and a life worth living, however parental empowerment and unity are critical forces in helping the patient to initiate change and sustain the changes made over the course of time.

The other major change you may have noted in the DBT-C treatment target hierarchy is the addition of three new secondary targets. The sense of self-love refers to loving oneself as one is, without any caveats or conditions. The sense of safety refers to the ability to accurately assess dangers in one's environment and to have confidence in one's ability to effectively navigate situations as they arise. Finally, the sense of belonging is the feeling of being wanted and being accepted as part of a group. The goal with regard to these secondary targets is to work with parents to instill these three core senses within their child.

Discipline-Specific DBT Treatment Target Hierarchies – An Alternative Approach

While we have taken the approach of suggesting the use of a single DBT treatment target hierarchy shared among multidisciplinary team members, it is worth noting that other scholars in the field have proposed the use of discipline-specific DBT treatment target hierarchies. As an example, the following DBT treatment target hierarchy was created specifically for use by pharmacotherapy providers (Witterholt, 2020):

1. Decrease behaviors likely to destroy treatment.
2. Decrease specific symptoms known to be effectively managed by medication.
3. Increase self-management of health-related behaviors.
4. Decrease pharmacotherapy-interfering behaviors.

There is no literature to date that provides guidance as to whether the use of a multidisciplinary DBT treatment target hierarchy is preferred over a discipline-specific DBT treatment target hierarchy, although each likely have their own distinct benefits. While a multidisciplinary DBT treatment target hierarchy encourages multidisciplinary collaboration and case conceptualization, discipline-specific DBT treatment target hierarchies provide clearer guidance as to targets within a specific discipline's scope of practice. These may be factors to take into account when considering which approach might work best within your practice setting.

Bringing DBT to Life – Megan's DBT Treatment Target Hierarchy

We'd like to revisit our patient Megan, who has now been in treatment at a residential level of care for a little over a month. Since you first learned about Megan, she has made progress with regard to decreasing restriction and purging behaviors and she has begun to restore weight. However, she has returned to engaging in self-injurious behaviors on a somewhat regular basis via scratching through use of her fingernails, as well as other objects she is able to obtain by disassembling items on the unit. Other patients are finding Megan's self-injurious behaviors to be "triggering" and she has had difficulty cultivating meaningful relationships with other patients on the unit. Although she is going on passes occasionally, she is underreporting eating disorder symptoms when she is on pass from the facility, which include restricting food, throwing food out, hiding food, and occasionally engaging in purging behaviors. She has been refusing her prescribed antipsychotic on occasion, as she is fearful that taking her medication as prescribed will result in additional weight gain. There is also some lack of alignment occurring among providers on Megan's treatment team. Megan's therapist has been relying heavily on validation during her sessions with Megan and has been avoiding discussing Megan's self-injurious behaviors. Megan's psychiatric provider is frustrated with both Megan, due to her medication noncompliance and fluctuating progress in treatment, as well as Megan's therapist for "not being focused in sessions." He has started to use judgmental language about Megan during treatment team meetings and when he speaks, Megan's therapist becomes quiet and assumes a defensive body posture. Megan's therapist is newer to eating disorders work and feels insecure about her abilities as a provider, yet has been unwilling to display vulnerability and solicit input from the team, in part because of her interactions with Megan's psychiatric provider. Let's take a peek at what Megan's DBT treatment target hierarchy might look like at this point in treatment.

Level 1 Target Behaviors:

- Life-Threatening Behavior:
  - Suicidal ideation of an average intensity of a one on a five-point scale
  - Holding suicide-related beliefs, including thinking that suicide would be a way to escape her hopeless and intolerable life
  - Scratching via fingernails and other relatively blunt implements found on the unit, resulting in skin irritation and occasional skin breakage

Level 2 Target Behaviors:

- Patient Treatment-Interfering Behavior:
  - Not being forthcoming about eating disorder behaviors on passes, including underreporting restricting food, throwing food out, hiding food, and occasionally engaging in purging behaviors
  - Filling out meal logs in a way that leaves out the behaviors mentioned above
  - Not following meal plan
  - Responding to questions in a way that feels rehearsed rather that genuine
  - Intermittent medication noncompliance with prescribed antipsychotic
  - Occasional therapy homework noncompliance
  - Engaging in behaviors that "trigger" other patients, including self-harm that occurs in areas visible to other patients
  - Intermittent lack of collaboration around working toward weight restoration
  - Disassembling items on the unit to create objects that are used for self-injurious behavior
- Patient Treatment-Enhancing Behavior:
  - Likable personality (e.g. good sense of humor)
  - Perfectionism that can be channeled in adaptive ways
  - Attention to detail that can be channeled in adaptive ways
  - Knowledge of DBT skills
  - Expresses appreciation for her treatment team, even when she is frustrated
- Family Treatment-Interfering Behaviors:
  - Parents refusing to participate in family programming and family therapy (specifically, parents have indicated that they've been involved in Megan's treatment before and it "wasn't helpful," so they have refused to participate to date)
  - High expressed criticism toward Megan, including communicating to Megan that they feel with all the treatment she's had that she "should be better by now" and implying that she is using her eating disorder to avoid adult life

- Provider Treatment-Interfering Behavior:
  - Not doing DBT (e.g. Megan's therapist is not targeting Level 1 behaviors consistently in session when they have occurred)
  - Provider focused on change to the point of invalidation (e.g. Megan's psychiatric provider not recognizing progress she has made with eating disorder behaviors and weight restoration, and instead solely focusing on progress still to be made with eating disorder behaviors and return of self-injurious behaviors)
  - Provider focused on acceptance to the point a patient is not learning new behavior patterns (e.g. Megan's therapist focusing on validation above all other therapeutic strategies in session)
  - Provider avoidance of challenging therapeutic tasks (e.g. Megan's therapist avoiding discussing self-injurious behavior in session)
  - Provider referring to patient using judgmental terms (e.g. Megan's psychiatric provider using judgmental terms to describe her during treatment team meetings)
  - Insecurity about one's skills as a provider (e.g. Megan's therapist does indeed have skills deficits that could be addressed through training and supervision, however she has been unwilling to discuss these skills deficits thus far)
- Team-Interfering Behavior:
  - Defensiveness (e.g. Megan's therapist has assumed a defensive body posture and attitude when Megan's psychiatric provider is speaking)
  - Speaking in an overly critical manner toward other team members (e.g. Megan's psychiatric provider has publicly criticized Megan's therapist for not being "targeted enough" in her sessions with Megan)
  - Not balancing acceptance and change (e.g. Megan's therapist and psychiatric provider appear to be at opposite ends of the dialectic of acceptance versus change)

Level 3 Target Behaviors:

- Eating Disorder Behaviors:
  - Restricting (occurring intermittently and primarily on passes)
  - Purging via vomiting (occurring intermittently and solely on passes)
  - Hiding food (occurring intermittently and solely on passes)
  - Throwing out food (occurring intermittently and solely on passes)
  - Avoidance of fear foods
  - Fear of weight gain
  - Body checking
- Co-occurring Mental Health Symptoms:
  - History of alcohol dependence (not a current target, but being monitored by patient's treatment team, given history of alcohol use as symptoms of eating disorder improve)

- Symptoms of depression, including depressed mood, anhedonia, cognitive impairment, feelings of worthlessness, suicidal ideation, and hopeless
    - Symptoms of posttraumatic stress disorder (not a current target, but being monitored by patient's treatment team, given patient's report that eating disorder behaviors may have "numbed out" her trauma-related symptoms)
- Serious Dysfunctional Interpersonal Behaviors:
    - Significant conflict with parents
    - Making others feel uncomfortable to the extent that cultivating friendships is difficult, including engaging in self-injurious behavior openly and engaging with peers in an awkward way during interpersonal interactions
- Employment-Related Dysfunctional Behaviors:
    - History of sporadic employment (being targeted by patient's case manager, even though not immediately relevant)
- Maladaptive Overcontrol Behavior:
    - Aloof and distant relationship behaviors, including only maintaining a small circle of friends outside of treatment and maintaining belief that other patients "don't understand" her

Level 4 Target Behaviors:

- Increasing Behavioral Skills:
    - Although Megan has intellectual knowledge of DBT and RO DBT skills, she is not always able to translate this knowledge into practical application in her day-to-day life and thus would benefit from a continued support in the context of DBT skills groups around how to put what she is learning into practice

In reviewing Megan's DBT treatment target hierarchy, you likely noticed that many of Megan's treatment targets are fair game for all of her providers to varying degrees. Let's take a look at "not following meal plan" as a target, for example. Megan's therapist is likely to target this extensively by examining emotions, thoughts, events, and bodily sensations that are hypothesized to be related to Megan's difficulty in following her meal plan and targeting these through various therapeutic interventions. Megan's psychiatric provider is likely to explore similar territory, however in addition to therapeutic interventions, her psychiatric provider may look at medication-based interventions as well. Megan's dietitian would also be heavily involved in addressing this therapeutic target, however is likely to focus less on emotion-related content and more on content specifically related "to the plate" and addressed through dietetically-focused therapeutic interventions. Megan's medical provider would be focused on monitoring and addressing medical ramifications associated with not following her meal plan. All team members, including frontline staff, may target Megan's meal plan noncompliance through meal coaching. Even Megan's case manager may have work related to Megan's meal plan noncompliance if the noncompliance is related to something within her scope, like financial barriers that are getting in the way of Megan meeting her nutritional needs while on pass. Other targets are addressed primarily by specific disciplines. For example, while it is important that all members of Megan's treatment team are aware of her self-injurious behaviors, these behaviors will be addressed primarily by Megan's therapist and psychiatric provider. However, other disciplines are still responsible for communicating information they learn about these behaviors with members of the treatment team and certainly for intervening, either directly or by seeking help from other treatment team members, if Megan is at imminent risk of self-harm. As you begin to explore the use of DBT treatment target hierarchies within your work, give consideration as to which targets and methods of intervention are within your scope of practice.

Provider Exercise – Constructing a DBT Treatment Target Hierarchy

Think of a patient with whom you currently work for whom you think creating a DBT treatment target hierarchy would be helpful. This exercise tends to be most useful to complete for patients who have a complicated clinical picture (e.g. multiple comorbidities, challenging dynamics with their families or supports). Review each target listed below and place an "X" in the box next to any targets that are relevant for your specific patient. If your patient does not have any targets in any of the levels listed, place an "X" next to the last box in the category (e.g. "I have no patient or provider Level 1 target behaviors."). Of note, if you work with a specific comorbidity regularly in the context of your work with patients diagnosed with eating disorders, the below DBT treatment target hierarchy can be modified to include a greater degree of granularity with regard to target behaviors associated with that comorbid diagnosis. For example, substance use disorders commonly co-occur with eating disorders, so you may want to add more specific targets related to those diagnoses, if you see this commonly in your practice (e.g. showing up to session intoxicated or hungover, maintaining drug dealer contact information, driving while intoxicated). As you are completing this exercise, you may also want to make note of which targets are within your scope of practice and which targets should be addressed by another member of your multidisciplinary team.

Level 1 Target Behaviors:

☐ Life-Threatening Behavior:
  • Eating disordered behaviors that put patient at imminent risk of death, as determined and defined by a medical provider (e.g. significantly low heart rate, electrolyte abnormalities)

- Suicide-related behaviors, thoughts, and urges
- Self-injurious behaviors and urges
- Other: _____

☐ Parent/Caregiver/Partner/Family/Support Life-Threatening or Treatment-Destroying Behavior:
  - Physical, emotional, and/or sexual abuse
  - Neglect
  - Behaviors that actively and intentionally directly contradict multidisciplinary team recommendations, such that patient progress in treatment is near impossible
  - Other: _____

☐ Milieu- or Treatment-Destroying Behavior:
  - Violence or aggression toward other patients
  - Bullying of other patients
  - Unwanted sexual behaviors toward/with other patients
  - Other: _____

☐ Provider Unethical, Severely Irresponsible, or Treatment-Destroying Behavior:
  - Sexual behaviors toward/with patients
  - Utilizing iatrogenic/harmful treatment approaches
  - Extreme interpersonal discord among staff
  - Creating false documentation (e.g. documenting sessions that did not occur, making inaccurate statements about what did/did not occur during a service)
  - Violations of license specific ethics codes, state or federal laws, and/or critical policies and procedures
  - Other: _____

☐ I have no patient, family/support, or provider Level 1 target behaviors

Level 2 Target Behaviors:

☐ Patient Treatment-Interfering Behavior (Including Milieu-Interfering Behavior When Providing Treatment at Higher Levels of Care):
  - Nonattentive behaviors
  - Noncollaborative behaviors
  - Noncompliant behaviors
  - Behaviors that interfere with other patients
  - Behaviors that burn out providers
  - Behaviors that push organization or company limits (when working in a setting other than an individual private practice)
  - Behaviors that decrease the provider's motivation
  - Other: _____

☐ Patient Treatment-Enhancing Behaviors:
- Making progress toward clinical goals
- Completing assigned therapeutic homework
- Participating actively in sessions
- Other: _____

☐ Family/Caregiver/Support Treatment-Interfering Behaviors:
- Arriving late or missing sessions
- Not bringing food to a family meal when asked
- High expressed criticism toward the patient in session
- Not following through with medical recommendations
- Reinforcing ineffective behaviors
- Not providing adequate supervision of meals, snacks, and physical activity when clinically indicated
- Significant interpersonal conflict and/or communication difficulties between family members
- Frequent invalidation of the patient
- Other: _____

☐ Alliance-Ruptures
- Provider Treatment-Interfering Behavior:
- Non-adherent behaviors
- Behaviors creating therapeutic imbalance
- Behaviors showing lack of respect for the patient
- Personal factors that can impact professional effectiveness
- Other: _____

☐ Team-Interfering Behavior (If You Are Working With a Group of Providers and Team Meetings Are Part of the Work You Do):
- Missing team meetings
- Showing up late to team meetings
- Not communicating about expected or unplanned absences with the team
- Not following through on assigned action items from team meetings
- Refusing to participate in team meetings and/or showing up to team meetings unprepared
- Breaching confidentiality of team
- Not adhering to the DBT Consultation Team Agreements, if relevant
- Doing two things at once and/or engaging in side chatter
- "Fragilizing" team members and/or refusing to address an issue that needs to be targeted
- Defensiveness
- Offering solutions before the target of a discussion is clearly defined
- Speaking in a judgmental and/or overly critical manner toward other team members

- Not balancing acceptance and change
- Other:_____
□ I have no patient, family/support, provider, and/or team-related Level 2 target behaviors

Level 3 Target Behaviors:

□ Quality-of-Life Interfering Behavior:
  □ All eating disordered behaviors and urges that do not meet the threshold for Level 1 or Level 2 Target Behaviors:
  - Restricting
  - Purging by vomiting
  - Purging by use of laxatives
  - Bingeing
  - Diuretic abuse
  - Emetic abuse
  - Enema abuse
  - Compulsive exercise
  - Avoidance of exercise
  - Chewing and spitting
  - Hiding, sneaking, stealing, and/or hoarding food
  - Eating too rapidly
  - Eating too slowly
  - Food rituals
  - Other: _____
  □ All behaviors associated with comorbid physical and mental health conditions that do not meet the threshold for Level 1 or Level 2 Target Behaviors
  - Interpersonal problems
  - Financial difficulties
  - Legal problems
  - Housing difficulties
  - School or employment-related difficulties
  □ Maladaptive overcontrol behaviors:
  - Inhibited emotional expression
  - Overly-cautious and hypervigilant behaviors
  - Rigid and rule-governed behavior
  - Aloof and distant relationship behaviors
  - Envy and bitterness
  □ My patient has no Level 3 target behaviors

Level Four Target Behaviors:

☐ Increasing Behavioral Skills:
   • Mindfulness
   • Interpersonal Effectiveness
   • Emotion Regulation
   • Distress Tolerance
   • Radically Open Skills
   • Self-Management Skills
   • Dietetic Skills (e.g. portioning, meal planning, grocery shopping, food preparation)
   • Medical Skills (e.g. self-administering medication, taking one's vital signs)

Secondary Targets:

• Emotional Vulnerability
• Self-Invalidation
• Active Passivity
• Apparent Competence
• Unrelenting Crises
• Inhibited Grieving
• My patient has no Secondary Targets

Dialectical Dilemmas Unique to Eating Disorders

• Rigid, Overcontrolled Eating
• Absence of an Eating Plan
• Apparent Compliance
• Active Defiance

Adolescent Dialectical Dilemmas (If Relevant):

• Excessive Leniency
• Authoritarian Control
• Normalizing Pathological Behaviors
• Pathologizing Normative Behaviors
• Forcing Autonomy
• Fostering Dependence
• The Adolescent Dialectical Dilemmas are not relevant for my patient

DBT-C Target Hierarchy (If Relevant)

Level One Targets: Decrease Risk of Psychopathology in the Future

- Life-threatening behaviors of the child
- Treatment-destroying behaviors of the child
- Treatment-interfering behaviors of parents
- Parental emotion regulation
- Effective parenting techniques

Level Two Target Behaviors: Target Parent-Child Relationship

- Improve parent-child relationship

Level Three Target Behaviors: Target Child's Presenting Problems

- Risky, unsafe and aggressive behaviors
- Quality-of-life interfering problems
- Skills training
- Treatment-interfering behaviors of the child

Secondary Targets: Three Core Senses DBT-C Aims to Help Parents Instill in Their Child

- Sense of self-love
- Sense of safety
- Sense of belonging

Chapter 13

Constructing and Using a Multidisciplinary DBT Diary Card

Now that you have created your patient's DBT treatment target hierarchy, you might be wondering how this tool can be used in the context of clinical care. One of the ways in which the DBT treatment target hierarchy can be helpful is in the construction of a multidisciplinary DBT diary card. For those of you who are familiar with self-monitoring as a component of cognitive-behavioral therapy, diary cards are a sophisticated form of self-monitoring. They are a tool that you can use with patients that assists them in self-monitoring behaviors, emotions, thoughts, urges, events, and skill use on a day-to-day basis. In most circumstances, the targets that you and your patient choose to track will draw directly from the highest priority targets in the patient's DBT treatment target hierarchy.

There are a number of reasons why diary cards are a key component of DBT. First, there is evidence that shows that simply by tracking behaviors, people tend to make changes in a positive direction, so one purpose diary cards serve is helping to promote behavioral change. Second, diary cards can help providers to quickly and efficiently set a session agenda based on the DBT treatment target hierarchy. We'll show how this can be done in more detail a little bit later, however in short, if your patient is tracking the most relevant targets from their DBT treatment target hierarchy on their diary card, you can quickly see which targets came up since your last appointment and triage them accordingly. Finally, because diary cards provide a wealth of information, they can be used to develop hypotheses about factors that influence our patients' behaviors and assist our patients in increasing their insight.

Now that you have an understanding of the benefits of diary cards, let's talk about how you would go about constructing one with a patient. If you are working within the context of a multidisciplinary team that is utilizing DBT principles and strategies, it is typically the therapist's role to orient the patient to diary cards, construct an initial diary card with the patient, and then circulate the diary card to the rest of the patient's treatment team for feedback around targets to add or modify. If you are working independently or as part of a treatment team that is not interested in using DBT principles and strategies in their work, you become

DOI: 10.4324/9781003495604-13

the individual responsible for orienting the patient to diary cards and guiding them through constructing one.

The first step in incorporating diary cards into your work with a patient is to provide your patient with education about diary cards. This includes orienting your patient in detail to what a diary card is, which may include showing them examples and explaining how diary cards can be beneficial, all in an individualized way that helps to get your patient's buy-in. It is important to note that orientation is not always a one-time event. If you've used diary cards in your work for some time, it can be easy to forget that the first time you saw a diary card, it was probably overwhelming and confusing and took you a bit of time to fully understand. It can be helpful to keep in mind that this is likely the experience of many of your patients as well, particularly if they are younger, malnourished, or have other cognitive or learning impairments. Once you have provided education about diary cards and obtained your client's buy-in around utilizing diary cards, it is important to ask your patient about what they are interested in tracking, with an emphasis on targets that tie into their goals for treatment. After you've gotten your patient's input about what they would like to track, you can then go about sharing your input as well. My (AHK) experience has usually been that my patients and I share a similar perspective about the majority of targets that seem like a high priority to track, although in many circumstances there will be notable omissions. For example, I've worked with patients who were willing to track information about self-injurious behaviors, restricting behaviors, and so forth, however when it came to tracking bingeing or purging behaviors, they were adamantly opposed due to shame they experienced associated with these behaviors. If you find that there are behaviors you would like to track that your patient is reluctant to track, it is important to have an open dialogue where their experience can be validated, while also exploring whether there are ways to problem-solve around barriers.

In order to show you how orienting a patient to a diary card and collaboratively determining what behaviors to track could look, we want to provide two examples of patient dialogue:

Orienting a Patient Who is New to Diary Cards. This example dialogue is between a therapist and a patient (Kara), who is undergoing treatment for the first time for Bulimia Nervosa with no other known comorbidities.

Therapist:	"So I wanted to use some of our session today to talk with you about diary cards. Are these something that you've heard of?"
Kara:	"Nope, they don't sound familiar to me."
Therapist:	"Okay, so a diary card is a tool that you can use to track different behaviors, thoughts, emotions, events, and so forth that come up for you in a week. Any ideas as to why this could be a helpful tool for us to use in our work together?"

Kara:	"I guess so you can see what's happened over the past week?"
Therapist:	"Totally! I know that you mentioned that you are really motivated to stop bingeing and purging, so this will give you and I exactly the type of information we need to work on those targets together. It will also help us figure out what's most important to work on when we meet, particularly if a lot of things have happened during the week. Finally, since I know you are really motivated to work on these behaviors, there's actually research that shows that just by tracking your behaviors, they tend to change in the direction you want them to go!"
Kara:	"Okay, cool."
Therapist:	"So are you willing to spend some time with me today coming up with what we want to track on your diary card?"
Kara:	"Sure."
Therapist:	"Awesome. So based on what you know about diary cards so far, what do you think it could be helpful to track?"
Kara:	"Definitely something to do with purging, and maybe something related to body image distress?"
Therapist:	"I think both of those sound like excellent things to track. Anything else that comes to mind?"
Kara:	"Nothing I can think of at the moment."
Therapist:	"That's totally okay. Your diary card is a living document, so we can always add, remove, or change things as we go along. So based on what I know about you so far, there's one other target I think it could be helpful to track. You didn't mention bingeing and I'm wondering if that's something we could include as well?"
Kara:	(pauses) "...I really don't want to track that."
Therapist:	"Talk to me a bit about that. How come?"
Kara:	"I feel so ashamed about bingeing. It's so gross and out of control. My roommates know that I've purged before because they've heard me, but they don't know that I binge and I don't want them to know that I binge. I'm afraid that I might accidentally leave my diary card out and that they might see it and know all my stuff, you know?"
Therapist:	"Okay, I think I understand where you are coming from and I can understand why it would be hard to put bingeing on there. We can talk about some strategies for helping to keep your diary card confidential a bit later, but I'm wondering...if you and I were able to come up with some other way to label your bingeing that wasn't just 'bingeing,' would you be willing to track it then?"
Kara:	"If we could figure something out that they weren't likely to guess means bingeing, then yes, I'd be willing to track it."

Therapist: "Excellent, thank you. So now let's figure out the specifics of how to track each of the things we talked about."

At this point in the process, the therapist and patient would figure out collaboratively how to track each of these targets. If I (AHK) was the therapist working with Kara, some specific suggestions I might make to track the targets she brought up include, "Purged? (Y/N)," "Urges to Purge (0–10)," and "Body Image Distress (0–10)." For bingeing specifically, I might suggest "BE (Y/N)" and "Urges (0–10)" as a starting point for Kara, although I would likely let her take the lead on the labels she wants to use at this point. Because shame around tracking bingeing behaviors is actually unjustified shame, I would also have the eventual goal of having her be able to track her bingeing behaviors and urges using an accurate rather than coded label, however early in treatment I would want to focus more on rapport building and being flexible, meeting Kara where she is at. Now let's take a look at how orientation dialogue might look for a patient who has been through treatment before by looking at a snippet of dialogue with Megan.

Reorienting a Patient Who Has Completed Diary Cards Previously. Orientation to diary cards is important not only for patients who are new to DBT, but also for patients who report having a course of DBT treatment previously and who are returning to treatment. Below is an example dialogue between a therapist and a patient (Jose), who has completed a couple of courses of DBT-informed treatment previously. Jose is diagnosed with Anorexia Nervosa – Binge/Purge Type and also struggles with self-injurious behavior in the form of scratching.

Therapist: "So I wanted to spend some of our session today talking about diary cards. I know you've done some DBT before. Are diary cards something that is familiar to you?"

Jose: "Yeah, I've completed diary cards before."

Therapist: "Awesome! Just to make sure we're on the same page, what's your understanding of why we would want you to complete diary cards as part of our program?"

Jose: "I mean, I know they are supposed to be used to track my behaviors, but I really didn't find them to be useful before."

Therapist: "Oh? How come?"

Jose: "Well, my last therapist didn't really look at them often, so I just kind of stopped doing them after a while, since I didn't really see the point."

Therapist: "I see. I can understand why you might not have found diary cards to be helpful. Can I share a bit about how we use diary cards in our program?"

Jose: "Sure."

Therapist: "So we view diary cards as an integral part of our program for a number of reasons. One of the reasons is that there is scientific evidence that shows that just by tracking your behaviors on a diary card, you are likely to start making changes to your behaviors in a way that is consistent with your goals for treatment. Also, even though we're just getting to know each other, I can tell you have a lot going on! Diary cards are a way for you and I to get a quick snapshot of your past week so we can figure out what's most important to talk about when we meet. You can expect that not only will I ask to see your diary card at the beginning of each time we meet, you can expect that your dietitian, psychiatric provider, and medical provider will be asking to see it as part of their meetings with you as well. I'm curious if this changes your perspective on diary cards at all?"

Jose: "I'm definitely willing to give them a shot for now."

Therapist: "Excellent. Can you and I plan to chat if you find yourself thinking that you're not finding them to be useful at any point in the future? I definitely want to make sure we talk if you're finding that to be the case."

Jose: "Sure, I'll let you know."

Therapist: "Great. So let's talk about what we might want to track on your diary card. Do you have any thoughts about things you've tracked previously that we would want to track on your diary card now?"

Jose: "I definitely remember tracking restricting and urges to restrict, and I think I might have tracked purging, too? Also, I think we tracked something related to staying safe."

Therapist: "I think tracking restricting, purging, and self-injurious behaviors and urges all make sense. Anything else you can think of that might be useful to track?"

Jose: "Maybe something about body image? I can't stand my body right now."

Therapist: "I think tracking body image distress makes a lot of sense. Anything else?"

Jose: "Nothing I can think of."

Therapist: "I noticed you didn't mention tracking anything about tracking body movement..."

Jose: "...well, that's because I don't think how much I exercise has anything to do with my eating disorder. It's totally normal and healthy to work out regularly."

Therapist: "If I remember correctly from our first meeting together, you said you are working out about two hours per day?"

Jose: "Yep. And that seems normal to me."

Therapist: "I'm hearing that you don't feel like your exercise has anything to do with your eating disorder. I think a spot where you and I might find some agreement is that physical movement is an important part of a life worth living for most people. I also know that many people with whom I've worked before have discovered over time that while some of their physical movement is simply about enjoyment, other times their physical movement ties into their disorder in ways they might not have thought of before. I wonder if you might be willing to track your physical activity, even if it's not something we decide to target at the moment?"

Jose: "I mean, I guess so?"

Therapist: "Okay. I really appreciate your willingness."

There are a couple of things to note about this dialogue between Jose and his therapist that highlight the importance of orientation to diary cards and collaboration around constructing diary cards for patients who have completed a course of DBT or DBT-informed treatment previously. First, it is not uncommon to find that patients who have been through DBT or DBT-informed treatment may not have been properly oriented to diary cards or even if oriented properly, that diary cards have not been effectively incorporated into treatment. As such, even for a patient who has been through a course of DBT or DBT-informed treatment previously, it is important to make sure that there is both understanding of and buy-in to completing diary cards as part of treatment. Second, although patients who have used diary cards before are more likely to be able to list reasonable treatment targets, it is still important that as a provider you are sharing your input about diary card targets as well. In the example above, had the therapist not been aware of Jose's DBT treatment target hierarchy, they may have omitted tracking physical activity on Jose's diary card. Given the likelihood that Jose's physical activity ties into other treatment targets, this omission could interfere with case conceptualization, treatment planning, and treatment interventions.

Once you've agreed upon targets for the diary card, you and your patient must then work to translate those targets into quantifiable or recordable data. Most targets lend themselves well to simple yes/no responses, Likert scale responses, number of times or number of minutes a behavior occurred, or fill-in-the-blank responses. For example, compulsive exercise-related targets could be measured as a yes/no question (e.g. "Engaged in compulsive exercise? (Y/N)"), as a Likert scale response (e.g. "Urges to engage in compulsive exercise? (0–5)"), or a specific amount (e.g. "Number of minutes engaged in exercise"). An example of a fill-in-the blank response would be having a patient record specific fear foods they had throughout the week. In creating a diary card with your patient, you'll find that some targets will be relevant across disciplines, whereas others will be discipline specific. When working with a patient diagnosed with an eating disorder, all eating disorder behaviors will have relevance to each provider on a patient's treatment team, although how each provider chooses to address eating disorder behaviors will be different. There are other behaviors that will have relevance to only certain disciplines. For example, self-injurious behavior is a critical target for a psychotherapist and psychiatric provider to address, however would not be an appropriate behavior for a dietitian to target. Because diary cards can be useful across disciplines, it is important once you have created a diary card with your patient to share this diary card with the other members of the patient's treatment team for feedback. Let's take a look at how this discussion might go:

Therapist:	"Here's a first pass at a diary card that Kara and I came up with in session. What do y'all think?"
Dietitian:	"I'm so glad she was willing to track binge behaviors and urges to binge. I wasn't sure she was going to be willing to do that, since she endorses so much shame about those behaviors. Overall I think it looks good, and I was wondering if we could add a column that says "Saved Up Calories (Y/N)?" Kara reported to me that sometimes she will restrict less preferred foods as a way to "counteract" calories of a strongly preferred food that she eats later."
Therapist:	"That totally makes sense. I'll talk with Kara about adding that. Marcie, how about you? Anything you're noticing?"
Psychiatric Provider:	"I don't know if she mentioned this to y'all when you did your assessments, but she has a history of abruptly discontinuing her mood stabilizers, so I think it could be helpful to have her track medication compliance. Can we add that somehow?"
Therapist:	"She didn't mention that to me at all. I'm glad you caught that! Yes, I'll absolutely add that in! Anyone else have feedback?"
Medical Provider:	"Looks fine to me."
Nurse Manager:	"Nothing on my end."
Case Manager:	"I don't think we need to add this in at this point, since it's early in treatment, but Kara did mention to me that she wants to start taking steps to get a different job. Maybe we could add that in when she transitions to IOP?"
Therapist:	"That sounds great, Sam. Thanks for putting that on the radar, even if it is a little ways out."

Once a diary card has been constructed, there are two other important steps in orienting a patient to a diary card. First, it can be useful to have the patient complete diary card information for the day prior during your session with them. The primary rationale for doing this is that often patients will verbalize understanding how to complete a diary card, however upon actually doing so they find that they have additional questions. Finally, once a patient has had an opportunity to complete a day's worth of their diary card, it is important to troubleshoot any barriers to completion that they anticipate arising. Common barriers to diary card completion include lack of comprehension of the rationale for diary cards, not understanding how to complete the diary card, lack of adequate cues to remind the patient to complete the diary card, difficulties with motivation and/or emotional reactions to completing the diary card, challenges with time management around creating time to complete the diary card, and concerns about diary card confidentiality.

There are a few other important points to make about constructing diary cards. First, when it comes to diary cards, function is more important than form. There are dozens of variations on diary card formats, so it's more important to find or create one that works for your patient, while also capturing what you need in terms of data about key targets. Second, be sure to adapt your diary card format and degree of complexity to take into account things like your patient's age, nourishment status, cognitive capacity, and so forth. Feeling too overwhelmed to complete a complex diary card is one of the most common barriers to diary card compliance we have encountered, so it's important to make sure what you are asking your patient to do feels reasonable and achievable to them. Third, it is important to remember that diary cards can track not only behaviors to decrease, but behaviors to increase as well. For patients who find being praised for engaging in adaptive behaviors to be reinforcing, this can be a particularly useful strategy. Finally, it is important to note that multidisciplinary team members play an important role not only in the construction of the diary card, but also in reinforcing it's usage and completion through incorporating it into individual provider appointments or in the case of frontline staff members, providing reminders and encouragement to assist with diary card compliance.

Using Diary Cards to Assist in Creating a Session Agenda. Before we take a peek at a couple of Megan's diary cards from various points in her treatment, we'd like to talk briefly about using a diary card to create a session agenda. If you are using a diary card with your patient, it is strongly recommended that you begin your session by asking your patient for their diary card and reviewing it together in a collaborative fashion. As part of reviewing the diary card together, it can be helpful to both celebrate patient successes (e.g. "It looks like you were able to complete the ice cream exposure we had planned this week! Awesome work!"), as well as validate patient struggles (e.g. "It looks like Saturday was a really challenging day for you. I definitely want to hear more about what happened during our session today."). Once you've reviewed the patient's diary card, you'll want to set a session agenda based on the information you reviewed. The agenda you set should be guided by the DBT treatment target hierarchy, with life-threatening behaviors being targeted first, treatment-interfering behaviors being targeted second, and quality-of-life interfering behaviors being targeted last. For therapy sessions, I (AHK) aim to cover no more than two to three targets per session, although what you are able to cover in a given session may vary by discipline. Your patient's input should be considered when creating a session agenda, although not to the extent that it detracts from focus on key treatment targets. For example, if I (AHK) had a patient who had engaged in self-harm and had a significant episode of bingeing and purging during the previous week, both of these targets would take priority over the patient's stated desire to process a conflict that had occurred with their partner.

Bringing DBT to Life – Megan's Diary Card

Now we are going to take a peek at two of Megan's completed diary cards; one that is from earlier in her residential admission and one that is from the latter half of her partial hospitalization admission after stepping down from residential. Our rationale for sharing two diary cards is to show how diary cards can evolve over treatment and to give you additional exposure to how each provider might use information from Megan's diary card to assist in setting a discipline-specific session agenda.

What you see on the following page (Figure 13.1) is a diary card from an earlier week in Megan's admission at a residential level of care. Before you read further, take some time to consider what you might prioritize for your session if this was a diary card you received from a patient. What sticks out to you as being most important? If we keep the DBT treatment target hierarchy in mind, on page 169 (Table 13.1), you will see how individual providers working with Megan might prioritize their sessions.

In reviewing Table 13.1, what you may have noticed is that there are both distinct and shared targets among Megan's providers and as we will discuss shortly, there can be benefit to multiple providers addressing the same target, as each discipline will approach a shared therapeutic target from different angles.

Now please turn to page 170 to take a look at Megan's diary card from PHP (Figure 13.2). What do you notice about Megan's diary card from this level of care? First, remember that diary cards are a living document that evolve over the course of time. What you might notice is that while certain targets have remained on the diary card, other targets have been removed and replaced with new targets that are relevant to where Megan finds herself in her overall course of treatment. Second, you'll notice that some of these targets directly relate to interventions that may be used with increasing frequency as a patient enters into lower levels of care, like exposure-based procedures and increased work around living in

Name: Megan										Date Started: 11/6/2023		Was the card filled out daily? Yes						
				Target Behaviors										**Emotions**				**Skills**
Day:	SI 0-5	SIB? Y/N	SIB Urges 0-5	Restricted? Y/N and If Yes, When?	Urges to Restrict 0-5	Purged? Y/N	Urges to Purge 0-5	Frequency of Body Checking 0-5	Honest w/ Team? Y/N	Took Meds? Y/N	Tried Pleasant Activity? Y/N and If Yes, What?	Anger 0-5	Sad 0-5	Joy 0-5	Shame 0-5	Fear 0-5	Loneliness 0-5	How they were used
Mon	1	N	2	Y – B	5	N	4	5	Y	Y	N	2	5	0	5	3	1	1
Tue	0	N	1	N	3	N	2	4	Y	Y	Y – Walk	0	3	3	5	3	0	5
Wed	0	N	0	N	5	N	2	5	Y	Y	Y – Puzzles and Knitting	3	3	2	4	3	0	5
Thu	0	N	0	N	3	N	1	4	Y	Y	Y – Watched a Movie	0	1	3	4	3	0	5
Fri	1	N	3	Y – ES	5	N	5	5	Y	Y	N	4	2	0	5	5	0	4
Sat	0	N	1	Y – B, MS, AS	5	N	2	5	Y	N	N	3	2	0	5	5	1	1
Sun	1	N	0	N	3	N	3	5	Y	Y	Y – Art Project	1	2	2	5	3	0	7

How were the skills used?

0=Not thought about or used

1=Thought about, not used, didn't want to

2= Thought about, not used, wanted to

3=Tried, but couldn't use them

4=Tried, did them, but they didn't help

5=Tried, Could use them, THEY HELPED!!!

6=Didn't try, used them, didn't help

7=Didn't try, used them, THEY HELPED!!!

Important events from the week:

Monday: Feeling super-depressed today. Not sure why. Had a hard time getting going this morning.

Tuesday: Had a good therapy session and got to go on a walk today. Still feeling a lot of body image distress.

Wednesday: It was a pretty quiet day. Had a session with my dietitian. My ED voice is really loud today.

Thursday: Movie night was fun. I liked spending time with everyone.

Friday: PIZZA NIGHT. Really wanted to restrict but was sitting at a table where everyone else was eating. Felt disgusting afterward. Didn't touch evening snack.

Saturday: Still feeling disgusting from pizza night. Didn't eat most of the day to make up for last night and didn't take my Zyprexa.

Sunday: Another quiet day. Worked on my art project. Was pretty tired a lot of the day.

Figure 13.1 Megan's Residential Diary Card.

Table 13.1 Session Targets

Therapist	Dietitian	Psychiatric Provider	Medical Provider
#1 – Heightened SIB urges (Friday) #2 – Significant restriction (Saturday)	#1 – Significant restriction (Saturday) #2 – Heightened urges to purge (Friday)	#1 – Heightened SIB urges (Friday) #2 – Medication noncompliance (Friday) #3 – Symptoms likely to be effectively treated by medication (e.g. heightened negative affect)	#1 – Medical concerns that have emerged or worsened due to eating disorder behaviors #2 – Any other medical concerns #3 – Medication noncompliance (Friday)

alignment with one's values on a day-to-day basis. Let's also take a peek at what Megan's providers might have as their session agendas, keeping in mind the DBT target hierarchy, by turning to page 171 and reviewing Table 13.2.

Once again, you'll notice that there are both shared and independent targets that are addressed by each member of the multidisciplinary team, again speaking to the value of multidisciplinary collaboration.

Provider Exercise – Constructing a Diary Card

For this provider exercise, you will need the DBT treatment target hierarchy you constructed for the previous provider exercise. Based on this DBT treatment target hierarchy, do your best to construct a DBT diary card that captures the most essential of your patient's Level One, Level Two, and Level Three target behaviors. Keep in mind that if you actually decide to use a DBT diary card with your patient, you should construct a DBT diary card with them collaboratively rather than showing up with the DBT diary card you create in hand. The purpose of this activity is simply to give you practice creating a DBT diary card and showing how the DBT diary card and DBT treatment target hierarchy are connected. Once you have completed a draft DBT diary card, you may consider sharing your DBT treatment target hierarchy and DBT diary card (ensuring they are both appropriately de-identified) with a trusted peer for feedback, ideally someone who is familiar with DBT. As a bonus activity that you may find helpful, consider creating a DBT diary card that tracks targets related to your own life and complete your DBT diary card daily for at least one month. I (AHK) found this activity to be invaluable in getting a sense as to what it is like for

Name: Megan   Date Started: 2/5/2024   Was the card filled out daily? Yes

Day:	SI 0-5	SIB? Y/N	SIB Urges 0-5	Restricted? Y/N and If Yes, When?	Purged? Y/N	Urges to Restrict 0-5	Urges to Purge 0-5	Home st w/ Team? Y/N	Motivation for Recovery 0-5	Completed Assigned Exposure? Y/N or N/A	Engaged in Values-Consistent Activity? Y/N	Anger 0-5	Sad 0-5	Joy 0-5	Shame 0-5	Fear 0-5	Loneliness 0-5	How they were used
																		Skills
					Target Behaviors							**Emotions**						
Mon	0	N	0	N	N	3	3	Y	3	Y	Y – Self-Care	0	2	2	3	4	0	5
Tue	0	N	0	N	N	2	1	Y	3	N/A	Y – Walk	0	2	4	2	2	0	5
Wed	1	N	1	Y – ES	N	5	3	Y	1	N/A	N	5	4	0	5	5	2	4
Thu	0	N	1	N	N	3	2	Y	1	N/A	Y – Spent Time w/Mom	2	2	2	3	3	1	5
Fri	0	N	0	N	N	2	2	Y	3	Y	Y – Read Book	1	2	3	3	5	0	5
Sat	1	N	0	N	Y	3	5	Y	3	N/A	Y – Movie	0	1	3	4	4	0	4
Sun	0	N	1	N	N	3	4	Y	3	N/A	N	0	3	0	3	3	2	2

Important events from the week:

Monday: Just a pretty typical Monday. Did casserole exposure like I had planned and felt kind of gross and worried about what was in it, since my mom made it. Did self-care afterward.

Tuesday: Pretty good day overall. The weather was really nice so I went for a walk in the evening.

Wednesday: REALLY BAD DAY. Made a mistake at work and my boss gave me a verbal warning. Totally unfair. Felt really angry and really ashamed. Went to bed before evening snack.

Thursday: Still feeling pretty upset from Wednesday, but talked about it in programming. I also talked to my mom and that helped.

Friday: Was pretty exhausted from the week, so didn't really do much after programming. Had a good therapy session. Spent time reading a new book that I like in the evening.

Saturday: Felt rushed all day. Went to the movies with friends. Ate too much banana bread. Purged.

Sunday: Felt pretty blah today. Kind of had to force myself through the motions artwork. Feeling upset that I purged but also having urges to do it again.

How were the skills used?

0=Not thought about or used

1=Thought about, not used, didn't want to

2= Thought about, not used, wanted to

3=Tried, but couldn't use them

4=Tried, did them, but they didn't help

5=Tried, Could use them, THEY HELPED!!!

6=Didn't try, used them, didn't help

7=Didn't try, used them, THEY HELPED!!!

Figure 13.2 Megan's PHP Diary Card.

Table 13.2

Therapist	Dietitian	Psychiatric Provider	Medical Provider
#1 – Instance of purging (Saturday) #2 – Instance of restriction (Wednesday) #3 – Difficulties with implementing skills (Sunday) #4 – Decreases in motivation for recovery (Wednesday and Thursday)	#1 – Instance of purging (Saturday) #2 – Instance of restriction (Wednesday)	#1 – Symptoms likely to be effectively treated by medication (e.g. heightened negative affect)	#1 – Medical concerns that have emerged or worsened due to eating disorder behaviors #2 – Any other medical concerns

our patients to complete DBT diary cards, with the added benefit of helping me to make some positive changes in my own life! Should you choose to do this bonus activity, you may consider making some notes about what you found to be helpful and what you found to be challenging, as well as additional insights you gained from the process.

Chapter 14

Chain Analysis and Behavior Analysis

Now that you have a fairly detailed summary of your patient's previous week, as well a session agenda with priorities triaged, you may be wondering what to do next. While DBT offers a fair amount of latitude with regard to interventions used during individual provider sessions, one of the most commonly utilized interventions is the chain analysis, which has been described by some as the "centerpiece of most individual therapy sessions." (Swenson, 2016) Chain analysis is a moment-to-moment examination of the antecedents and consequences surrounding a target behavior. Metaphorically, chain analysis is almost like working together with your patient to get such a detailed account of their experience that a screenwriter could create a script and provide it to an actor and that actor would be able to depict what transpired with a fairly high degree of accuracy. For those of you who are familiar with the ABC (Antecedent-Behavior-Consequence) Model from CBT or the ARC (Antecedents-Response-Consequences) of Emotions from the Unified Protocol for Transdiagnostic Treatment of Emotional Disorders, these interventions may sound fairly similar to chain analysis. While there is a decent amount of overlap, as we review chain analysis further, you are likely to observe some subtle yet important differences as well.

There are a number of different components to a chain analysis. The target behavior is the specific behavior that you and your patient would like to explore. Examples of target behaviors could include purging once immediately after dinner, doing one hundred situps, restricting afternoon snack, cutting superficially a dozen times with a razor on the stomach, running on a treadmill for two hours, and so forth. With target behaviors, you want to be sure to define specifically what the behavior was (topography), how many times it happened in a specific episode (frequency), how severe the behavior was (intensity), and how long the behavior lasted (duration), if relevant. With rare exceptions, chain analyses start by defining the target behavior.

Chain analyses can go a number of different directions after defining the target behavior and many providers have found it helpful to then identify the

DOI: 10.4324/9781003495604-14

prompting event. The prompting event is an external (e.g. seeing one's weight on a scale) or internal (e.g. experiencing a trauma-related flashback) event that sets a series of things in motion that ultimately lead to the target behavior occurring. Metaphorically speaking, the prompting event is a bookend of sorts when thinking about a chain analysis as a whole. Examples of some questions that might help in identifying a prompting event include, "When do you think the train first started down the track toward purging?" or "When did you first notice an urge (or if your patient says urges are always present, a notable uptick in the intensity of their urges) to do sit ups?"

The next component of a chain analysis is vulnerability factors, which some individuals choose to examine prior to identifying the prompting event. Vulnerability factors are any factors that increase the patient's overall susceptibility to engaging in the target behavior. Some categories of vulnerability factors include physical illness, imbalanced eating, unbalanced sleep, substance use, stressful events, and intense emotions. Specific examples for patients with eating disorders might include a migraine that is causing nausea, restriction of intake that sets the stage for an instance of bingeing, food-oriented holidays like Thanksgiving, or high baseline negative affect. Of note, vulnerability factors can be both acute or chronic in nature.

With the target behavior, the prompting event, and vulnerability factors identified, the next step in conducting a chain analysis is to identify all of the granular links that connect the prompting event to the target behavior. These links can include actions the patient took, body sensations they were feeling, thoughts they had, urges they noticed, events that occurred in the environment, or feelings or emotions they experienced. When gathering information about urges and emotions in particular, it can also be helpful to have patients rate the intensity of these urges and emotions on a Likert scale (e.g. 0 to 10), as this can help to identify particularly salient points on the chain. As you are gathering information about what transpired, it is critical not to make assumptions or jump to conclusions, but rather to assume no understanding of the situation at hand and let the story tell itself. Rather than asking questions like, "What caused that?" or making assumptions like, "So then you restricted because you were feeling anxious," simply ask questions that allow the story to unfold, like, "So tell me what happened next?" and "Did you have any emotions or thoughts come up at that time? If so, what were they?"

Once you have completed the chain analysis up to the point in time where the target behavior occurs, it is then important to explore both immediate consequences of the behavior, as well as delayed or long-term consequences of the behavior. It can be helpful to inquire about emotions, thoughts, and bodily sensations that came up for the patient immediately, as well as later on, in addition to exploring the impact of the patient's behavior on others and on the environment. When reviewing consequences, there are three types of effects of consequences that are of particular interest. First, you are looking for consequences that may have a role in maintaining a target behavior. For example, if a patient experiences a significant decrease in anxiety after an instance of purging, one hypothesis you might explore is that purging is being maintained by negative reinforcement. Second, you are looking for consequences that may weaken the target behavior. Working with the same example, if a patient experiences significant shame immediately after purging, it is possible that this reaction will weaken the target behavior. Finally, you are looking for consequences that may inhibit behaviors that would be more adaptive than the target behavior. For example, if your patient engages in restriction at a meal and then overhears a peer making negative comments about a patient who completed their meal, this could inhibit your patient's willingness to make efforts to complete meals in the future.

There are a number of ways in which chain analyses can be useful interventions in treatment. First, they help to gain a deep level of understanding and insight with regard to a patient's experience. It is rare in our day-to-day lives that we hear an account of an event in as detailed and nuanced a fashion as you get with chain analysis. Second, chain analyses can help to generate hypotheses about the purpose a target behavior may be serving for a specific patient. By having a working hypothesis about the function of a target behavior, in addition to understanding other factors that might be influencing the likelihood of the target behavior occurring, the problem-solving process can then begin. As we will discuss shortly, there are four groups of interventions that solutions generated from the problem-solving process tend to draw from in DBT. For a more eloquent description on the benefits of chain analysis, Charlie Swenson summarized them as follows: "Behavior chain analysis can help patients move from chaos to order, from confusion to insight, and from helplessness to planful behavior change. It provides a counterpoint to passivity and dyscontrol for both therapist and patient. It provides structure and direction in therapy, supplementing a mindful and compassionate, empathetic and validating approach. It provides a ladder for descending into the patient's hell, and a ladder for helping the patient to climb out. It helps a therapist to think clearly amidst the chaos." (Swenson, 2016)

As with the majority of procedures used in DBT, patient orientation prior to using the procedure is crucial, as this increases the likelihood of patient buy-in and demonstrates transparency as providers. Orientation to chain analysis should include describing what chain analysis is as a whole, in addition to describing the specific components, providing a rationale for why chain analysis is used, and describing situations under which chain analyses may occur. It is also important to remember that you may need to reorient your patient to chain analysis at various points in treatment.

If you are doing family or couples' work as part of your work with a patient, it is also worth mentioning that chain analyses can be conducted in a way that includes more than one person's perspective. Double chain analyses are chain analyses that can be conducted on an unfavorable interpersonal interaction that has occurred (e.g. a partner verbally attacking their partner or withdrawing from their partner), in which both parties involved in the interaction contribute to links in the chain. The goals of double chain analyses are two-fold. One goal is to have each person involved in the double chain analysis gain a better understanding of the other person's experience, with the other goal being for each person involved in the double chain analysis to commit to working on specific links in their part of the chain (e.g. regulating their emotions, challenging their judgments). When doing a double chain analysis, some links in the chain will be publicly observable (e.g. overt behaviors or verbalizations made by one of the two parties involved in the interaction), whereas other links are covert yet important in understanding the interaction (e.g. thoughts, particularly those taking the form of judgments or assumptions, emotions). While double chain analyses look similar to chain analyses done with an individual, one important element of doing double chain analyses is ensuring that each person participating validates the other person's experience as they share relevant links in the chain. This helps in achieving the first goal of double chain analyses mentioned above. We will be discussing solution analysis in much greater depth later in this text, but in short, solution analysis is focused on targeting specific problem links identified in the chain analysis through various clinical interventions. This is an important follow-up to double chain analyses as well. Once each person involved in the double chain analysis has shared their chain, each person should identify something they would like to try to do differently and ideally, practice this new skill or approach in session (Fruzzetti & Payne, 2015).

Once you have completed numerous chain analyses with a patient or with a patient and a family member in the case of double chain analyses, this can assist in further refining the initial case conceptualization and treatment plan you have for a patient. As you complete each additional chain analysis, it can be helpful to identify emotional, behavioral, cognitive, and environmental patterns that emerge, as well as to consider interventions that can effectively address concerns that are arising within these patterns. The take-home point here is that chain analyses can be helpful both in understanding a specific situation that transpired, as well as informing your bigger picture understanding of your patient.

Bringing DBT to Life – Megan's Chain Analysis

In order to better understand how chain analyses can be used across disciplines, we will look at a chain analysis of the instance of purging that you saw on the second of Megan's completed diary cards. To demonstrate how the application of principles of chain analysis can vary by provider, we will show you dialogue from both a therapist perspective and a dietitian perspective when conducting a chain analysis. Let's start by taking a look at how an exchange between Megan and her therapist might look when conducting a chain analysis of her instance of purging.

Therapist: "Exploring the instance of purging this past week definitely seems like our top priority for today. So talk to me – when did you first notice you were having urges to purge?"

Megan: "I'd say it was probably when I was about three-quarters of the way through the second piece of banana bread that I was having for evening snack."

Therapist: "Sounds like I might need a bit more backstory here. Maybe let's start right before you got started with evening snack. Do you remember about when that was?"

Megan: "It was probably around 10:15pm."

Therapist: "Oh, that's much later than usual…"

Megan: "Yeah, I had gone to see a movie at the mall and I hadn't checked how long the run time was and it was definitely longer than I expected, so I didn't get home until after 10:00pm."

Therapist: "Gotcha. So what happened next?"

Megan: "Well, I noticed I was feeling pretty hungry, especially because I had dinner on the earlier side of things. I had planned to have a slice of banana bread, so I went and plated that and then sat down on my couch and turned on the TV. The evening news was on and I should have known better and changed the channel, but I can't pull myself away from everything that's going on these days. So I definitely got sucked into that a bit."

Therapist: "Any emotions that were coming up for you at that moment in time?"

Megan: "Oh, definitely anger. Some of the things going on in our country right now make me livid. I also noticed that I was enjoying the taste and the texture of the banana bread, which brought up some mixed feelings for me. You know, like one hand I really do want a normal relationship with food. On the other hand, foods like banana bread feel like forbidden foods to me. Like, I don't deserve to have a food like that, especially if I have eaten normally that day."

Therapist: "I hear you – on one hand, a part of you recognizes that incorporating banana bread into your diet is a totally normal thing. On the other hand, your eating disorder is telling you that banana bread is off limits, especially if you haven't compensated in some way in order to "earn" it. Was there a specific emotion that was coming up for you at that point?"

Megan: "Maybe some guilt or shame?"

Therapist: "Gotcha. So what happened after that?"

Megan: "Well, I was getting near the end of my piece of banana bread and I couldn't tell if I was still hungry or not. And so I was feeling pretty indecisive about what to do. Do I get another piece of banana bread, do I wait a few minutes, do I just tell myself that one piece of banana bread was all I need and move on with my night?"

Therapist: "Any emotions come up for you at that point?"

Megan: "I think I was feeling a bit anxious, although I probably didn't recognize it at the time."

Therapist: "As you're reflecting on things now, what information do you have that suggests it was anxiety you were experiencing?"

Megan: "It definitely felt like my thoughts were racing and I remember my heart feeling like it was going pretty fast."

Therapist: "Yup, definitely things you would experience if you were feeling anxious. So what happened next?"

Megan: "So I decided to get another piece of banana bread so I went and got one and came back to the couch and I was definitely eating it more quickly than the first piece of banana bread for some reason. And it felt like my mind was still racing. Like, I wasn't sure I actually needed the second piece of banana bread and I was definitely starting to feel guilty and disgusted with myself. And then I noticed some crumbs had fallen onto my shirt and my pants and I noticed how flabby and gross my stomach and thighs look. And at that point, I was just feeling really out of control and sloppy."

Therapist: "It sounds like a whole lot was coming up for you at that moment. Where were your urges to purge at that point?"

Megan: "Maybe like a three out of ten. They had definitely started to creep in, but were still manageable."

Therapist: "Okay, so keep going…what happened after that?"

Megan: "So I was almost done with the banana bread and I started noticing that I was feeling full and I could feel my stomach going over my waistband and I just had this thought that I needed to get the banana bread out of me."

Therapist: "Where were your urges to purge at that point?"

Megan: "Probably at a six out of ten."

Therapist: "Definitely a substantial jump. What happened next?"

Megan: "It felt like my whole body was shaking and I realized things were kind of spiraling out of control, so I decided I needed to try to distract myself."

Therapist: "That was really wise-minded of you! What did you do next?"

Megan: "Well, I was feeling really overwhelmed and the only thing I saw around me that I could use to distract myself was my crocheting stuff, so I picked that up and tried to crochet. But my hands were shaking so bad, I really couldn't get it to work."

Therapist: "I imagine that was really rough. Trying to use a skill and then not being able to use it because your emotions were running so high."

Megan: "Yeah, I honestly think it made the situation worse. I got super-frustrated and threw my crocheting stuff across the room and then really just started berating myself."

Therapist: "Can you elaborate on that further?"

Megan: "Yeah, I remember just telling myself how fat I've gotten, how I've really let myself go. That I didn't deserve that banana bread, especially with everything I ate earlier in the day. Then I got really stuck on ruminating about the nachos I had and at that point, I just decided I had to purge. That there was no way I was going to feel better if I didn't."

Therapist: "What happened next?"

Megan: "I went into the bathroom and purged. It was actually a bit hard to do since I hadn't purged in a while, but once I did I had such a sense of relief. I stopped shaking and just felt this wave of calm."

Therapist: "I see. Were there any other short-term consequences that happened?"

Megan: "I did have this brief moment while I was glancing at the toilet where I did think, 'Ugh, this is gross.' But I also was so thankful to feel such a sense of relief. That feeling of anxiety was just unbearable."

Therapist: "Got it. Were there any long-term consequences you can think of?"

Megan: "I think for me the biggest thing is this fear I have that now that I've purged, the floodgates have opened for purging. Which I absolutely don't want to do. But it's made me feel like I'm on shaky ground. And I have some lingering shame and guilt."

Therapist: "It sounds like purging has really brought up some concerns for you."

Megan: "Yeah, it has."

Therapist: "Well, I definitely want to go back through everything we covered and see where there might be opportunities to prevent something similar in the future, and before we do that, I totally forgot to ask earlier – do you think there is anything that made you more vulnerable to the possibility of purging that day?"

Megan: "Well, I definitely had some challenging foods earlier in the day, and my sleep schedule has been a little off. I didn't think it was something that was impacting me, but as we're talking now, I wonder if it has made me more vulnerable…"

Therapist: "Knowing what you've shared with me before, that's definitely a possibility. Shall we spend some time going back through this chain a bit together?"

Megan: "Sure."

The same event chained by another provider, in this case the dietitian, looks a lot different.

Dietitian: "I'm noticing something I haven't seen in a while on your diary card... it looks like you purged this week. Are you open to discussing what happened?"

Megan: "I feel like I just did with my therapist. I'm not sure it's gonna help to do it again."

Dietitian: "Maybe it won't, but let's give it a shot. I want to understand what happened. Walk me through that evening."

Megan: "I went to the movies with some friends, came home, ate a snack and purged. That's really all there is to it."

Dietitian: "Take me back further. Let's start from the beginning of the day."

Megan: "I woke up late, maybe around ten. I was scheduled to work at noon, so I didn't need to wake up early. I just messed around on social media before I left."

Dietitian: "What about breakfast?"

Megan: "I had a bagel and cream cheese."

Dietitian: "I know that's a challenge! Good for you! Didn't meet the full meal plan, as you know, but we can celebrate this win. What size was the bagel?"

Megan: "... it was one of those thin, reduced carb bagels my mom always keeps when she's 'trying to be good.' I can't believe you thought to ask about the size of the bagel. Nothing gets by you!"

Dietitian: (smiles) "Well, we both know your eating disorder can be a little slippery at times. So, you didn't quite meet your meal plan...got it. What happened next? Did you eat at work?"

Megan: "I took your suggestion and picked up a sandwich and chips on the way in. I had the sandwich and a Diet Coke. Honestly, I thought about having the chips, but I kept thinking about early dinner plans with friends and that I would definitely make up exchanges at the restaurant."

Dietitian: "And how were you feeling about going out to eat? You've mentioned restaurants are extremely challenging for you."

Megan: "You'll be proud though! We went to that Overtime Bar and Grill place before the movie and I shared some nachos for an appetizer.

	Ordered a salad for the meal though because the calories for the burger were almost 2,000! All-in-all, I think I met my needs."
Dietitian:	"Mmmhmm. Fast forward a little for me…on your diary card you purged after evening snack."
Megan:	"Well we saw a movie, and by the time I got home, it was almost ten. I was having some binge urges come up, actually…I don't think I put that on my diary card."
Dietitian:	"Stop there for me. When did you first notice those?"
Megan:	"…I guess it was during the movie, now that I think of it. Alex got a huge thing of buttered popcorn and it smelled so good. It didn't fit my meal plan though, so I didn't touch it. I think then my mind started to think about bingeing later in the evening. Anyway, the movie was super long so I was tired when I got home but knew I needed to eat a snack. See? I'm trying my best here."
Dietitian:	"I can see that, I really can. Keep going."
Megan:	" I foolishly put on the news when I got home." (laughs) "Yeah, I should know better with everything going on right now. I was going to eat yogurt and granola for snack but my mom made banana bread because she knows I love it. I still had a nagging sensation to binge but I *really* didn't want to. Luckily there were only two pieces of banana bread left. I ate the two pieces of the banana bread pretty quickly. I had to purge, I felt so gross."
Dietitian:	"Got it. When did you first have the thought to purge?"
Megan:	"I was pretty worked up watching the news and I felt so gross in the pants I was wearing. I knew they were tighter after eating the banana bread. I was shaking and it was all I could think about. I tried to distract myself, but it didn't help. I know I'd instantly feel better if I purged. And guess what? I did. I immediately felt more calm."
Dietitian:	"I hear you. Were there any long-term consequences that happened?"
Megan:	"I'm definitely still feeling shame and guilt around bingeing and purging, so I guess there's that?"
Dietitian:	"Gotcha. Thanks for sharing all of this with me, Megan. Would you be cool with us going back through your chain together? I see some places where we might be able to do some work together to prevent something similar from happening in the future."
Megan:	"Sure."

When diary cards are regularly completed and reviewed, patients and providers alike can quickly identify the most relevant target behaviors that have occurred over the prior week. As you can see above, both of Megan's providers completed chain analysis for one single purging event. While it may seem like overkill to have multiple providers spend a significant session time on one event, we believe it presents an opportunity to enhance patient and provider understanding of a problem behavior. You likely noticed that while Megan's overall narrative was consistent in the chain analysis conducted with each provider, there were important nuances that were unearthed in each chain analysis that added further richness to the overall understanding of what transpired. Even working alongside adherent DBT therapists, I (ETM) have gathered additional useful information from a chain analysis led from a dietitian's perspective. I also want to stress that, as a non-therapist, I believe it's more important to embody the spirit of DBT when chaining a single event than to carefully explore therapeutic nuances of emotions, cognitions that are unrelated to dietetic topics, and so forth, as this runs the risk of drifting out of scope of practice. Rather, the chain analysis of a dietitian reads almost like a diet recall and is crafted around thoughtful questioning. By not getting in the emotional weeds and staying focused on the patient's intake, we can learn about the physiology and psychology of food selection throughout the day that may have contributed to the target behavior. Not only does this prevent drift from scope of practice, it also contributes different information that a therapist may not have unearthed in their chain analysis. When providers then communicate about information gained through their respective chain analyses, this can help to develop a more robust clinical picture, which informs both case conceptualization and treatment planning.

There are a few other nuances worth mentioning about the chain analysis examples you see above. First, you'll notice that both providers take a curious, nonjudgmental, and conversational tone, and that they weave validation into their chain analysis as appropriate. The process by which a chain analysis is conducted can have a significant impact on the extent to which your patient engages in the process and finds the process to be beneficial. Second, you'll notice that both providers also make an effort to highlight adaptive behaviors and patient successes throughout. This can help to counterbalance the focus on maladaptive behaviors and cognitions that are identified throughout the chain analysis. Lastly, you'll notice that while both providers took a relatively linear approach in conducting their chain analyses, there are moments where both deviate from a linear structure. Taking a nonlinear approach from a conversational standpoint is absolutely permissible when conducting a chain analysis and it is important that as a provider, you ultimately do get a linear picture of the sequence of the chain analysis as it transpired.

Provider Exercise – Chain Analysis

Think about a recent session you had with a patient where you discussed a behavior that occurred and see if you can construct a chain analysis focused on that behavior based on the information you can recall from your session. Now that you know more about chain analysis, make notes of questions you would want to ask at specific points in the chain where it feels like more information is needed to have created a chain analysis that has an adequate amount of detail. If you want to expand upon this exercise further, consider conducting a chain analysis during an upcoming session and if possible, getting feedback about your chain analysis (ensuring it is appropriately de-identified) from a trusted peer, ideally someone who is familiar with DBT. As a bonus activity that you may find helpful, you might also consider doing a chain analysis of your own behavior, like making a rude comment to your partner or making an impulsive purchase online. Doing a chain analysis of your own behavior is a great way to get a sense as to what it is like for our patients to complete chain analysis, as well as an opportunity to learn where our patients may encounter challenges in completing them.

Chapter 15

Missing-Links Analysis

A closely related procedure to chain analysis is missing-links analysis, which is a strategy for methodically exploring barriers to engaging in effective behaviors (Linehan, 2015). In other words, rather than conducting a chain analysis of a target behavior that occurred, missing-links analysis examines the factors that got in the way of an expected or needed behavior occurring.

Missing-links analysis begins by exploring whether the patient knew what behavior was needed or expected. Sometimes our patients may not actually know what was expected of them. For example, as a therapist, there have been times where I (AHK) have not spent sufficient time orienting a patient on how to complete a diary card, only to have the patient come to our next session with their diary card incomplete. Looking more at a situation relevant to a dietitian's role, a patient who is still new to a menu planning approach such as an exchange system for meeting their nutritional needs may inadvertently restrict part of a meal due to lack of understanding about what food choices would be necessary to meet all of their needs. In cases where lack of knowledge is the issue at hand, further education is the solution.

In the event that a patient understands what was needed or expected, the next step in missing-links analysis explores whether the patient was willing to engage in the expected or needed behavior. This is a particularly common barrier that arises when a patient has been tasked with engaging in therapeutic exposures, like eating a fear food or dining in a restaurant. When willingness is the barrier at hand, many of the commitment strategies we discussed earlier in this text can be helpful in the context of a conversation focused on enhancing willingness to engage in the expected or needed behavior in the future.

In the event that neither knowledge or willingness are a barrier, the next area for exploration is whether the thought of engaging in the needed or expected behavior ever entered the patient's mind. In some cases, the patient may simply have forgotten what was expected of them. For example, a patient may make themselves a note about therapy homework for the coming week, but then store this note in a location that they do not access in between sessions, thus preventing

DOI: 10.4324/9781003495604-15

them from being cued visually to complete the assignment they agreed to do. In other cases, a patient may remember that they are supposed to do something, but are unable to access the specifics about what exactly it is they are supposed to do. For example, a patient may commit to practicing certain skills when faced with a difficult mealtime situation, however once they are in the situation they find that their anxiety interferes with their ability to recall what skills they had agreed to try.

Finally, in situations where a patient knew what was needed or expected, was willing to do what was needed or expected, and had thought about doing what was needed or expected, it can be helpful to explore whether there was a delay in engaging in what was needed or expected. For example, a patient may find themselves in the middle of an activity at the time they are supposed to eat their afternoon snack and instead of stopping their activity to eat the snack, they continue on with the intention of eating it later. By the time that they are done with their activity, they may have forgotten about snack entirely, or may decide to skip afternoon snack because of fears it will make them too full to complete dinner.

Bringing DBT to Life – Missing-Links Analysis With Megan

Let's take a look at what a missing-links analysis could look like for someone like Megan. In this example, we'll be exploring different factors that could get in the way in terms of compliance with a new psychiatric medication regimen.

Psychiatric Provider: "So, how has the quetiapine been working for you at night?"

Megan: "...was I supposed to be taking that every day?"

Psychiatric Provider: "Yes, you're supposed to be taking it every night before you go to bed."

Megan: "Oh, I thought it was just something I was supposed to take as needed. Like, times when my mood gets really bad."

Psychiatric Provider: "Gotcha! I'm sorry that wasn't clear based on our last conversation. It's a medication where taking it each night before bed will be important in order to have its intended effect. Does that make sense?"

Megan: "Yes. Every night before bed. Got it."

In this example dialogue, the issue at hand was that Megan didn't understand what was expected in terms of her medication and simple education was sufficient to resolve the issue moving forward. Let's take a look at a scenario where this might not have been the case:

Psychiatric Provider:	"So, how has the quetiapine been working for you at night?"
Megan:	"I'm going to be honest, I haven't been taking it."
Psychiatric Provider:	"I appreciate you being up front with me. What's been getting in the way?"
Megan:	"I've taken so many different medications before that haven't worked, so I can't say I'm particularly hopeful this one will work, either. Also, I looked up some of the side effects and increased appetite and excessive weight gain are two of the ones that are most common. So yeah, that's a no-go for me."

In this example dialogue, Megan understood what was expected, however the willingness to do what was expected wasn't present. This would be an excellent time for her psychiatric provider to use commitment strategies. Evaluating the pros and cons, playing devil's advocate, and highlighting the freedom to choose and the absence of alternatives are all strategies that could be particularly helpful here. Now let's assume that Megan knew what was expected and was also willing to do what was expected, however the thought of following through on taking her medication never entered her mind:

Psychiatric Provider:	"So, how has the quetiapine been working for you at night?"
Megan:	"Okay, so I totally meant to take it this past week, and I keep forgetting! All my other medications are in the morning, so I'm not in the habit of taking nighttime medications."
Psychiatric Provider:	"Gotcha. Any thoughts come to mind about what might help you remember?"
Megan:	"Well, I keep my morning meds in a pillbox right by my coffee maker and that helps me to remember to take them in the morning, so maybe I need a separate pillbox that I can put in my bathroom by my toothbrush to help me remember to take them at night."
Psychiatric Provider:	"I think that's an excellent solution. Anything else you can think of that might help you remember?"
Megan:	"Nothing immediately comes to mind for me."

Psychiatric Provider:	"Can I offer one other suggestion I think could be useful, at least for now while you're getting used to a new routine?"
Megan:	"Sure."
Psychiatric Provider:	"I'm wondering if you'd be willing to set a daily reminder alarm on your phone. This way, in case you're somewhere other than home or in case you decide not to brush your teeth at night for some reason, you'll still have something that will help you to remember to take your meds."
Megan:	"I can do that."
Psychiatric Provider:	"Awesome. You want to take a minute or two now to set that alarm up?"

Now let's take a look at one final scenario. In this scenario, Megan knew what was expected, was willing to do what was expected, and had thought about doing what was expected, but still encountered a situation where she did not ultimately take her medication.

Psychiatric Provider:	"So, how has the quetiapine been working for you at night?"
Megan:	"It's sort of hard to say."
Psychiatric Provider:	"What do you mean?"
Megan:	"Well, I've probably only taken it three or four times in the past week. I actually set that alarm that you and I talked about, but a few nights it went off in the middle of this new show that I'm watching and so I silenced the alarm and then I totally forgot to take it later."
Psychiatric Provider:	"I see. It sounds like that delay is really getting in the way when it comes to your meds. Any thoughts about a solution we could put in place?"
Megan:	"I guess for now it might make sense for me to keep my meds on the side table by my couch instead of in my bathroom. That way if my alarm goes off during my show, I can just grab them, rather than having to pause to go take them."
Psychiatric Provider:	"That sounds like a solid plan to me. Why don't you give that a shot during the next week and if you're still struggling with staying consistent, we can talk about it in more detail next week. Sound good?"

Provider Exercise – Missing-Links Analysis

Think about a recent session you had with a patient where they encountered difficulty in engaging in a needed or expected behavior. Walk through each of the steps in a missing-links analysis to see if this helps you in getting a better understanding as to what got in the way and what strategies you might be able to use to help your patient engage in the needed or expected behavior in the future. If you want to expand upon this exercise further, consider conducting a missing-links analysis during an upcoming session and if possible, discuss your experience conducting a missing-links analysis, ideally with someone who is familiar with DBT. As a bonus activity that you may find helpful, as you may have done with the chain analysis provider exercise, you might also consider doing a missing-links analysis of your own behavior, like missing a dose of a prescribed medication or missing a deadline at work. Doing a missing-links analysis of your own behavior is a great way to get a sense as to what it is like for our patients to complete missing-links analysis, as well as an opportunity to learn where our patients may encounter challenges in completing them.

Chapter 16

The Four CBT Procedures Embedded Within DBT

Once you've completed a chain analysis with your patient during a session, your work is only partially done. A reasonable next step after ensuring you have a good understanding of antecedents and consequences surrounding the patient's behavior is to come up with treatment strategies that directly address factors that increase the likelihood of the target behavior occurring again in the future. There are four questions you can ask yourself that can help you to figure out which interventions may be most useful:

- *Does the patient have the skills necessary to both tolerate and regulate their emotions, navigate interpersonal situations effectively, and manage their own behavior?* If the answer to this question is no, the behavioral skills training procedures outlined below may be of help.
- *Are ineffective behaviors being reinforced and/or are effective behaviors being punished or reinforced with a delay?* In situations where the answer to this question is yes, contingency procedures may be an appropriate intervention.
- *Are there patterns of avoidance or is the patient unable to engage in effective behaviors due to intense, unwarranted emotions, like anxiety, guilt, or shame?* In cases where the answer to this question is yes, exposure-based procedures may be a helpful treatment approach.
- *Is the patient unaware of the contingencies at play in the environment or are effective behaviors being inhibited by beliefs or assumptions that do not align with the facts?* When the answer to this question is yes, cognitive modification procedures may be useful interventions.

With these questions in mind, let's review each of these four sets of interventions.

DOI: 10.4324/9781003495604-16

Behavioral Skills Training Procedures

Behavioral skills training procedures may be relevant solutions when a patient cannot emit a skilled response even under the most ideal of circumstances, or when a patient has a skilled response in their repertoire, however cannot engage in this skilled response at times when it is most needed.

We will go into further depth around specific DBT skills that are taught to patients later in this text, and it is important to note that with eating disorder work in particular, the skills taught to patients must extend beyond the DBT skills themselves. A list of other potentially relevant skills and the providers responsible for teaching them can be seen in the table on the next page.

There are four tasks to be accomplished in the context of behavioral skills training (see Linehan, 1993, pp. 329–343 for additional information regarding these tasks). First, it is important to orient your patient to skills training and ensure they have at least some degree of buy-in around learning a new skill. This includes providing a rationale for why you think a specific skill would be helpful for the patient to learn and use, as well as cultivating hope in the patient's ability to learn the skill and apply it in a way that brings them closer to their goals and life worth living. As part of the process of orienting your patient, it can also be helpful to share if you personally have found the skill to be helpful or have examples of other people using the skill to good effect.

The second of these tasks is teaching the patient the new skill, known in DBT as skill acquisition. As a precursor to skill acquisition, it can be helpful to take a brief moment to assess what, if any, components of a skill a patient already has in their repertoire. For example, a patient may have the ability to make a request of someone, however in the context of role-playing making a request, you find that your patient immediately backs down from their request when you demonstrate reluctance to honor it, or that your patient gets drawn into a discussion about an entirely different topic when you attempt to divert their attention away from the request they are making. By taking time to assess their existing abilities with regard to components of a skill, you are now able to be more targeted in helping them to acquire the components of the skill they do not already have in their repertoire.

There are a couple ways that you can assist patients in acquiring new skills. The first of these methods is through providing them with instructions. Instructions provided should be broken down into easy-to-understand steps and supported with written materials or other visual cues, as well as specific examples when feasible. For example, if a dietitian is teaching a patient about appropriate portioning, a patient is more likely to be able to acquire the skill if the dietitian not only discusses appropriate portion sizes, but supplements this information with visual cues and other tips for remembering portion sizes. For example, the patient might benefit from seeing actual portioned food or pictures of portioned

Table 16.1 Discipline-Specific Skills

Nutrition	Medical	Case Management	Culinary
- Meeting nutritional needs in general (e.g. using an exchange system) - Meeting nutritional needs under circumstances of increased or altered need (e.g. physical activity, illness) - Meeting nutritional within context of school, work, or travel - Creating a balanced plate - Proper portioning - Assessing hunger and satiety - Menu planning - Grocery shopping - Shopping on a budget	- Checking vital signs at home - Checking and administering insulin - Properly responding to signs you are at risk of falling or passing out - Managing medication side effects	- Locating and accessing resources, including medical, dental, food, financial, legal, housing, transportation, employment, and education resources - Finding a job appropriate for someone with an eating disorder - Ensuring basic needs are met	- Basic knife and prep skills - Learning how to stock a pantry - Figuring out how to cook on a budget - Learning to cook specific types of meals (e.g. one-pot) or learning specific cooking techniques (e.g. grilling, broiling)

food, as well as other ways to remember portion sizes, like comparing specific portion sizes to specific items (e.g. a portion of meat being about the size of a deck of cards). The other method of helping patients to acquire skills is through modeling. Modeling can be done through demonstrating the skill yourself, either independently or in the context of a role-play with the patient, as well as through examples provided through audiovisual means. For example, if a patient was recently discovered to have a severe food allergy, a medical provider could model for the patient how to self-administer epinephrine through the use of the mock auto-injector used in First Aid classes. Once a skill has been modeled for a patient, they should be asked to see if they can identify other examples of individuals modeling effective behaviors in their day-to-day lives or in the context of books, television shows, or movies. This can help patients to see there is often more than one way a skill can be applied to good effect.

The third task in behavioral skills training is helping the patient to develop fluency in engaging in the skill, which is referred to as skill strengthening. For those of you who are familiar with the "see one, do one, teach one" method of training in medicine, skill strengthening falls into the "do one" category. The first component of skill strengthening involves having the patient actually use the skill. This can be done via role-play (e.g. having the patient practice asking for help), practicing the skill in-session (e.g. doing a paced breathing exercise in the office), practicing the skill in imagination (e.g. imagining effectively navigating a grocery shopping trip), or practicing the skill in vivo (e.g. going with a patient to an ice cream shop to do an exposure and having the patient practice opposite action). It is critical that as part of the process of the patient practicing a skill with you present that you are taking any opportunity to reinforce their efforts and improvements in skillfulness. Particularly if you have strong therapeutic rapport, reinforcing patient efforts can have a powerful impact on future behavior. Finally, it is important to provide coaching if and when you notice your patient struggling to use a skill effectively. Coaching in this context refers to providing nonjudgmental feedback about what you are observing, coupled with instructions about what the patient can do to improve their use of the skill they are working on strengthening. In the event that there are many elements of the patient's skill use that would benefit from feedback, it is important to be mindful to provide feedback on only the most critical elements. This helps the patient to keep their focus on what aspects of the skill are most important, while also preventing them from becoming overwhelmed or discouraged. Keep in mind that additional feedback can be provided at a later time and after the patient has been able to make improvement with regard to the most critical elements initially identified.

The final task in behavioral skills training is helping the patient to apply the skill they have just learned across all relevant contexts in their life, known in DBT as skill generalization. One way to assist with skill generalization is to collaborate with your patient in coming up with a homework assignment that involves intentional practice of the skill they just learned, ideally across a variety of contexts if relevant and feasible. Another way to assist with skills generalization that is focused on the specific skill just learned is to encourage your patient to take notes during your session or even consider allowing your patient to record your sessions, if permitted in your specific work environment. Thinking about skills generalization more broadly, there are three other strategies that can be helpful. First, it is important that our patients have a wide range of skills to draw from in any given situation, which is known as response generalization. For example, when faced with a challenging meal, it is important that our patients have both acceptance-focused and change-focused skills to draw from, rather than just a single skill they default to, like deep breathing. Second, in-the-moment coaching, which involves providing a patient with support in applying skills in between sessions, is another strategy that can help with skill generalization. We devote a whole chapter to this mode of treatment later in this text. Finally, you can provide your patient with guidance around how to create an environment that reinforces skillful behaviors. On the side of self-management, you can teach your patient how to create structure, prompt skillful behaviors, and reinforce adaptive behaviors. For example, perhaps you are working with a patient whose historical relapses are accounted for in part by a busy and chaotic workday schedule that resulted in skipped meals. You might work with your patient to help them figure out how to meal prep for a whole work week on Sundays and how to use interpersonal effectiveness skills to advocate for time to eat during his workday. On the side of managing others in their environment, you might teach your patient how to advocate for what they need from others in order to increase skillful behavior. For example, if a patient's eating disorder behaviors serve the function of communicating distress, working with supports in their environment to be more proactive in terms of noticing signs of distress and actively intervening while also helping the patient to simultaneously develop more effective ways to communicate their distress is likely to shift contingencies in play to ones that are more adaptive.

It is important to note that, particularly when working with patients who display a great deal of apparent competence, providers can make the faulty assumption that skill acquisition alone naturally leads to skill generalization. It is necessary instead to assume that skill strengthening and skill generalization procedures are necessary each time you have selected behavioral skills training as a solution and treatment intervention. Patients who tend to be more perfectionistic and achievement-oriented may avoid acknowledging that they don't actually understand how to put a skill into practice or admitting that they tried to use a skill but were unable to do so. Increasing your intentionality with the behavioral skills training process helps to prevent patients from finding themselves in this type of situation.

Bringing DBT to Life – Behavioral Skills Training Procedures With Megan

As mentioned earlier, there are many other skills that are relevant to eating disorders that do not fall under the umbrella of DBT skills to which behavioral skills training procedures can be applied. We will discuss Megan's skills deficits in terms of DBT skills a bit later, so we thought it could be beneficial to explore how behavioral skills training procedures can be applied to skills outside of specific DBT skills. One area that Megan experiences a skills deficit is with cooking and kitchen skills. As a child, her often overworked mother would rely heavily on fast food and convenience foods. After her parents' divorce, Megan would eat foods prepared by her grandmother. Megan doesn't remember participating in food preparation at this age and doesn't recall having anyone else in her life model basic cooking skills. A lack of confidence in the kitchen coupled with memories of engaging in eating disorder behaviors has greatly contributed to a pattern of avoidance.

As an adult, Megan has avoided hot meals and anything that requires preparation in the kitchen. Her kitchen is not well-stocked and lacks key basic ingredients, like cooking oils and spices. Even in periods of stability, she has difficulty investing her time and energy into preparing food for herself, feeling deeply unworthy of the effort it takes to create a meal that will only make her feel guilty.

Megan's treatment team has recognized that increasing Megan's kitchen skills is a critical component of her treatment and Megan's dietitian has been spearheading efforts to increase Megan's kitchen skills during her residential admission. Claire started with orienting Megan to the goal of increasing comfort and confidence in the kitchen. She was able to get some buy-in by tying this back to Megan's life worth living, which includes building meaningful relationships. Megan noted, "I'd like to learn how to cook for my friends. They like to host potlucks and I'd like to actually bring something that's not a store-bought, premade item." Next, they explored some of the skills Megan already had in the kitchen. Megan reported moderate confidence in her ability to make scrambled eggs, quesadillas, and grilled cheese, stating, "Anything that doesn't require lots of steps or measuring and that's hard to mess up. That's where my skill level is." Claire reflects back that Megan does have some basic skills, even though they may not be too obvious, stating, "Feeling comfortable making those foods tells me you have careful management of the temperature of your skillet and timing, including handling and flipping the quesadilla or grilled cheese and managing the eggs."

Claire then explored Megan's willingness to engage in cooking chicken, which Claire noted can be the basis of many meals and can be the springboard for learning lots of culinary techniques such as stir frying, pan frying, deep frying, baking, poaching, and grilling. She decided the next step would be to connect Megan with the sous chef, Manny. Manny was able to show Megan how to cook chicken a few ways, including roasting, pan frying, and baking. Although begrudgingly, Megan agreed to work beside him on her own skillet. In addition to the hands-on practice, Manny provided her with recipes and encouraged her to take detailed notes and even videos on her phone, so she can recall the techniques they practiced.

After the session, Claire and Megan set goals around cooking chicken using the techniques learned with Manny. Megan agreed to Claire's goals to cook a chicken dish two ways this week, but initially rejected the idea of a method involving frying the chicken. However, eventually Megan comes around and learns to even like the taste of pan fried chicken. Claire worked with Megan on a weekly basis through the rest of residential and partial hospitalization care, setting goals around food preparation with the intention of skill strengthening and skills generalization. Towards the end of her partial hospitalization stay,

Megan was able to join in on her friends' potluck by contributing a casserole she made from scratch, demonstrating skills generalization in a context that is an important element of Megan's life worth living.

Provider Exercise – Putting Behavioral Skills Training Procedures Into Action

Think about a skill that you have had to teach a patient before or one that you anticipate having to teach a patient in the future and consider the questions below. If you are willing, once you have completed this exercise, discuss it with a peer for additional feedback or ideas.

1. How might you go about using instructions and/or modeling to teach this skill? Are there supporting materials that would be helpful to create to use as part of the skill acquisition process?

2. What activities could you do with your patient to assist with skill strengthening for this specific skill?

3. What homework assignments could you give your patient that focus on skill generalization? What in-between session support might be necessary to assist your patient with skill generalization?

4. What barriers do you anticipate encountering with behavioral skills training? How might you go about addressing these barriers?

Contingency Procedures

Contingency procedures are focused on examining how behavioral principles, like reinforcement, punishment, extinction, and shaping, may be at play as they relate to responses to a patient's behavior. In any given day of our lives, we encounter hundreds of contingencies, all of which influence our future behavior. Many of these contingencies are so subtle that they likely fade into the background of our awareness, like increasing the amount of chores you do around the house in response to expressions of gratitude from a partner or decreasing how much you go to a coffee shop because they regularly make mistakes with your order. What contingency procedures do is bring awareness to contingencies relevant to your patient's eating disorder, which then opens up the possibility to consider whether there are changes that can be made to support more adaptive behaviors moving forward. These changes should be focused on reinforcing adaptive behaviors and extinguishing maladaptive behaviors, ideally while simultaneously helping your patient to strengthen adaptive replacement behaviors.

Contingency procedures tend to be easier to understand if one has a working knowledge of basic behavioral principles, so before we get into the specifics of contingency procedures, we wanted to spend a bit of time elaborating upon reinforcement, shaping, extinction, and punishment. A reinforcer is any consequence that increases the frequency of a behavior. What is important to note here is that reinforcers aren't defined by what one might perceive is a reinforcer, but rather are defined by the impact that the reinforcer has on behavior. For example, if I am writing a blog on a quarterly basis for free as part of my job and my boss offers to pay me fifty dollars for every blog that I write beyond my quarterly minimum and my blog writing behavior does not increase, then money is not actually functioning as a reinforcer in this circumstance. Now that we've defined what a reinforcer is, let's take a look at various types of reinforcement. Positive reinforcement is typically what people think of when they think about reinforcement and is defined as increasing a behavior by adding a reward. Had my boss' financial incentive in the previous example resulted in an increase in the number of blogs I was writing, then this would be an example of my boss utilizing positive reinforcement. Negative reinforcement is defined as increasing a behavior by removing something aversive or unpleasant. For example, if I am experiencing acid reflux and I take an antacid and my acid reflux resolves, I will be more likely to take an antacid in the future when faced with similar circumstances. For many of our patients, their eating disorder behaviors are maintained by negative reinforcement. For example, if a patient completes a meal and is experiencing a great deal of anxiety as a result, and then they purge and their anxiety immediately decreases, this is a form of negative reinforcement that unfortunately increases the likelihood they will engage in purging behavior in similar situations in the future.

In addition to understanding the two types of reinforcement mentioned above, it's also important to have an understanding of schedules of reinforcement. Continuous reinforcement is a schedule under which a reinforcer is provided after each instance of a behavior. For example, if a teenager is doing a car wash fundraiser and they receive ten dollars for every car they wash, this is an example of continuous reinforcement. The other schedules of reinforcement are called intermittent schedules of reinforcement. A fixed ratio schedule involves a reinforcer being provided after a fixed number of instances of a behavior have occurred. For example, when I (AHK) was in kindergarten, my kindergarten teacher had a program where students received badges for every twenty-five books they read. I thought these badges were incredibly cool and as such, I greatly increased the amount of reading that I was doing in order to earn as many badges as possible. A variable ratio schedule is one in which reinforcement is provided after an unpredictable number of instances of a behavior. Slot machines in a casino are set up on variable ratio schedules, such that there is no set number of pulls that will result in a payout, although if one plays the slot machines enough, eventually there will be a payout. Of note, variable ratio schedules of reinforcement are the most powerful type of reinforcement schedule. A fixed interval schedule of reinforcement involves a reinforcer being provided after a set amount of time has elapsed. For example, paychecks for many jobs are on a fixed interval schedule, with paychecks being distributed every two weeks. Finally, a variable interval schedule of reinforcement involves reinforcement being provided after an unpredictable amount of time has elapsed. For example, the behavior of checking one's email inbox will eventually be reinforced by an unread email showing up, however the amount of time that elapses before a new email arrives is variable in nature.

Now that you are familiar with different types of reinforcement, we wanted to briefly discuss shaping. Shaping involves reinforcing small changes in behavior that are moving in the direction of a larger goal with regard to behavior change. For particularly time-consuming tasks (like writing a book, for example!) or tasks that involve multiple steps (like learning a complicated piano piece), waiting to reinforce only the ultimate desired behavior does not leverage behavioral principles in an optimal manner. Rather, it can be helpful to find ways to reinforce smaller behaviors to assist the person in achieving a larger goal or change in behavior. Using the examples above, one might consider providing reinforcement after each page of a book that is completed or after a person demonstrates mastery of the first few lines of a piano piece. For many patients who are diagnosed with eating disorders, it is not reasonable to expect instantaneous, wholescale change when it comes to entrenched patterns of behavior. In these circumstances, looking for incremental progress and ways this progress can be reinforced is critical.

A third behavioral principle to be aware of is extinction, which involves decreasing a behavior by withholding reinforcement for that behavior. For example, a parent may find themselves in a situation where each time they take their child to a video game store, their child throws a tantrum if they are told they are not allowed to purchase a game and in response to the tantrum, the parent ultimately relents and allows the child to select a game to purchase. Recognizing this is a problematic pattern, the parent may make the decision to no longer allow their child to select a game for purchase when they throw a tantrum, which is putting tantruming behaviors on extinction. What is often observed when extinction is utilized is that an extinction burst occurs, where the behavior that is being put on extinction temporarily intensifies before declining in frequency and intensity. What this parent may experience in this circumstance is that their child's tantrum may become louder or more intense in nature, however it is critical that the parent maintains their boundary in order to see a reduction in the frequency and intensity of these behaviors. So how does this apply to eating disorders? Many family members of loved ones with eating disorders find themselves in situations in which they are accommodating their loved one's eating disorder behaviors, which results in temporary relief for both themselves and their loved one, but has the long-term impact of worsening of eating disorder symptoms. For example, if a parent of an adolescent child has historically purchased fat free dairy products for them, however decides they will no longer be engaging in this accommodating behavior and instead purchases full fat products, they may see a temporary worsening of eating disorder behaviors and symptoms, like threats to restrict or actual restriction of meals that utilize the full fat products. However, it is critical in this circumstance that the parent continues to refuse to purchase fat free products and make their best effort to support their loved one around meeting their nutritional needs, while their loved one's treatment team also works in tandem in addressing the eating disorder behaviors and symptoms that have arisen.

The last behavioral principle we would like to cover is punishment. Punishment is defined as a consequence that decreases a behavior by adding something aversive or removing something positive. Punishment is an approach that should generally only be used as a last resort, like in circumstances where you as a provider do not have control over the factors maintaining a maladaptive behavior and there are no other adaptive behaviors that can be reinforced or in situations in which the maladaptive behavior is interfering with being able to make progress on any other adaptive behaviors. The rationale for avoiding the use of punishment is threefold. First, punishment tends to only lead to temporary suppression of behavior, rather than sustained behavior change. Second, punishment conveys to a person what not to do, however does not result in them learning alternative adaptive behaviors. Finally, punishment tends to damage therapeutic rapport.

Now that you are familiar with basic behavioral principles, we want to show how these principles are used in the context of contingency procedures in DBT. There are two types of contingency procedures within DBT. The first of these procedures are contingency management procedures. Contingency management procedures are focused on examining and modifying contingencies that are relevant to behaviors that are part of a patient's DBT treatment target hierarchy. These are behaviors that, by virtue of entering treatment for their eating disorder, the patient has agreed to work on. A patient with Anorexia Nervosa – Restricting Type may not express motivation to decrease instances of restricting, yet in seeking treatment for their eating disorder, this is undeniably part of the process. Observing limits is the other type of contingency procedure within DBT and is focused on patient behaviors that cross a provider's personal limits. While the deciding factor about whether to use contingency management procedures is determined by whether doing so is in the best interest of the patient, whether to use observing limits procedures is determined by how the patient's behaviors interact with a provider's personal limits. In other words, the provider's personal limits are the primary consideration here, above the patient's preferences and well-being. We will elaborate on observing limits procedures in considerably greater detail in a bit, and the take-home point at this moment is that it is necessary to be aware of your personal limits and boundaries, communicate these to patients, and adhere to them over the course of time in order to prevent burnout and to have the capacity to provide high-quality patient care. Observing limits procedures metaphorically parallel the instructions to put your own oxygen mask on first before helping others if you are on a plane flight where this is needed.

There are both formal and informal contingency procedures. Formal contingency procedures include token economies and level systems that commonly exist within inpatient and residential settings, as well as treatment contracts that can be used across all levels of care. With formal contingency procedures, desired behaviors and the consequences for both engaging and not engaging in these behaviors are clearly specified and communicated to the patient and their treatment team. Informal contingency procedures are more organic in nature and involve moment-to-moment responses to patient behavior that are conscious, strategic, and intentional. The therapeutic relationship is often a powerful tool and our moment-to-moment responses as providers can have a significant influence on patient behavior within the context of a strong therapeutic relationship. Informal contingencies outside of the therapeutic relationship can also present themselves in treatment. For example, I (AHK) was once conducting a DBT skills group with a milieu of adolescents who were having a difficult time on that specific day, which was leading to them struggling to engage with the group. After trying a few of my usual methods to increase group engagement, which had no effect on this particular day, I offered up the following contingency to the group: if they could give me thirty minutes of a reasonable degree of group participation, the definition of which I described in further detail, then we could end the group with enough time that they could have fifteen minutes to relax or engage in a fun activity prior to transitioning to their next therapeutic activity. This was a reinforcing consequence for the majority of group members, so group engagement increased, in turn helping patients to learn about a skill that could help them in achieving their goals of treatment.

There are a number of types of contingencies that can be at play that may be interfering with our patients making progress toward their goals. In some circumstances, maladaptive behaviors may be reinforced. For example, if an adolescent patient says to their parents that if they don't prepare meals that are vegan, they will stop eating altogether and the parents relent and prepare only vegan meals, a maladaptive behavior has been reinforced. Using contingency procedures in this case would involve supporting parents in preparing meals they had previously cooked for the family, while simultaneously considering other contingencies they can use to ensure their child meets their nutritional needs, like not permitting their child to go to soccer practice in the event they begin restricting meals or snacks. Neutral or punishing responses to adaptive behaviors is another type of contingency that can impact our patients' behaviors. For example, if a patient diagnosed with Anorexia Nervosa is working on being more flexible with food and takes an extra dessert at work gathering and has a coworker who is unaware of her diagnosis makes a comment about it, this might be experienced as punishing by the patient and decrease her likelihood of engaging in behaviors demonstrating food flexibility in the future. Having reinforcement occur in a way that is too distant from the behavior one intends to reinforce is another example of a contingency that can interfere with patient progress. For example, if an adolescent says their primary motivation for completing treatment is to get out of the hospital so they can go back to school, however completing treatment will require multiple months of care, the reinforcing consequence of going to school is likely too distant in the future to impact current behavior. A workaround for this type of situation, particularly for younger patients, can involve the use of sticker charts, which provide immediate reinforcement (a sticker) for a desired behavior (completing a meal or snack) that gets them closer to their long-term goals. Finally, there may be situations in which a goal has been set with a patient that is beyond the capacity of their current skills repertoire, necessitating a change in the goal to something that is more reasonable for the patient to achieve. For example, if you are working with a patient on increasing their assertiveness around support they need from their partner, your patient may genuinely lack the interpersonal skills to communicate her needs. A more reasonable goal in this circumstance might be to set the expectation that the patient initiates a conversation around this during a couples' therapy session, with you supporting the patient in communication of her needs beyond that point. The goal would be to gradually increase the patient's ownership of these discussions over the course of time.

Now that we've provided an overview of the types of faulty contingencies that may be in play for our patients, let's discuss specific contingency management procedures rooted in behavior therapy that you can apply (for a more extensive review of these procedures, readers are encouraged to read Linehan, 1993, pp. 297–319). The first of these is reinforcing target-relevant adaptive behaviors. In order to use reinforcement to assist with behavior change, you need to both have a clear understanding of what patient behaviors you are trying to increase, as well as what your patient will experience as a reinforcing response to these behaviors. For example, if meal completion is a behavior you would like to increase, the cheerleading and encouragement that you might provide to one patient may be experienced as reinforcing by that individual, whereas another patient may find the same approach to be aversive. There are a few things to keep in mind when using reinforcement. First, reinforcement tends to be most effective when it occurs immediately following the behavior that one would like to increase. For example, if a young adolescent patient at a residential level of care has a contingency in place where they can earn a pass out of treatment if they complete 100% of their meals and snacks for three consecutive days, you may want to devise a method where a smaller form of reinforcement can occur following completing behaviors (e.g. putting a sticker on a sticker chart, receiving praise), rather than relying solely on a more distant reinforcer. Second, it is important to provide frequent reinforcement of target-relevant adaptive behaviors early on in treatment and then gradually fade your schedule of reinforcement over the course of time, as intermittent reinforcement helps to make behaviors more resistant to extinction and because an intermittent reinforcement schedule is more likely to parallel what a patient may experience in their life outside of treatment. Third, keep in mind principles of shaping. It is possible that you may need to reinforce smaller improvements in behavior rather than waiting for a patient to engage in the ultimate adaptive behavior you would like them to emit. Fourth, use natural over arbitrary consequences whenever possible. While token economies and other forms of behavior management can play an important role in treatment, particularly when working with younger patients or when working at higher levels of care, natural consequences are more reflective of life outside of treatment and tend to be more effective in creating lasting behavior change. Finally, be mindful that every single moment spent with a patient is a potential opportunity to reinforce adaptive behaviors. In an individual provider session, behaviors like expressing willingness to follow-through on an assignment discussed in the session, disclosing difficult information instead of shutting down, or displaying engaged and cooperative body language are all small, but potentially meaningful and adaptive behaviors one might choose to reinforce. In milieu-based settings, following rules, treating staff kindly, participating in groups, and engaging with peers instead of isolating are also positive behaviors that any staff member present could reinforce. The take-home point here is that there are ample opportunities for any individual interacting with a patient to assist in shifting their behavior in an adaptive direction.

Another contingency management procedure involves extinguishing target-relevant maladaptive behaviors. In order to use this procedure, one must first identify what is reinforcing the maladaptive target behavior. Once these reinforcers are identified, they must be consistently withheld. Two other actions should be taken concurrently to this. First, alternative adaptive behaviors should be identified and reinforced on a consistent basis, with the ultimate goal of these behaviors becoming more reinforcing than the maladaptive behaviors targeted for extinction. Second, extinction should be coupled with soothing and validation. Often what our patients want is valid in some way, even if the methods by which they have gone about attempting to get these wants met is not.

The final contingency management procedure involves the use of punishment. As mentioned previously, punishment is an approach that should only be used as a last resort, when all other approaches to behavior change have been exhausted. As with extinguishing target-relevant maladaptive behaviors, any opportunity to reinforce adaptive behaviors that occurs in the context of utilizing punishment should be capitalized upon.

Contingency Contracting in the Context of Eating Disorders Treatment

Many unique characteristics of eating disorders, like their associated medical consequences and challenges with personal accountability in the context of substantial ambivalence, mean that individuals diagnosed with eating disorders may require treatment at higher levels of care during the course of their illness in order to ensure safety and help them to make progress in their recovery. Many treatment programs have used a combination of the APA Practice Guideline for the Treatment of Patients With Eating Disorders, internal program criteria, and insurance company criteria to determine appropriate levels of care, however Wisniewski and Ben-Porath (2015) suggest that there can also be value in proactively involving patients in a discussion around what criteria they believe would suggest they need to step-up in levels of care or are ready to transition to lower levels of care. The goal in these discussions is for the provider and the patient to establish criteria that both parties can agree upon as reasonable. When the provider and patient find they are not on the same page, discussion is continued until a synthesis can be reached or until one of the parties involved can convince the other of the wisdom of their perspective. The rationale for this approach is that it is believed to decrease apparently compliant or actively defiant behaviors and allow patients to take more ownership of their goals and whether they are moving closer toward them.

Bringing DBT to Life – Using Contingency Procedures With Megan

Let's take a peek at how the use of contingency procedures with a patient like Megan might look. Megan and her mother went on a day trip and en route to their destination, they stopped for lunch and discovered that the only restaurant nearby is a local diner that primarily serves foods that Megan still considers to be challenging. Megan ordered a burger and fries and when the waitress brought the food to the table, Megan noticed a spike in her anxiety, as the burger and bun were both larger than other burgers she is accustomed to and the fries were thick cut rather than thin cut. Megan found herself perseverating about portion sizes, however was still able to meet her nutritional needs. However, later in the day, Megan restricted her afternoon snack. Here, she recounts what transpired with her psychiatric provider:

Ayesha: "I had a chance to take a peek at your diary card and overall, it looks like you had a great week! I did notice that you skipped afternoon snack on Saturday, though. Can you share a bit about what happened?"

Megan: "Well, my mom and I had gotten lunch at this local diner and the burger and fries I ordered were both huge. I'm pretty sure that I probably ate more than what I needed and I was still pretty full when afternoon snack came around, so I just skipped it."

Ayesha: "Actually, a burger and fries sounds totally appropriate to meet your nutritional needs. It's also completely normative to have above your exchanges on occasion. But I want to go back to what happened that afternoon, since I'm not sure I follow how you ended up skipping afternoon snack, particularly with your mom around. Can you give me a bit more detail about what transpired?"

Megan: "Well, when afternoon snack rolled around, my mom was like, 'We should probably figure out what we're going to have for a snack…' and I told her that I was still feeling full from lunch and didn't think I needed a snack. Then she said that she thought that even if my body wasn't hungry, I still needed to meet my nutritional needs. I told her that I was feeling bloated and gross from lunch and that it was definitely more than my exchanges and that having a snack would just make that worse and that I didn't want to ruin the rest of our trip together. So then she just kind of relented and said something like, 'You know, that was an awfully big burger and fries, and I bet you're right. Plus I know how hard having a burger and fries is for you in general.' And so she just kind of dropped the snack thing and we went about our way."

Ayesha: "I see. What are your thoughts as you look back on the situation now?"

Megan: "I probably needed to have afternoon snack, but it felt like my mom was confirming that I ate too much and kind of giving me permission to skip it, you know?"

Ayesha: "Totally. I imagine her comments felt at odds with what we've been telling you, and I can imagine it would be hard to not just go along with not having afternoon snack when it felt like you were off the hook for it from an accountability standpoint. What do you think would be more helpful for your mom to say and do in a similar situation in the future?"

Megan: "I think I needed her to validate that I was feeling uncomfortable, while also reminding me that it's normal to feel uncomfortable at this point in the process and that I need to trust you guys. I think it also could have been helpful to hear that what I ate for lunch was appropriate for my needs."

Ayesha: "That all sounds spot-on to me. I'm also trying to put myself in your mom's shoes…I imagine it might have been hard for her to continue to try to encourage you to eat afternoon snack when it felt like she was being met with some resistance. How would you want her to handle that situation, if it comes up again?"

Megan: "I guess it could have helped if she had maybe taken a step back and asked me more about how I was feeling in that moment and then maybe asked how she could be of help. I didn't think about this at the time but honestly, I think if she had just picked something out that met my exchanges, that could have helped too. I imagine that even if she had gotten me to be more willing to have snack, I would have felt a bit paralyzed about selecting something."

Ayesha: "Everything you said makes sense. So here's the deal...I don't think this is likely to be the last time you encounter a situation like this."

Megan: "You're probably right."

Ayesha: "I'm wondering if you might be willing to put together a DEAR MAN of sorts to communicate to your mom about how she might be able to support you in similar situations in the future. What do you think?"

Megan: "I think that's doable, and it makes sense."

Ayesha: "Awesome, I'll be curious to hear how it goes!"

What you see in the example above is a situation where faulty contingencies are at play. In this example, Megan's verbal resistance to snack is reinforced when her mother backs down on holding the boundary around meeting her nutritional needs. Ayesha's conversation with Megan is intended to help Megan take ownership of intervening to prevent a similar contingency from playing out in the future, which would likely further reinforce verbal resistance around meeting her nutritional needs, followed by subsequent restriction.

Provider Exercise – Contingency Procedures

For this provider exercise, start by identifying a patient for whom you think faulty contingencies are at play. Use the prompts below to guide you through applying contingency procedures in your work with this patient. Once you have completed the below, consider discussing your reflections with a trusted colleague for feedback.

What is the Faulty Contingency at Play For My Patient?

- ☐ Ineffective behavior(s) are being reinforced
- ☐ Effective behavior(s) are being punished
- ☐ Reinforcement of adaptive behavior(s) is delayed
- ☐ The degree of behavior change that has been identified for reinforcement is beyond what my patient's current abilities

□ Other:

How do I plan to go about altering this contingency?

After the new contingency had been implemented for a period of time, did you notice any changes in your patient's thoughts, behaviors, or emotions as a result?

What do you think went well in using contingency procedures? What would you do differently in the future?

What other reflections do you have about your experience?

Provider Exercise – Contingency Procedures Bonus Activity

Another way to learn more about how behavioral principles work is through a fun activity that can be done as a group. For this activity, you will need one person to volunteer to have their behavior shaped by the group. The remainder of participants will be the ones helping with the shaping. Once you have a volunteer to have their behavior shaped, ask the volunteer to leave the room. The remaining group members should decide on a behavior they want to shape, like having the volunteer write their name on the whiteboard, sit in a specific chair, or pick up a certain object in the room. Remember, be kind! Once the target behavior has been selected, have the volunteer come back in the room. Group members should then cheer or clap if the volunteer gets closer to engaging in the target behavior (e.g. in the example of writing their name on the whiteboard, moving closer to the whiteboard, picking up a dry erase marker) and become quiet or even playfully boo a little if the volunteer is engaging in behaviors that do not align with the target behavior (e.g. walking to a part of the room that is far away from the whiteboard). Once the volunteer engages in the target behavior, be sure to celebrate and then discuss any take-aways the group had from the activity as it relates to contingency procedures, behavioral principles, and behavior change.

Observing-Limits Procedures

As was mentioned earlier, the other contingency procedures in DBT are observing-limits procedures (Linehan, 1993). These procedures focus on the provider identifying, communicating, monitoring, and adhering to their own personal limits. Given the high acuity and complex comorbidities with which patients diagnosed with eating disorders often present, in addition to the ego syntonic nature of certain eating disorder diagnoses, observing-limits procedures are particularly critical to prevent burnout as well as treatment intervention missteps that may occur in the context of burnout.

The first step in observing-limits procedures is becoming familiar with your own personal limits, knowing that certain limits may change over the course of time. It is important to note that there are few arbitrary limits in DBT, most of which are defined by your licensing board. Regardless of your own personal limits, all licensing boards have limits around certain provider behaviors. This means that the majority of limits set in DBT are your own personal limits. It is also important to note that while many patients with eating disorders find consistency to be comforting, personal limits will vary from provider-to-provider, meaning that some work may be necessary to help our patients effectively tolerate and navigate different provider limits. If you have not taken time before to consider your personal limits, this can actually be a challenging exercise. Some signs that we have seen that are potential indicators that a provider's personal limits may be being crossed by a patient include negative affect around that specific patient (e.g. feelings of frustration or fear), behavioral avoidance associated with a specific patient (e.g. being slow to return phone calls or e-mails, being unwilling to schedule an extra session even though you have time and think it would be beneficial to the patient), applying overly rigid treatment interventions you wouldn't typically utilize with other patients, and difficulties cultivating empathy for your patient. In order to help you in further exploring your own personal limits, here are some categories of personal limits we have regularly seen:

• Limits around frequency of contact (e.g. number of sessions per week, number of phone calls or emails) and time of contact (e.g. limits around times of day you will respond).
• Limits around methods of contact and the conditions under which they can be utilized (e.g. limits around use of texting, phone, and e-mail, limits around topics permitted via email).
• Limits around the degree of risk you are willing to tolerate in working with a patient (e.g. having limits around severity of eating disorder symptoms or suicidality that would prompt a referral).
• Limits around patient interpersonal behaviors (e.g. yelling at a provider, saying "yes, but..." to any intervention suggested, lack of participation in sessions).

Bringing DBT to Life – Observing-Limits Procedures With Megan

In order to show the variety of ways in which observing-limits procedures can be relevant across disciplines, we wanted to share a couple of examples below. The first of these examples occurs when Megan is on a residential level of care. After numerous experiences of having patients ask for last-minute changes to planned meals or snacks, Claire has discovered that one of her personal limits is that patients must give her at least a day's notice if they would like to make changes to a planned meal or snack, so she can discuss potential changes with them in a thoughtful manner. Although Megan is aware of Claire's personal limit, she is struggling with willingness to follow-through on a planned meal, and asks Omkaar if he can speak to Claire about a change in plans. Here is how Claire navigates maintaining her personal limits:

Omkaar (Psychiatric Technician):	"Hey Claire, do you have a quick second to chat?"
Claire (Dietitian):	"Sure, what's up?"
Omkaar:	"Megan said that she had a plan to eat pizza for lunch today, but she's having a bad day and doesn't think she can do it. She asked me to check-in with you to see if she could switch up to a PB&J and some veggies and dip for lunch instead. What do you want me to tell her?"
Claire:	"Please let her know that we need to stick to the plan we discussed earlier this week. I imagine she may not be pleased with that answer. Is there any support you need from me to support her?"
Omkaar:	"Nothing I can think of at the moment, but I'll let you know if that changes!"

About ten minutes go by, and Omkaar returns to speak to Claire again:

Omkaar: "So I let Megan know what you said around sticking to plans and she definitely wasn't happy. I tried to support her, but she's saying she's just not going to eat unless you allow her to have PB&J and veggies and dip. What do you want me to do?"

Claire: "Please let her know that we are still sticking with the plan that we discussed previously and that we can chat more about what came up for her during our session tomorrow. Is there any support you need in supporting her around this meal?"

Omkaar: "I feel like I have some good ideas of skills I can suggest if she actually gets started with the meal, but I really worry that she isn't going to touch anything at all. Any ideas?"

Claire: "I think first off, remember that you can be providing the best support possible, and someone still may not complete or even attempt a meal. So give yourself grace! But in terms of skills that might be helpful, if she's open to doing a pros and cons list with you before the meal, that's the first thing that comes to mind. I also know that she has been wanting to earn a pass in order to spend some time with friends, so I think reminding her that this meal is one of the steps in the direction of earning a pass could be useful. Lastly, I think looking at some of the thoughts and beliefs that are coming up for her and asking her what her Wise Mind says about whatever is coming up might help. Does that give you some starting points?"

Omkaar: "Sure does. Thanks for the help, Claire."

The above vignette demonstrates how Claire can respect her personal limits, while also working effectively with her coworker to make sure he feels supported.

In this second example, Megan is in the latter half of her time in IOP. Although she is generally doing well, she has only been intermittently completing her diary card and often comes to session without an idea of what she would like to discuss. Her therapist has been working to target these treatment-interfering behaviors as part of their sessions. During today's session, Megan asks her therapist (Serena) if they can start meeting twice per week. Serena notices that she has a strong negative reaction to this request and recognizes that she has a personal limit around how frequently she is willing to meet with a patient if they are not coming prepared to session. Here is how she navigates this request in session:

Serena (Therapist): "...so I'm noticing the time and we need to start wrapping up for today..."

Megan: "...but we haven't even had a chance to talk about what came up with my mom yesterday! Could we meet again on Friday this week? I feel like there's so much left to discuss."

Serena (Therapist): "I totally understand wanting to meet again, and one of the things that we've been working on together is helping you use our existing time together as effectively as possible. I really enjoy working with you Megan, and I'm finding it hard to have the willingness to have additional sessions when you're spending the first fifteen minutes of our existing sessions completing your diary card and coming up with what you want to talk about."

Megan: "I promise I've been working on being better and that I'll bring my diary card and some ideas of things to talk about in the future. But could we *please* meet again on Friday?"

Serena (Therapist): "Megan, I know it feels like I'm being inflexible here and I'm really not up for scheduling additional sessions until you are able to complete your diary cards and come with a bit of an idea about what you want to talk about in our sessions on a more consistent basis. I'd be happy to revisit

	the idea of a second weekly session once that happens, if it seems like a second session would be beneficial."
Megan:	(looking a bit upset) "Fine."
Serena (Therapist):	"I get that this is disappointing, Megan. Recognizing that, how can I support you in completing your diary card this week?"

Provider Exercise – Personal Limits

In the space below, write your top ten personal limits. Consider discussing your personal limits with a trusted peer, ideally someone who knows you well enough as a provider that they may be able to provide feedback about limits you may have missed.

Now that you have clarified your personal limits, in the space below, write out your individual warning signs that your personal limits may have been crossed.

Finally, write out a list of personal (e.g. physical illness, birth of a child) and professional (e.g. increase in caseload acuity, changes in company policies and procedures) events that might result in a change to your existing personal limits.

Once you've clarified your personal limits, it is important to consider the mechanisms by which you will communicate your personal limits to your patients moving forward. Information about a subset of your personal limits may be appropriate to include as part of your consent documents and discussed briefly as part of your intake process, whereas other limits may be more appropriate to include as part of verbal discussions over the course of treatment. Remember that personal limits often fluctuate over time, so it is important to monitor shifts in your personal limits and proactively communicate these to patients as they occur, when appropriate. It's also important that you take ownership of your personal limits. It can be tempting to want to place the ownership of your personal limits on other entities, including the patient themselves, particularly when you think the patient won't respond favorably to the limit you are setting. However, our patients can often detect dishonesty and our patients deserve the respect that being honest conveys.

Another component of observing-limits procedures is monitoring your limits routinely over the course of time. DBT consultation team, the fourth mode of DBT, can be a helpful venue in which to solicit and receive feedback and support from other team members around monitoring and adhering to your personal limits. However, we imagine that not everyone reading this text will be part of a DBT consultation team or an equivalent meeting of providers that can serve the purpose of helping you to monitor and adhere to your limits. In these circumstances, it is critical that you are setting aside time on a routine basis to check-in with regard to how you are feeling in your work with each of your patients. Using the warning signs your personal limits might be being crossed that you identified in the previous provider exercise as a guide can be helpful in this process.

Finally, considering how the provider characteristics of unwavering centeredness and compassionate flexibility play out in the context of observing-limits procedures can be helpful. On one hand, it is critical to be consistently firm when it comes to limits. Choosing not to adhere to a personal limit in the context of a patient's persistence in trying to get you to change the limit only increases the likelihood that the patient will be equally or more persistent in trying to get you to change limits in the future. Instead, it is important to put efforts made by the patient on an extinction schedule through being compassionate and validating, yet firm, and through helping the patient figure out how to use acceptance-focused and change-focused skills to help them in being effective in responding to your personal limits. On the other side of the dialectic, it is also critical to consider times when extending limits might be appropriate and demonstrate willingness to do so. For example, I (AHK) was once working with a patient who was going through the excruciating process of slowly losing one of her pets to a chronic illness. Although I was someone who was fairly willing to take after-hours pages for assistance, I was not someone who was typically willing to meet for multiple therapy sessions per week. However, the nature of the situation was such that being temporarily flexible around my limits was the compassionate and clinically effective thing to do. It is also important to note that as my flexibility around frequency of therapy sessions increased, my limits around frequency of after-hours pages began to tighten. What resulted from this were ongoing discussions with my patient where we attempted to figure out what approach around therapeutic contact would be helpful for her, while also within my personal limits.

Exposure-Based Procedures

Exposure-based procedures are a set of procedures that are designed to help patients decrease the frequency and intensity of negatively-valenced emotions over the course of time. The emotions most commonly targeted through exposure-based procedures when working with patients diagnosed with an eating disorder are fear, guilt, and shame, although other emotions may be targeted as well. These emotions may specifically be related to a patient's eating disorder or may be related to common co-occurring illnesses, like anxiety disorders.

Exposure-based procedures entail repeated, non-reinforced exposures to stimuli that evoke the emotion the patient would like to reduce, coupled with blocking action tendencies associated with that same emotion. For example, if you've ever gotten over a fear, you most likely were able to do so through a combination of being routinely exposed to the situation that evoked fear, coupled with remaining physically and psychologically present during the fear-evoking situation. This is a simplified example of exposure-based procedures at work. While standard DBT tends to use exposure-based procedures in a more informal manner, like having a patient continue to discuss a situation that evokes shame for them rather than "shutting down" in session, we believe that in eating disorders work there are advantages to taking a more formal approach to exposures as well.

The timing of the use of exposure-based procedures in the treatment of eating disorders is important to consider. For a patient who is at an inpatient level of care or early in treatment at a residential level of care, your work may simply be focused on helping your patient meet their nutritional needs, even if this means using distraction or other skills that can be helpful in achieving this aim. As a patient progresses through treatment, the goal would be to help them to be more able to complete their nutritional needs without the aid of distraction or other strategies that impede their ability to be present with the meal or snack at hand, in the service of helping them to be able to reduce the intensity emotions they experience in the context of meals and snacks rather than relying on "white-knuckling" it through meeting their nutritional needs. While the use of exposure-based procedures for some patients may come at a later point during their course of treatment, it is also important to note that there is research that suggests exposure-based procedures can be implemented very early in treatment at the highest levels of care, as long as there is patient buy-in to utilizing exposures. For example, a case study series conducted by Farrell and colleagues (2019) found that adult inpatients who participated in food-based exposures experienced significant reductions in eating-related fears and avoidance behaviors and found exposures to be an acceptable intervention. The take-home point here is that while in some circumstances exposure-based procedures may need to be delayed to allow for a focus on nutritional rehabilitation and medical stabilization, we should not make the assumption that patients who are early in treatment or being served at higher levels of care do not have the capacity to do this critical aspect of their therapeutic work.

As suggested above and as with all procedures in DBT, orienting patients to the procedure before implementation is critical and this is a particularly important step with regard to exposure-based procedures. Exposure-based procedures are often experienced by patients as aversive, so it is critical to have their buy-in and understanding, as exposure-based procedures done incorrectly will likely produce no positive results and may actually heighten negative affect. Using metaphors, stories, or benign examples from your own life, like getting over a fear of flying or public speaking, can be helpful in introducing the topic of exposure-based procedures to patients. There are a number of important points to touch on as part of the orientation process. First, it can be helpful to orient your patient to what exposures are and why they are believed to be effective. There are two hypothesized mechanisms of action for exposure-based procedures. The habituation model hypothesizes that if a patient is exposed to a stimulus or context that evokes negative affect and that they remain in contact with that stimulus or context for an extended period of time, the intensity of their negative affect will decrease. Thus, the patient learns both that the stimulus or context is not harmful and that the negative affect they experience will eventually subside. The inhibitory learning model hypothesizes that through repeated exposures to a stimulus or context that evokes negative affect, safety learning begins to occur and compete with danger learning, and ultimately is able to inhibit danger learning associated with the stimulus or context (Becker, Farrell, & Waller, 2019). Second, it is important to note the circumstances under which exposures are an appropriate intervention. Exposures are intended to reduce unwanted, dysfunctional emotional reactions to a situation. They are not intended to reduce functional emotions even if they are unpleasant, like fear when faced with a legitimately dangerous situation or sadness experienced after the recent death of a loved one. Third, it is important to highlight that a common action urge in response to facing an exposure is to avoid the exposure, whether physically or mentally. Patients may notice urges to distract themselves during exposures or urges to terminate the exposure early. It is critical to provide education that these actions are likely to result in the exposure being ineffective and in some cases, engaging in these behaviors may actually make the patient feel worse than before. Thus, it is important that when a patient commits to doing an exposure, they are committing to do the exposure all the way. Finally, it can be helpful to discuss with patients that not only are we wanting them to be fully present during exposures, both mentally and physically, we also want them to be cognizant of how they are expressing their emotions outwardly. During exposures, an additional goal for patients is to display facial expressions and body postures that are incongruent with the emotion they are experiencing. For example, a patient who is experiencing intense fear may have urges to curl up as tightly as possible. The goal in this circumstance would be for them to be able to remain fully present, both mentally and physically with the stimulus or context that is evoking fear, while also maintaining an open and relaxed body posture.

Once you have oriented your patient to exposure-based procedures and obtained their buy-in around engaging with exposures, it can be helpful to create a comprehensive graded exposure hierarchy. The clinical potency of this step can be enhanced through multidisciplinary collaboration, in that providers of each discipline may have input about exposures that are relevant to their work with a specific patient. Understanding graded exposure hierarchies is typically a bit easier when you have a visual to work from, so let's take a peek at Megan's multidisciplinary graded exposure hierarchy.

On the next page, you will see an example of Megan's graded exposure hierarchy as it looked later in treatment. She initially created the first draft of an exposure hierarchy in session with her dietitian, Claire. This assignment came up naturally as Megan and Claire sat down to menu together for the upcoming

Table 16.2 Megan's Multidisciplinary Graded Exposure Hierarchy

Extremely Challenging	• Clothing shopping by myself (especially right after a meal) • Going out to dinner with the calories on the menu • Wearing tight-fitting clothing • Fast food drive-thru (especially places with burgers and milkshakes) • Halloween candy (candy corn) • Birthday Cake (yellow kind with chocolate frosting) • Thanksgiving foods (all) • Lasagna and other casseroles, my aunt's mac and cheese
Moderately Challenging	• Clothing shopping at the mall with my mom • Pizza, especially with thick crust • Beef cheeseburgers with the bun • Going out to dinner with my friends, appetizers • Restaurants that don't have calories on the menu • Mexican food such as tacos, burritos, chips and salsa • Full fat salad dressing • Fast food, going inside and ordering • Eating on campus, eating at work – eating around other people in general • Surprise meals and snacks that I don't plan for • Gas station food and road-trip food • Family-sized bags of snacks • Caloric beverages, especially lattes • Chocolate bars with lots of fillings • Eating any meal with my extended family • Wearing yoga pants, leggings, dresses
Easy	• Meals that are less than 200 calories • Black coffee, water, sparkling water and calorie-free flavor drops, artificial sweeteners • Sugar-free ice pops, fat free ice cream and peanut butter, fat free dairy and cottage cheese • Baked potato chips (not regular) • Eating by myself • Wearing baggier clothes like sweatpants, shopping for clothing online • Lean protein (fish that is baked, chicken without breading) • Eggs without the yolk • Smoothie bowls, avocado toast • When things go as planned and I feel in control • When I bring my own food to a friend's house • Fruits and vegetables generally OK (not the starchy kind) • Salad with dressing on the side, especially fat free dressing

Table 16.3 First Draft of Megan's Multidisciplinary Graded Exposure Hierarchy

Extremely Challenging (Absolutely Not Gonna Happen)	• Cake • Max and Cheese • Milkshakes
Moderately Challenging (Sometimes, Maybe)	• Pizza • Salad Dressing • Mexican food
Easy (Usually Fine)	• Diet soft drinks • Water (depending on how I am feeling about my weight, sometimes even water is scary)

week and Claire noticed that Megan continued to refuse to plan many different food items, becoming argumentative and tearful at times. Claire was mindful of the value of incremental exposure to challenges and asked Megan to work with her in creating a "fear food hierarchy." The first draft of this hierarchy can be seen above.

As you can see, the first draft of the hierarchy is sparse and vague in comparison to the final draft you previously reviewed. With the support of a patient's team, exposure hierarchies can evolve to include pertinent details that lead to highly specific exposures. In this case, Megan's dietitian and therapist worked alongside Megan to enhance the richness of her hierarchy, adding additional context and expanding beyond just food to include exposures focused on body image-related concerns as well. If you refer back to the final hierarchy, you'll see that "clothing shopping at the mall, especially with my mom" and "clothing shopping by myself, right after a meal" fall in two very different places in Megan's hierarchy. Exposures that you don't see listed in Megan's graded exposure hierarchy that may also be appropriate for patients diagnosed with eating disorders include weight-related exposures, interoceptive exposures, movement-related exposures, perfectionism-related exposures, emotion-related exposures, and exposures related to various diagnostic comorbidities for which exposures are appropriate interventions (e.g. substance use disorders, generalized anxiety disorder, posttraumatic stress disorder).

After completing the first comprehensive draft of the graded exposure hierarchy, it should be shared with the rest of the multidisciplinary team as there is usually clinical relevance across all disciplines, both in terms of exposures that may be more relevant to one discipline than others (e.g. exposures related to perfectionism or social anxiety), as well as exposures where multidisciplinary collaboration may be particularly beneficial. For example, Megan may recall "eating a muffin" as very challenging nutritionally due to the calorie and fat content. However when asked to explore further, she's able to differentiate "eating a muffin whole" as markedly more challenging than eating it by crumbling it, cutting it into smaller pieces, or using a fork because she believes that eating a muffin whole will result in her having crumbs on her face. Unpacking this even further, Megan shares that she has fears that others will perceive her as "messy" and judge her for being "gluttonous." This example speaks to the importance of therapist and dietitian collaboration in both planning and post-processing an exposure like this one.

There are a number of elements involved in successful implementation of exposure-based procedures. First, the exposure-based procedure must involve non-reinforced exposure to the stimuli that evoke the emotion the patient wants to change. To understand better what this means, let's take a look at a couple of examples. If a patient is planning to do an exposure involving going to an ice cream shop to eat an ice cream sundae, which is one of their fear foods, it is critical that they actually complete the ice cream sundae as planned. In the event that they go to the ice cream store and purchase the ice cream sundae, but either don't complete the ice cream sundae or complete the sundae and then purge immediately afterward, no new corrective information has been introduced. The ice cream sundae still remains a stimulus to be feared. This is why being thoughtful about graded exposures is so critical. For this patient, an ice cream sundae exposure may be too far up on their graded exposure hierarchy, however something like having a small scoop of ice cream with no toppings might be an exposure they are capable of doing that would help them progress toward being able to successfully complete an ice cream sundae exposure. Another situation that commonly arises in the treatment of eating disorders is that a patient communicates that they feel guilty asking others for support. Before tasking a patient with completing an exposure of asking for help to target their guilt, it can be important to assess how their supports have responded to them asking for help previously. If their supports have responded by unfavorably, like directly or indirectly communicating that they are "needy" or "a burden," having them complete an exposure where these responses are likely to occur again will probably result in increased guilt when asking for support in the future.

The next element involved in successful exposure-based procedures is ensuring the patient is actually engaging with the exposure. Continuing with the ice cream sundae example, if a patient is watching a distracting video on their phone or using another tactic to pull the majority of their attention away from the experience of eating the ice cream sundae, they are not likely to see a significant reduction in their anxiety in response to ice cream sundaes. Thinking back to graded exposure hierarchies, it could be that an initial planned exposure involves some distraction, like completing the ice cream sundae exposure with a friend who can keep the patient engaged in conversation. However for anxiety to decrease more substantially over time, the patient will need to work up toward exposures where their attention is more present with the feared stimulus.

The final element necessary for successful exposure-based procedures is blocking the patient from engaging in behaviors associated with the action urges they have in response to the emotion elicited by the exposure. For example, if the patient has a history of purging after eating ice cream sundaes as a method of decreasing the intense anxiety they feel when exposed to this stimulus, it is critical that you plan with your patient how they will cope ahead with urges to purge that arise. If they are someone who experiences the emotion of guilt in response to completing their ice cream sundae, it is important to help them plan for how they will block both overt actions, like engaging in self-injurious behavior, as well as covert actions, like engaging in caustic self-talk, as methods of self-punishment.

Next, we wanted to provide a clinical example of how preparation for an exposure might look in session. In this example, our patient is planning to eat with their family for the first time since treatment started, in a restaurant that specializes in New York style pizza slices, which is a big fear food for them. Here's how dialogue might look between the dietitian and patient in preparation for this exposure.

Dietitian: "So if I'm not mistaken, tonight you'll be going to the pizza place with your parents, right? That's pretty high on your exposure hierarchy!"

Patient: "Ugh. Don't remind me."

Dietitian: "Let's take a moment and talk about it. Tell me what it's going to be like."

Patient: "This is a place we always went to as kids, every birthday, every celebration. Most Fridays nights we ended up at this pizza place. The slices are enormous. It's New York style, whatever that means. The slices are bigger than my face and they add way too much cheese."

Dietitian: "Keep going. What will tonight be like?"

Patient: "Well, the owners know my parents and they always put us at the same booth, right near the window. It's downtown so everyone who walks by can see us. So yeah, I expect we'll be there. And they always give us free garlic knots when we sit down at the table. My parents will ask a million questions about my treatment and eating disorder and will undoubtedly make comments on my body. They'll also keep a close eye on me to make sure that I eat everything that's on my plate. It's going to be terrible."

Dietitian: "What are you anticipating is going to happen? What's the outcome you're afraid of?"

Patient: "...I'm afraid I'm going to eat it all. The garlic knots, the large pizza slices. I'll eat it and then feel terrible about myself. Also because of the location of the table, people will see me eating those big slices."

Dietitian: "What do you feel you won't be able to manage?"

Patient: "I can't sit with the fullness and disgust of that and not purge."

Dietitian: "Sounds like this is going to be a great exposure for you, completing the meal and tolerating the fullness while not acting on anxiety reduction techniques, like restriction or purging. I know this sounds really scary and I'm confident this is a great next step in helping to reduce anxiety, disgust, and shame long-term."

Now let's take a look at what post-processing this exposure might look like in a dialogue between the patient and her therapist.

Therapist: "So talk to me about how the pizza exposure went for you this week…"

Patient: "So I had the pizza that we talked about, as well as the garlic knot that we planned, even though I really didn't want to have it because it was over my exchanges."

Therapist: "I'm so proud of you! I know the garlic knot was above your exchanges and making the choice to eat garlic knots with your family is a completely normative thing to do. And it sounds like your fear of starting to eat and not being able to stop really didn't materialize. I know that you also mentioned that you were worried about other people watching you while you eat. How did that piece of the exposure go?"

Patient: "There were definitely a lot of people walking by the window the whole time we were there, since it was a Friday night, but most of them didn't even look in the restaurant. Even the people who did glance in didn't really seem to be looking at me specifically. More just looking into the restaurant in a non-focused sort of way."

Therapist: "So what did you learn from that element of the exposure?"

Patient: "I guess that people probably aren't paying as much attention to me specifically as I might think? It's not that I think people didn't see me eating. But I don't really think they thought anything after that, one way or another."

Therapist: "That sounds like a pretty accurate observation to me. So talk to me about the fears that you had about sitting with fullness and disgust without purging. How did that aspect of the exposure go?"

Patient: "So I definitely did feel incredibly full at first and felt a lot of disgust, but I was able to manage sitting with those feelings and didn't purge. And I will say that both the sense of fullness and sense of disgust went away quicker than I thought they would. When we were driving back home, the feelings were still there, but they weren't as intense."

Therapist: "I'm so glad you noticed that! You'll find that as we continue to do more exposures, these feelings will decrease both in terms of their intensity, as well as how long they tend to last. Speaking of, I know we've talked in the past about the importance of repeating exposures with different variations to help with safety learning. What do you think could be a good next step in terms of an exposure from your perspective?"

Patient: "I'm not thrilled about this as an idea, but I do think it could make sense for me to go back and do the same meal, but this time alone."

Before elaborating on specific exposures that might be helpful for Megan, we'd like to share a few additional tips for conducting effective exposures, beyond those mentioned above (Becker, Farrell, & Waller, 2019). In terms of intensity and pace of exposures, it is important to start with exposures that are as intense as your patient can tolerate and to move through exposures as rapidly as your patient is willing. While this may increase your patient's distress in the short-term, this can help with seeing positive outcomes materialize more rapidly and it also conveys the message that while distressing, exposures are not dangerous. Adding to the complexity of exposures can also assist with the pace of exposures by combining numerous exposures together. For example, if I have a patient who would benefit from exposures to eating in a college dining hall, wearing form-fitting clothing, and eating with friends, they could do an exposure where they eat in a college dining hall with friends while wearing form-fitting athletic clothes.

To help achieve more durable and robust results with exposures, it is also important to vary the stimuli and contexts to which a client is exposed. For example, if a client has a fear of consuming burgers and the only exposure you have them do around this fear is to go to the same restaurant and order the same burger over and over again, the learning that has occurred is not as robust as it likely will be if you have them vary stimuli and contexts. For example, you might have them try burgers with different ingredients (e.g. adding bacon, pimiento cheese, or a fancy aioli) from different types of establishments (e.g. a fast food restaurant, a fast casual restaurant, a high-end steakhouse) or in different contexts (e.g. eating a burger in their car, eating a burger at home, or eating a burger at a backyard cookout).

Lastly, exposures should resemble situations patients will encounter in the real world as closely as possible. This includes making some aspects of exposures unplanned over the course of time. For example, if you are working with a patient who has numerous fast food restaurants they avoid, all of which they would benefit from exposures to, you may have them put all of the restaurants' names on pieces of paper and place them in a hat and then randomly select a restaurant thirty minutes before their scheduled meal time. This mimics situations patients are likely to encounter in real life. For example, if a patient is doing a road trip through a rural area and makes plans to go to a restaurant and finds that restaurant is closed, they need to have the ability to meet their nutritional needs with whatever options are available, even if these options are limited and non-preferred.

Bringing DBT to Life – Exposure-Based Procedures for Megan

Revisiting Megan and her graded exposure hierarchy, we thought it could be helpful to provide some examples of specific exposures under broad categories that Megan might complete, in addition to showing how a provider-focused worksheet could be used to guide planning an exposure with Megan. You'll have an opportunity to complete this worksheet as well!

Some examples of broad categories of exposures, followed by specific examples of exposures, can be seen below:

1. *Eating around other people*: For Megan, the fear of eating around other people is partly driven by a fear of being perceived as gluttonous, messy, dirty, and out of control. Megan has also expressed concern that "if [my] friends or family see me eating, they'll think [I'm] doing better than I actually am, so I'd rather eat alone." Some sequenced exposures related to eating around other people could include:

   a. Having Megan eat safer food while on video chat with family or friends (if conducted more than once, consider varying which family members or friends are present)
   b. Having Megan eat a messy challenge food while on video chat with family or friends (if conducted more than once, consider varying the messy challenge food and/or which family members or friends are present)
   c. Having Megan eat a safer food at a dining hall (if conducted more than once, consider varying the dining hall)
   d. Having Megan eat a messy challenge food in a dining hall (if conducted more than once, consider varying the messy challenge food and/or dining hall)
   e. Having Megan eat a messy challenge food while no one else is eating (if conducted more than once, consider varying the messy challenge food and/or context in which the exposure is conducted)

2. *Eating when I don't have a plan:* Megan reports needing a plan for upcoming meals and snacks, as this helps her feel in control and allows her to plan in foods she feels comfortable eating and to avoid challenges she anticipates

encountering. Some sequenced exposure related to unplanned eating could include:

    a. Providing Megan an unplanned component of her meal (if conducted more than once, vary the types of foods that are unplanned)

    b. Providing Megan an entirely unplanned snack (if conducted more than once, vary the contexts in which the snack is completed)

    c. Providing Megan an entirely unplanned meal (if conducted more than once, vary the context in which the meal is unplanned)

    d. Having Megan navigate meeting nutritional needs at a potluck without gathering information about the food that will be served in advance

    e. Having Megan navigate meeting nutritional needs at a large buffet without gathering information about the food served at the buffet in advance

    f. Having Megan navigate meeting nutritional needs while on a road trip without researching options available in advance

3. *Clothing shopping when I'm feeling full:* Megan avoids clothing shopping at all costs, especially when she is feeling full and bloated following a meal. She reports the fullness leads to intolerable body image distress and a desire to avoid her body.

    a. Having Megan go to the mall and eat a meal and then browse clothes without trying anything on (if conducted more than once, consider varying how challenging the meal is)

    b. Having Megan go to the mall and eat a meal and try on a less distressing clothing item (if conducted more than once, consider varying how challenging the meal is)

    c. Having Megan go to the mall and eat a meal and try on difficult clothing items (if conducted more than once, consider varying how challenging the meal is)

    d. Having Megan go to the mall, eat a meal, try on clothes, and then ask another person for feedback about the clothes (if conducted more than once, consider varying how challenging the meal is, what clothing items are tried, and/or who is asked for feedback)

    e. Having Megan go to the mall, eat a meal, try on clothes, purchase a clothing item, and then wear that clothing item while continuing to shop

4. *Uncertainty in general, especially around food:* Megan has always had difficulty tolerating uncertainty and often seeks information to reassure her, even when the feared outcome is low. In general, exposures to uncertainty are broad and lend themselves to multidisciplinary intervention.

    a. Having Megan practice tolerance of not knowing when her next provider session is (only applicable at higher levels of care)

b. Having Megan sit with a new food with nutrition information hidden
c. Having Megan attempt a new food with nutrition information hidden
d. Having Megan do an unplanned activity
e. Having Megan go out to a meal with friends and allow them to pick the restaurant and food that is ordered

Now that you've seen some examples of exposures Megan might participate in, we will use the below questions to show how you might implement this exposure.

1. *What is the exposure you would like to implement?*

Having Megan go to the mall, eat a meal, try on clothes, and then ask another person for feedback about the clothes.

2. *In what ways could you vary this exposure to enhance safety learning? How could you vary the features of the feared stimulus or context? What exposures could you combine with this one?*

Having Megan do this exposure multiple times and vary the cuisines she is consuming for the meal, the types of clothes she is trying on (including having her to try on clothes that are form-fitting and/or that she is likely to experience as somewhat uncomfortable when feeling bloated or full), or the types of people she is asking for feedback. This exposure could lend itself well to being done in combination with various food-related exposures (e.g. exposure to a fear food).

3. *What safety signals might you need to be on the lookout for? What avoidance or safety behaviors do you think your patient might have urges to engage in? How will you address safety signals, avoidance behaviors, and safety behaviors in the context of planning this exposure with your client?*

I would want to make sure Megan wasn't carrying any medications with her that she could use to reduce the sensation of bloating or fullness. In terms of avoidance behaviors and safety behaviors, I would want to make sure that Megan mindfully consumed her meal, wore reasonably fitting clothes (versus very loose clothes, which might lessen the intensity of sensations of fullness or bloating), and tried on clothing in a slow and intentional fashion, including spending time mindfully observing the fit of the clothing in a mirror. I would also want to make sure that Megan avoided asking reassurance-focused questions about the appearance of the clothing on her body (e.g. "Does this pair of jeans make me look fat?"). Given that this is not likely an exhaustive list of safety signals, avoidance behaviors, and safety behaviors that might be relevant for this exposure, I would want to ask Megan for her thoughts on this as well and then cope ahead for how she was going to navigate urges to utilize safety signals, avoidance behaviors, and safety behaviors.

4. *What sorts of topics might you want to discuss with your client in the context of post-processing the exposure?*

Prior to engaging in the exposure, I would want to talk with Megan about anticipated feared outcomes of the exposure and then when post-processing, talk about whether those feared outcomes occurred. I'd also like to discuss with Megan what she learned based on her experience and what she feels would be a good next exposure to build upon this one.

*Adapted from Graves & Kalata (2021)

Provider Exercise – Creating a Graded Exposure Hierarchy and Planning an Exposure

Using the graded hierarchy tool on the next page, create a graded exposure hierarchy for a patient with whom you have worked or are currently working. Remember that the creation of a graded exposure hierarchy should be a collaborative process, however we have found value in providers practicing creating them independently as a method of learning. Consider discussing your graded exposure hierarchy (ensuring it is appropriately de-identified) with a trusted peer for feedback.

Now that you've completed a graded exposure hierarchy, use the below questions to help you in planning an exposure to one of the stimuli or contexts listed, regardless of whether you plan to implement this exposure with a client. Consider discussing your planned exposure with a trusted peer for feedback.

1. *What is the exposure you would like to implement?*

2. *In what ways could you vary this exposure to enhance safety learning? How could you vary the features of the feared stimulus or context? What exposures could you combine with this one?*

3. *What safety signals might you need to be on the lookout for? What avoidance or safety behaviors do you think your patient might have urges to engage in? How will you address safety signals, avoidance behaviors, and safety behaviors in the context of planning this exposure with your client?*

4. *What sorts of topics might you want to discuss with your client in the context of post-processing the exposure?*

*Adapted from Graves & Kalata (2021)

Table 16.4 Graded Exposure Hiearchy Exercise

Exposure		Subjective Units of Distress (SUDS)

Cognitive Modification Procedures

Cognitive modification procedures (originally outlined in Linehan, 1993, pp. 358–370) are a set of both acceptance-based and change-based approaches for addressing cognitions that are impeding a patient's ability to move toward their goals and their life worth living. In general, cognitive modification procedures are focused on altering the content, form, and style of a patient's thinking. DBT is specifically concerned with cognitions that have a causal or mediating impact with regard to target behaviors. For example, if the thought, "I'm so fat and don't deserve this food" results in intense shame followed by restriction, this might be a cognition that is worth targeting. While this is an example of a cognition as a relevant antecedent to a behavior, there are also instances in which a cognition that occurs after a behavior may also be relevant in the maintenance of that behavior. For example, if a patient engages in self-injurious behavior after completing a meal and has the thought, "That was a good enough punishment for losing control and eating" and subsequently the emotion of shame sharply declines, this also might be cognition to target in order to reduce the likelihood of self-injurious behavior after completing meals in the future.

The first step in conducting any form of cognitive modification procedures is teaching patients how to observe and describe their thoughts. For many patients with eating disorders, their thoughts (especially those related to their eating disorder), are experienced as intense and unrelenting. In order to offer up the possibility of changing their thoughts or altering how they relate to their thoughts, patients first need to be able to establish enough space between themselves and their thoughts to notice and describe their thoughts as such. Although this may sound like a relatively easy task, it is not one to be underestimated. As part of teaching patients this component of cognitive modification procedures, it can be helpful to discuss specifically how they envision observing and describing their thoughts and perhaps even practicing this task in session. It can also be helpful to incorporate written self-monitoring into this process, through actions like including a space for thought recording on the patient's diary card or encouraging them to complete a supplemental handout or writing assignment focused on recording thoughts that come up for them throughout the day or week.

Once a patient has begun to develop the skill of observing and describing their thoughts, this opens up the possibility for the provider and patient to begin to identify, confront, challenge, and modify maladaptive cognitions that arise, with specific attention paid to non-dialectical thinking, faulty rules that influence behavior, inaccurate descriptions, and dysfunctional allocations of attention. One important aspect of this piece of cognitive modification procedures is approaching this process in a nuanced fashion. The goal of discussions around maladaptive cognitions is not to prove a patient "wrong," but rather to create space for a patient to consider other cognitive approaches that may be more adaptive and consistent with their long-term goals and life worth living. This often requires a dance between irreverence and confrontation and warmth and validation. It is important to note that our patients' behaviors often must shift before making substantial changes in their thinking become feasible. For example, challenging a patient's belief that they are not deserving of kindness and self-compassion is going to be awfully hard to do if they are actively engaging in behaviors like self-injurious behavior or saying nasty things to themselves that are wholly inconsistent with kindness and self-compassion. It is also important to remember that our patients' belief systems have often developed over the course of years and may have been or still may be being reinforced by their environment. The take-home point here is that it is important to be patient when targeting patients' thoughts and beliefs. Let's take a look at different types of thinking that may arise for patients and approaches one can take to target this thinking.

Examples of Non-Dialectical Thinking

Non-dialectical thinking refers to thinking that falls at extreme ends of a spectrum, like black-and-white thinking or always-never thinking. In the example below, the therapist is working with a patient diagnosed with Anorexia Nervosa – Restricting Type, who is very concerned about eating "healthy" and who struggles with understanding that foods of all types can be an appropriate part of one's diet. She is also very rigid with portioning, such that she only portions the bare minimum amount of food required by her meal plan.

Therapist:	"So, I'm noticing that it doesn't look like you completed the loaded tots challenge you had planned with your dietitian this week. It seems like you've been avoiding challenges like this one a lot lately."
Patient:	"Yeah…I guess I just don't know what's normal in terms of when you'd allow yourself those types of meals versus when you'd just eat something else. And I'm afraid that if I eat it and actually like it or feel hungry, that I'm completely going to lose control."
Therapist (said in a playful manner with a slightly irreverent facial expression):	"Okay, we've been working together for a while now…can you think of one single instance where you've actually lost control?"
Patient:	"No, although to be fair, I haven't actually tried this exposure. So I don't know if I would lose control or not."
Therapist:	"Totally valid point. And doing the exposure is the only way we'll get to the bottom of this. So can we talk about what it's going to take to get this to happen this upcoming week?"

In this next example, we have a patient diagnosed with Anorexia Nervosa – Restricting Type who is being seen in the outpatient setting and who is concerned with how she will be perceived by others for the choices around foods that she makes. At the time of the encounter with her dietitian, the patient is avoiding all foods that are processed, including minimally processed foods, and instead she is choosing to make everything from scratch.

Dietitian:	"I'm reviewing your food logs… and I have an observation. Mind if I share?"
Patient:	"Go for it. What's up?"
Dietitian:	"It looks like everything you've eaten in the last three to four weeks has been homemade."
Patient:	"Yeah! I make everything from scratch."
Dietitian:	"Wow…you even noted your granola bars are homemade. What's up with that?"
Patient:	"I don't buy processed food."
Dietitian:	"Huh, really? What's that about?"
Patient:	"Lazy people eat processed food. And I don't want to be seen as lazy."

Dietitian: "Tell me more about that."

Patient: "I don't buy into the big food industry. I have my own garden and I grow a lot of my own herbs and vegetables."

Dietitian: "Don't you think there's a time and a place for convenience products? Sometimes life is just too busy to make homemade granola bars!"

Patient: "People who can't find time to prioritize eating from scratch, knowing and sourcing all ingredients, are lazy. It's really not that hard. I take pride in the fact that I only buy raw ingredients from the grocery store."

Dietitian: "I'm really curious about this lazy piece. You literally can't think of someone who eats processed foods who *isn't* lazy?"

Patient: "Nope, can you?"

Dietitian: "Actually, I can think of hundreds of people."

Patient: "Really?"

Dietitian: "Sure! I know the Olympics just wrapped up, and I guarantee you most Olympic athletes are not making their own granola bars. Nor is someone making homemade granola bars for them! And while I can't say that I know the ins-and-outs of the day-to-day dietary choices of CEOs and the like, I have a hunch that their diets include processed foods as a component of what they eat..."

Patient: "I mean, so maybe not *everyone* who has processed foods is lazy. I just think *I* would be lazy if I started turning to processed foods. I've been doing this for years. I can't stop now and eat some packaged junk. That's *not* who I am. It goes against my values."

Dietitian: "If I had to guess, this black-and-white thinking is likely tied into your eating disorder. I do think it's worth further exploration and goal-setting to help you live more in the 'gray,' like someone who occasionally eats convenience foods. I know this is probably a hard sell and I'm wondering if you'd be willing to dig into this a bit further?"

Patient: "Not promising I'll be making any changes, but sure, we can chat about it more."

Examples of Faulty Rules That Influence Behavior

Now let's take a look at some examples of faulty rules influencing patient behavior.

Patient: (in the context of a larger discussion about ambivalence around giving up restriction) "I can just go back to restriction without engaging in other behaviors and be fine."

Therapist: (therapist has knowledge that patient's restriction has then led to subsequent binge/purge/restrict cycles that patient is motivated to stop) "Is that *actually* the case?"

Patient: "Yeah, I'm sure I can do it. It'll be fine."

Therapist: "Can we take a step back and see what history tells us?"

Patient: "Sure."

Therapist: "Walk me through how you ended up relapsing and returning to treatment this go round."

Patient: "Well, I started 'eating healthier' a few months after I left PHP last time and then I started restricting afternoon snacks because I felt like I didn't really need them. And that went on for a while and things were okay."

Therapist: "...and then?"

Patient: "And then I started restricting more and more and then I started to purge when I was eating and then eventually I started bingeing, too."

Therapist: "Okay, so what does history tell us?"

Patient: "That I really can't just engage in restricting. But I really want to. It's just not fair."

Therapist: "I recognize that even the thought of giving up restriction is hard and you've shared with me that you absolutely don't want to go back to bingeing and purging. I imagine that if we continue to work on targeting your restriction that the thought, 'I can just restrict and things will be fine' is going to come up. I'm wondering if you have any ideas about how you might challenge that thought when it does arise?"

Patient: "Well, I'm zero for three in terms of just restricting and not returning to other behaviors. So I guess I could remind myself that it's looking like the data is not just a coincidence at this point."

Dietitian: "I see that you've been underportioning a lot of your meals and snacks this past week."

Patient: "You said that I was getting close to being fully weight restored last week and so I worried that if my portions were accurate and I reached my EBW and I was still on this meal plan and I didn't see you until until today that I would go way over my EBW." (patient slowly begins to crack a smile as she says all of this out loud)

Dietitian: "I see that you started to smile. Tell me what you're thinking."

Patient: "...I get how this must sound, now that I'm saying it out loud."

Dietitian: "Okay, so what does your wise mind say might actually be more true than what you just shared?"

Patient: "It's taken me so long and has taken such a big meal plan just to get me close to my EBW that there is no way I could possibly go that much over my EBW in just a few days."

Dietitian: "Exactly what I was thinking."

Examples of Inaccurate Descriptions

In this first example of inaccurate descriptions, a therapist is working with a patient diagnosed with Bulimia Nervosa who is in college and who eats most of her meals in the dormitory cafeteria with her friends. She has been extremely reluctant to incorporate desserts into her diet. She had come up with a plan with her dietitian to eat a dessert as part of her dinner each day this week, however she has been struggling with following through on this plan.

Therapist: "I know that you made a plan with Sarah to have dessert with dinner every day this week and I'm noticing that hasn't yet happened. Care to share what's going on?"

Patient: "It's not that I haven't thought about it. But you know I do not eat desserts."

Therapist: "I know that this would be a big change for you. Help me understand what's getting in the way."

Patient: "Well, since I never eat desserts, it would be weird for me to suddenly start eating them. I know my friends are going to notice."

Therapist: "You know your friends are going to notice, and...?"

Patient: "...and I think they are going to think I'm gluttonous and out of control. Like, who eats a dessert with dinner every day?"

Therapist: "There are so many directions we could go here, but let's start with your friends. Assuming that they do notice a change in what it is that you're having for dinner, are there other things they might think besides that you are gluttonous and out of control?"

Patient: "I mean, I guess they could notice and just not really think much of anything at all. Like, 'Oh, that's a change?' and then just kind of move on from there. I guess maybe for me it feels gluttonous and out of control, or at least maybe that's what my eating disorder wants me to think, so it's hard not to imagine that others wouldn't think the same."

Therapist: "I can totally understand your brain taking things in that direction and having a dessert as part of dinner is a completely normative thing. I wonder if there is something you can tell yourself when you notice thoughts about what your friends might be thinking come up?"

Patient: "I'm not totally convinced that they wouldn't be having thoughts that I'm gluttonous and out of control and I know my eating disorder wants me to think that they are thinking those things. I guess where I could land is that I really don't know what they are thinking and it's genuinely possible they are thinking nothing at all."

In this second example of inaccurate descriptions, a dietitian is working with a patient to plan a meal that includes a serving of lasagna as part of the meal.

Patient: "There is no way I am going to eat this meal. This is a *massive* amount of food that is *totally* over my exchanges. Not happening."

Dietitian: "Let's slow it down for a moment. What's in the lasagna?"

Patient: (patient pushes food around with fork) "Looks like those long noodles, and cheese. So much cheese. And meat sauce. But seriously, the cheese alone is more calories than my entire meal plan."

Dietitian: "Haha...I doubt it. Pasta, cheese and meat sauce...all foods you've been successful with! What makes this different?"

Patient: "Yeah, but when it's all together it's *so much*. It's overflowing with cheese and sauce and more than my exchanges. It's got to be at least 800 calories per slice. What is that, like 8 starches and 14 fat exchanges?"

Dietitian: "It's not, actually. What I love most about this meal is it meets all of your exchanges! It has it all...starches, proteins, vegetables, fats. Plus, it's a food you used to eat before the eating disorder, so there's lots of positive memories. You're good to go."

Patient: "Promise it's not too much?"

Dietitian: "I think it's a perfect option for lunch."

Example of Dysfunctional Allocations of Attention

Finally, let's take a look at an example of dysfunctional allocations of attention.

Therapist: (speaking with a patient who was returning to campus after a residential treatment stay that required weight restoration) "So how did your first day back on campus go?"

Patient: "Well, I got to see one of my good friends and even though she didn't mention anything about my weight, I know what she was thinking."

Therapist: "What are you imagining that she was thinking?"

Patient: "That I had put on a *lot* of weight. And that I am unattractive. I imagine it was jarring."

Therapist: "Hmm...what gave you that impression?"

Patient: "Well, when we were first walking up to each other on campus and she was starting to say hello, I feel like she awkwardly paused once we got up closer. And I caught her looking at my body a couple of times."

Therapist: "Is there any other evidence that supports your hypothesis that she was having a lot of judgmental thoughts about your appearance?"

Patient: "I mean, none I can really think of."

Therapist: "Well, what was the rest of the conversation like?"

Patient:	"She seemed really happy to see me. We mainly just talked about school stuff…what classes we were taking, things we're excited about this semester."
Therapist:	"Huh. So it sounds like the conversation went really well. Can I take a step back and share with you what I'm noticing?"
Patient:	"Sure."
Therapist:	"So it sounds like there were a few moments where you are convinced that your friend was having some really judgmental thoughts about your appearance, and I'm noticing that the conversation as a whole went well and that your friend didn't verbally acknowledge your appearance at all. You know, I'm wondering if there are any alternative interpretations you can think of that might account for her awkward pause and these moments where you think she was looking at your body?"
Patient:	"I mean, I guess it's always weird when you haven't seen someone in a while. So maybe it was just weird to see me after a few months away. And maybe she was looking at my body, but wasn't necessarily thinking bad things about it."
Therapist:	"What other things do you think she could have been thinking?"
Patient:	"I mean, maybe that I actually look healthier. Or maybe just neutral things. Maybe she was actually thinking my body *hadn't* changed much or just noticing something else, like the clothes I was wearing or something."
Therapist:	"I think those are all potentially valid interpretations, too. What are you thinking now that we're looking back on that experience together?"
Patient:	"I don't know. It's definitely possible she was thinking other things. And I don't think she would want to be hurtful toward me. It's just hard to believe other people don't notice all these changes that have happened, because I definitely notice them."
Therapist:	"I totally get that. It's hard not to assume that others aren't having a similar reaction to the changes you've experienced because they definitely feel noticeable to you and you're definitely having a lot of judgments about them."

A Brief Word on Cognitive Modification Approaches From Other Empirically-Supported Treatments for Eating Disorders

For those of you who are familiar with other empirically-supported treatments for eating disorders, you may be wondering the extent to which cognitive elements of these treatments fit within a DBT framework. Perhaps the most empirically-supported treatment with cognitive components is CBT-E and the cognitive interventions within this treatment (e.g. addressing dietary rules, targeting overvaluation of weight, shape, and size) dovetail quite nicely with DBT cognitive modification procedures. Because DBT was not originally developed for the treatment of eating disorders, many of the foundational texts do not provide guidance around the application of cognitive modification procedures to eating disorder-related content. As such, it can be useful to review the cognitive interventions from these other treatment approaches and consider the ways in which these elements fit within a DBT framework.

Bringing DBT to Life – Cognitive Modification Procedures With Megan

While in treatment at a Residential level of care, Megan and her dietitian (Claire) have worked to create a fear food hierarchy. At the top of the list is a bagel sandwich; specifically, bacon, egg, and cheese on an everything bagel. Megan has acknowledged that she has many good memories with this food, including eating it out of the back of her dad's station wagon while watching the sun rise and driving her high school friends to the local bagel shop when she got her learner's permit. Like many things in her life, Megan's eating disorder took away the joy of this food, beginning in the form of restriction. She remembered when she calculated the total calories in this sandwich and exclaimed to Claire during a session, "There's like, 800 calories in one of those!" Once Megan had calculated the number of calories in the bagel sandwich, this led to her avoiding this food for many years, and instead opting to get a black coffee when she would go to the bagel shop with her friends. A few years later, the bagel sandwich became one of Megan's primary binge foods. In a recent session with Claire, she noted that she would often get two to three bagel sandwiches and binge and purge on Sunday mornings.

Claire has been working alongside Megan and coaching her with her fear foods and Megan has experienced a reduction in negative affect associated with previously feared foods. Lasagna, pizza, and cheeseburgers, all of which were extremely challenging foods at the start of treatment, are now foods she is successfully completing. However, Megan has stated that she feels that the bagel sandwich is outside of what she has the capacity to complete and has noted that she believes eating even half of a bagel sandwich would lead to purging. Let's take a look at a dialogue between Megan and Claire where Claire applies various cognitive modification procedures:

Megan (in the context of discussing a possible bagel sandwich exposure):	"There's something about that bagel sandwich...I just can't do it. It's not going to end well. The volume, the textures, the carbs...it's not going to happen. Even thinking about it is making me anxious."

Claire:	"So let me get this straight…you're okay having the foods separately…scrambled, cheesy eggs, bacon…but eaten together is a no-go."
Megan:	"Yes… I know my eating disorder logic is ridiculous, but it's a *completely* different thing. A bagel sandwich is the single most overwhelming food I can think of in this moment."
Claire:	"Hm… okay. Walk me through it…so, you regularly eat cheesy eggs…"
Megan:	"…almost every morning."
Claire:	"Right! And on the weekends, you plate bacon and sausage from the buffet and you eat it…"
Megan:	"Yes. Like I said, I know it makes no sense."
Claire:	"And I know you've had a bagel at least once in treatment because we ate it together in session! But for some reason, if you put it all together it's too much. Help me understand why?"
Megan:	"It's so condensed. High calorie. It's all mixed together, so it would take me like, five minutes to eat it. And it's just so many calories. I'd much rather eat those exact foods separately. Also, if I ate all of my exchanges that quickly, I would look and feel gluttonous. And I might want to eat even more because everyone at my table would still be eating and I would be sitting in front of an empty plate. So it would feel binge-y. I would be full and anxious and calorie counting everything I had just eaten in a few bites. That, plus the high associations of the meal would make me want to purge."
Claire:	"I really appreciate you talking me through all of that. I can see why it's a challenging food for you and it feels even more important that we keep our focus on it. It's remarkable how compelling your eating disorder is! I mean, you know it's not *more* calories to eat the foods together. And you know it's not *more* volume to eat the foods together as a sandwich. The portions are actually the same, the foods are just… configured in a different way. It's like if you traded me four quarters for a dollar. It's the same."
Megan:	"I know, I know…it sounds more ridiculous when you put it that way."
Claire:	"And what I'm hearing is that there are both a lot of past associations with this particular food, in addition to some fears and beliefs about what it would be like to eat this food now. In addition to continuing to explore some of your eating disorder logic, I think another way we can start to challenge your past associations and current fears and beliefs is through creating some new, corrective experiences. So what do you say?"
Megan:	"Okay, fine, I guess I can try it. Let's plan for a bagel sandwich tomorrow."

Provider Exercise – Cognitive Modification Procedures

What examples of non-dialectical thinking, faulty rules that influence behavior, inaccurate descriptions, and dysfunctional allocations of attention have you seen in your work with your patients? How might you go about exploring and challenging this cognitive content with patients? If you feel comfortable doing so, consider discussing your reflections with a trusted colleague for feedback.

If you are a provider who has previous training in cognitive treatment strategies in the treatment of eating disorders, in what ways are the strategies outlined in DBT similar and different to what you have previously learned? In what ways might the DBT cognitive modification strategies influence your work in the future?

Chapter 17

Solution Analysis and Tips for Closing Your Session

Solution Analysis

Now that you have awareness of the various solutions that DBT most commonly draws from in addressing target behaviors, let's take a look at how a solution analysis ties into the chain analysis process. The process of assessing a target behavior and generating insight around it is rarely sufficient in leading to sustained behavior change. Identifying potential solutions and making a plan for implementing them is needed. Solution analysis is a specific form of problem-solving that uses the wealth of information gained from a chain analysis to generate targeted and specific solutions, critically evaluate these solutions, select a solution that is most likely to be beneficial, and create a plan for implementing the solution.

The first step in solution analysis is to work collaboratively with the patient to brainstorm as many potential solutions as possible, particularly solutions that are relevant to specific links in the chain analysis. At this point in the process, no solutions suggested by either the patient or the provider should be evaluated or rejected. The more solutions that are generated, the more likely the patient and provider are to find a greater number of quality solutions. Of note, the patient should be encouraged to take the lead on solution generation, with the provider only stepping in when the client finds they are having difficulty coming up with potential solutions. The rationale behind this is that we ultimately want our patients to develop the skills they need to solve their own problems independently, while also not assuming and acting as though they have these skills already.

Once a lengthy list of potential solutions has been created, the provider and patient must then evaluate each solution, both in terms of anticipated effectiveness and feasibility. Short-term and long-term effectiveness should both be given consideration. Feasibility should also be examined, with particular attention being paid to anticipated barriers to successful implementation of the solutions identified. Common barriers include skill deficits, problematic contingencies in the environment, emotions (e.g. anxiety, shame) inhibiting adaptive responses,

DOI: 10.4324/9781003495604-17

or faulty beliefs impeding in implementation of an identified solution. What you might notice is that all of these barriers can be addressed through the use of the four CBT based procedures we recently reviewed!

After each solution has been evaluated, a solution should be selected and troubleshooting around this solution should occur. The primary factors that should be prioritized when selecting a solution are a greater likelihood of long-term value versus short-term value and the likelihood of a positive effect on a patient's life worth living goals. It is important to keep in mind that there is no "right" answer when completing a solution analysis, but rather a menu of potential choices, many of which will have a reasonable likelihood of being viable options. Once a solution is selected, the last step in solution analysis is to work with the patient on identifying where implementation of the solution could go awry and devising a plan for addressing those situations, should they occur.

Provider Exercise – Solution Analysis

For this provider exercise, you have one of two options. If you completed the chain analysis provider exercise, please revisit what you put together and make note of specific solutions you might suggest for various links on your chain below. If you did not complete this exercise or you completed this exercise but do not have sufficient information to conduct a solution analysis, please revisit the chain analysis we did with Megan and make note of specific solutions you might suggest for various links we identified in her chain analysis. After you complete this exercise, we'll share our solution analysis for Megan, and you can see how your solution analysis compares and contrasts with ours!

Bringing DBT to Life – Completing a Chain Analysis and Solution Analysis With Megan

If you remember back to the chain analysis dialogue you read in Chapter 14, what you see on the following page is a summary of the chain analyses that Megan's therapist and dietitian completed on the left, coupled with a solution analysis on the right that is focused on specific skills that Megan could have implemented at specific links within her chain analysis. Let's take a peek at what she came up with.

What we know from Megan's history is that she has an intellectual knowledge of each of the DBT skills, which means that the focus with regard to the skills listed in the solution analysis would be on skills strengthening and skills generalization. However, there are other therapeutic interventions that may be beneficial for Megan as well. We have now become aware that Megan is continuing to struggle with urges to binge, which suggests that exposure-based procedures involving exposures to binge foods may be beneficial. Megan also struggles with a variety of maladaptive cognitions that appear to be relevant variables in increasing her likelihood of engaging in eating disorder behaviors. Therapeutic work utilizing cognitive modification procedures would also be important to incorporate into Megan's treatment plan.

When utilizing DBT principles and strategies in a multidisciplinary way, solution analyses also become a time where consideration should be given to other multidisciplinary interventions. For example, Megan's dietitian might focus on the following solutions:

Ways to Reduce My Vulnerability in the Future

1. Identifying and preventing physiological vulnerability factors to binge eating and purging including eating balanced meals and snacks at regular intervals and avoiding low blood glucose
2. Identifying compensatory thoughts and behaviors (e.g. planning to "make up" the exchanges at dinner with friends, which contributed to restriction at lunch) and more skillful responses
3. Improving food selection to more closely aligned with patient's taste preferences (e.g. a regular bagel and not a reduced carbohydrate bagel; choosing an entree Megan actually wanted at Overtime Bar and Grill instead of the salad; sharing a snack at the movies instead of avoiding it all together)

Ways to Prevent Precipitating Event From Happening Again

1. Coping ahead for expected nutritional challenges and anticipating urges that might come up
2. Increasing awareness of schedule by anticipating how long events will last (e.g. check movie listing for duration of film) and planning to meet nutritional needs accordingly (e.g. having evening snack at the movies versus waiting until 10pm to have a later evening snack and/or packing a balanced snack for schedule challenges)

Skillful Behaviors

1. Wise Mind (e.g. trying to achieve a more holistic perspective on nutritional intake for the day versus perseverating on one or two distressing moments such as sharing nachos)
2. Check the Facts (e.g. the banana bread, which increased guilt and shame, is likely nutritionally-equivalent to another, "safer" choice)
3. Opposite Action (e.g. using Opposite Action in response increasing thoughts to purge and obsessing over nachos eaten earlier in the day)

Table 17.1 Megan's Chain Analysis and Solution Analysis

Vulnerability Factors
1. Disrupted sleep schedule.
2. Various food-related challenges during the day (ate a bagel and cream cheese; shared nachos with friends in a restaurant).
3. Urges to binge in the hours before evening snack.

Ways to Reduce My Vulnerability in the Future
PLEASE to address disrupted sleep schedule. Cope Ahead for food-related challenges. Observe, Describe, and Mindfulness of Current Thoughts to be more cognizant of urges to binge and thoughts related to bingeing. Using targeted skills to address whatever is leading to increased urges to binge.

Precipitating Event
Arrived home later than expected (10:00pm), so I started evening snack late (10:15pm). Urge to binge (6/10). Anxiety (6/10). Felt hungry (8/10).

Ways to Prevent Precipitating Event From Happening Again
Be more attentive to my schedule to ensure that I can meet my nutritional needs in a timely fashion. Keep a snack available in my purse in case my plan for a snack goes awry.

Links in the Chain
1. Plated one piece of banana bread, sat on couch, and turned on TV. Evening news was on. Anger (7/10).
2. Started eating banana bread. Noticed I was enjoying it. I don't deserve to eat this because I ate normally today. Guilt (6/10).
3. Got near the end of piece of banana bread. Couldn't tell if I was still hungry or not. Do I get another piece of banana bread, do I wait a few minutes, or do I just tell myself that one piece of banana bread is all I need? Heart beating rapidly. Anxiety (7/10).
4. Get another piece of banana bread and sit back down on the couch. Eating more rapidly. Guilt (8/10). Disgust (4/10).
5. Notice some crumbs had fallen onto my shirt and pants. My stomach and thighs look so flabby and gross. Felt out of control and sloppy. Urge to purge (3/10).

Skillful Behaviors
- Wise Mind (Links #1, #2, #3, #6, and #10)
- Nonjudgmentally (Links #5 and #9)
- One-Mindfully (Links #4, #5, and #6)
- Effectively (Link #10)
- DEAR MAN (Link #8)
- Thinking and Acting Dialectically (Link #3)
- Check the Facts (Links #2, #5, #6, and #9)
- Opposite Action (Links #1, #2, #9, and #11)
- Mindfulness of Current Emotions (Links #1, #3, and #8)
- STOP (Link #10)
- Pros and Cons (Link #10)
- Self-Soothing (Links #7 and #8)
- Improving the Moment (Links #3, #7, and #8)
- Mindfulness of Current Thoughts (Links #2, #3, #5, #6, #9, and #10)
- Burning Bridges (Links #1 and #10)

Table 17.1 (Continued)

6. Notice I'm feeling full at about 3/4ths of the way through the second piece of banana bread (6/10). Felt my stomach going over my waistband. I need to get this banana bread out of me. Urge to purge (6/10).
7. Body started shaking. Felt out of control. I need to distract myself.
8. Overwhelmed. Had difficulty finding something to distract. Found crochet materials and tried to crochet, but my hands were shaking too bad. Frustration (9/10).
9. Threw crochet stuff across the room and started berating myself. You've gotten so fat, you've really let yourself go. You don't deserve this banana bread, especially with everything you ate today.
10. Started ruminating about nachos specifically. Decided I needed to purge.
11. Went to the bathroom and purged (1x).

Consequences
Immediate relief (less anxiety [1/10], wave of calm [8/10]), followed by looking in the toilet and thinking, "Ugh, this is gross." Worried that this has opened the door back up for purging. Lingering guilt and shame (5/10).

Plans to Repair, Correct, and Overcorrect Harm Caused By My Behavior
I'm going to practice Dialectical Abstinence to recommit to abstinence from all behaviors, even restricting, and Burning Bridges to address ways in which I'm keeping the door open for behaviors (e.g. asking my mom to buy regular bagels instead of low carbohydrate bagels). I also plan to use Nonjudgmentally coupled with Opposite Action for shame as a way to be more compassionate toward myself.

4. Pros and Cons (e.g. weighing the Pros and Cons of plating entire evening snack versus one piece of banana bread which may not meet nutritional needs)

Plans to Repair, Correct, and Overcorrect Harm Caused By My Behavior

1. Burning Bridges (e.g. eliminating options to engage in eating disorder behaviors)
2. Building New Bridges (e.g. making the banana bread next time to create new associations)

Tips for Closing Your Session

What we have covered over the past number of sections of this book are all strategies you would employ in the context of an individual provider session, organized in a way where we started by discussing how to open a session and effectively set a session agenda and then summarizing a wide range of interventions that you might use throughout the majority of your session. How to close a session is not a topic that usually gets a significant amount of attention, yet approaching how you close a session thoughtfully can have positive effects for both the therapeutic relationship and clinical outcomes.

The first thing to keep in mind when you are closing a session is allowing for sufficient time and space to close the session effectively. When I (AHK) was first starting out as a provider, I wanted to cover so much ground with a patient during a session that it got in the way of a number of things, including allowing for sufficient space for ending a session effectively. Especially when working with patients whose ability to retain and process information may be adversely affected by malnourishment and symptoms of comorbid psychiatric conditions, it can be helpful to remember that perhaps less is more.

Each of your patients will have individual needs and preferences around what feels appropriate to them in terms of the amount of time they would like to wrap up a session, as well as how they would like that time to be used. Some patients may want space to regulate their emotions and prepare for transitioning to whatever activity is next for them. I've (AHK) found this to be particularly true when working at higher levels of care, where patients have to enter back into a milieu and may not feel comfortable doing so if they will appear visibly emotionally dysregulated to their peers. Other patients may find the routine of a specific ending ritual to sessions to be helpful in making effective transitions.

Independent of the above, there are three components of ending sessions that we feel are critical in most circumstances. First, closing the session with some form of cheerleading or praise honors the hard work our patients are doing and expresses our belief in their ability to create a life worth living. It is an incredibly vulnerable act to share the types of things our patients share with us, particularly thoughts and behaviors that evoke guilt and shame. Cheerleading and praise can both reinforce behaviors we want to see continue in future sessions, like being open and honest, and help our patients to build a little momentum to carry forward what they have taken from a session into their day-to-day lives. Second, in many cases it can be helpful to collaboratively summarize key points from your session with the patient. It can be useful to hear what they took from your session, as well as to share what you found to be key take-home points. Summarizing sessions can be particularly useful in situations where a patient has a more limited cognitive ability or where a number of topics were discussed and your patient might feel overwhelmed. Session summaries can lead nicely into the final component of ending a session effectively, which is agreeing upon some type of homework for the upcoming week. The primary goal of our work with patients in our sessions is to increase our patients' motivation and ability to create meaningful change outside of sessions. In-between session homework assignments are one way to approach this task. Ideally, agreeing upon homework should be a collaborative process. This is a form of treating your patient as an equal, and in many cases, allowing a patient to have input into the homework assignment will increase their buy-in around actually completing it. As a final note about homework assignments, it can be helpful for both you and your patient to make note of the assignment and it is critical that you follow-up about how their assignment went prior to or during your next appointment.

Chapter 18

The Second Mode of DBT

Skills Training

The second mode of DBT is skills training and the primary function of this mode is to enhance our patients' capabilities. Each of the DBT skills modules will be reviewed below, in addition to other skills that are not neatly captured in the core DBT skills modules, however, but have relevance to the treatment of eating disorders. Please note that there are two existing DBT skills manuals, one for adults and one for adolescents (Linehan, 2015 and Miller, Rathus, and Linehan, 2007), that provide an excellent description of each skill in detail. Additionally, a RO DBT skills manual also exists (Lynch, 2018) that covers each RO DBT skill in-depth. As such, descriptions below are not exhaustive and readers are encouraged to reference these texts for further information about specific skills.

The Mindfulness Module

The Mindfulness module in DBT is a compilation of acceptance-focused skills, many of which have their origins in Eastern spiritual practices. There are a few broad areas of focus within the Mindfulness module. First, there is an emphasis on teaching patients to access their wise mind, which is a synthesis of all of our different ways of knowing – knowing through reason and logic, knowing through emotion and feeling, and knowing through intuition and instinct. Teaching our patients wise mind helps them to make decisions and act from a place of centeredness that aligns with their goals and their life worth living.

A second area of focus in the Mindfulness module is on teaching patients how to observe their behaviors, urges, thoughts, and feelings and attach accurate and nonjudgmental labels to their behaviors, urges, thoughts, and feelings as appropriate. This area of focus has relevance to eating disorders in a number of different ways. For patients who are diagnosed with Anorexia Nervosa, alexithymia is a common co-occurring issue that can impede our patients' ability to effectively navigate their lives. There is evidence that being able to accurately label our emotions in and of itself can help us to better regulate them and for individuals who struggle with alexithymia, the process of observing and describing an

DOI: 10.4324/9781003495604-18

emotional experience is one that has to be both taught and practiced. For patients who experience urges to engage in more impulsive behaviors, like bingeing or purging, being able to take a step back and notice urges and associated emotions is a necessary precursor to making behavioral change.

Third, the Mindfulness module places an emphasis on engaging in day-to-day life wholeheartedly and effectively. Many of our patients struggle with ruminating and engaging in negative self-talk. The Mindfulness module provides guidance around how to be more present with life moment-to-moment. This module also discusses how to let go of "shoulds" and the notion of something being fair or unfair, and instead focusing on being as effective as possible regardless of opinions and feelings about a given situation.

Finally, the Mindfulness module helps our patients to find balance in behaviors, thoughts, and emotions, rather than operating at extreme ends of the spectrum. One way that this is approached is through helping patients examine where they fall in terms of doing mind and being mind. Doing mind is a state of mind that is focused on achieving goals and completing tasks, whereas being mind is focused on being fully immersed in the present moment. For patients who are more goal-oriented and perfectionistic, being mind can be a hard sell, and striking the balance between these two states of mind is critical for long-term happiness and wellness.

The Interpersonal Effectiveness Module

The Interpersonal Effectiveness module is primarily change-focused, with an emphasis on helping our patients to develop and improve a wide range of skills necessary for cultivating and sustaining healthy interpersonal relationships. There are three primary areas of focus in the Interpersonal Effectiveness module. First, patients are taught how to ask for what they need or want or say no to unwanted requests in a way that also maintains a positive relationship and their self-respect. Many individuals with eating disorders struggle with the assertiveness skills necessary to ask for what they need from family members and friends, which can hinder their eating disorder recovery process. The Interpersonal Effectiveness module provides concrete guidance for patients around how to advocate for their needs, like asking family members to eat meals and snacks with them or to refrain from diet talk when they are around.

Second, the Interpersonal Effectiveness module teaches patients how to initiate and sustain positive relationships and terminate negative or unhealthy relationships. There is evidence that suggests that interpersonal difficulties, such as difficulties cultivating and maintain meaningful friendships, is associated with maintenance of eating disorder behavior and poor eating disorder treatment outcomes (e.g. Carter, Kelly, & Norwood, 2012; Eldredge, Lock, & Horowitz, 1998; Ung, et al., 2017). This speaks to the importance of providing patients with guidance around how to go about making friends. The Interpersonal Effectiveness module gives concrete instructions around how to identify people who could be good fits as friends, initiate and sustain engaging conversations, effectively enter into social groups, and increase mindfulness skills in the context of interpersonal interactions. Many of our patients may also have relationships that are impeding their recovery process, and this particular module provides information about how to end those relationships in an effective manner.

Finally, the Interpersonal Effectiveness module covers skills for "walking the middle path." The overall aim of walking the middle path is to move away from patterns of extreme actions, emotions, and thoughts to a balance where actions, emotions, and thoughts are more balanced, flexible, and appropriate to the situation at hand. There are numerous ways in which patients with eating disorders can struggle with walking the middle path. Cycles of restricting, bingeing, and purging are representative of vacillating between extremes. For other patients, there is a need to move away from rigid patterns of thinking and behavior in order to make progress in the treatment and recovery process. Walking the middle path helps our patients to begin to identify and examine the ways in which extreme actions, emotions, and thoughts play out in their life, and initiate the process of exploring ways in which they can make changes to take a more balanced approach.

The Emotion Regulation Module

The Emotion Regulation module is also primarily change-focused, with the overarching goals of helping our patients to decrease the frequency and intensity of emotions they find to be unpleasant, like anxiety, shame, and sadness, and increase the frequency with which they experience emotions they find to be pleasant, like calmness, pride, and joy. This module is the largest skills module and the content can be broken into four major themes.

First, the Emotion Regulation module focuses on helping patients to understand the purpose of emotions and to increase their ability to observe and label their emotional experiences. It can be helpful for patients to understand that the goal of emotion regulation is not to eliminate experiencing emotions, but rather to teach them skills that can help them to change their emotional reactions. Our emotions serve a variety of functions, including communicating to others, influencing our own and others' behaviors, and alerting us to important information. Given that our emotions serve important functions, working to eliminate them would be unwise. Rather, understanding their function and using this information to help guide our responses is a more effective approach. The other important component of the first part of the Emotion Regulation module is helping patients to observe and label their emotional experiences. Many patients with eating disorders, particularly individuals with restrictive illnesses, experience alexithymia. This doesn't mean that our patients don't experience intense emotions, but rather that they lack the ability to be able to identify and label what they experience. What we also know is that being able to observe and label our emotional experiences increases the likelihood we will be able to shift our emotions in a desired direction. One phrase that I (AHK) have heard other members of the DBT community use is, "If you can name it, you can tame it." In other words, if you can label your emotion, you are more likely to be able to regulate it. Thus, this becomes an important area of focus early on in the Emotion Regulation module.

Second, the Emotion Regulation module teaches patients skills for decreasing unwanted emotions. This is accomplished through changing thoughts and interpretations around a situation, changing a behavioral response to a situation, or using problem solving to come up with a solution to a problem at hand. Many patients with eating disorders struggle with eating disorder thinking that does not align with the facts of a given situation. For example, a decrease in a meal plan can be interpreted by a patient as meaning they have gained a significant amount of weight in a short period of time and are now outside of their weight range, rather than that they have reached a point where shifting from a meal plan focused on weight restoration to one focused on weight maintenance is appropriate. Patients with eating disorders also often struggle with problematic behavioral responses to situations that result in an immediate decrease in unpleasant emotions, but with the long-term effect of increasing the intensity and pervasiveness of these emotions over time. For example, avoidance of fear foods, feared eating situations, form fitting clothing, and so forth all usually result in an immediate decrease in anxiety, coupled with a worsening of anxiety associated with these stimuli over the course of time. Effective emotion regulation requires that patients learn how to inhibit ineffective behavioral responses and engage in responses that may be more immediately unpleasant and that will help them to shift their emotional reactions over the course of time. If you remember the exposure-based procedures we discussed in Chapter 16, some of the skills taught in the Emotion Regulation module dovetail nicely with exposure-related strategies. Finally, problem solving can assist in situations in which a person's emotional response is justified by the situation and where the emotions associated with the situation can be changed by putting a solution into place. For example, if a patient is feeling justified anger after a conflict with a friend, they might use problem solving and arrive at the conclusion that they could use interpersonal effectiveness skills to address the situation, which in turn likely would reduce the anger they are experiencing.

Third, the Emotion Regulation module covers skills that can help reduce the likelihood of experiencing unwanted emotions and increase the likelihood of experiencing desirable emotions. One way this is accomplished is through helping patients to engage in activities that evoke immediate pleasant emotions, connect them with their values, or evoke a sense of mastery. For many patients diagnosed with an eating disorder, their eating disorder begins to take up an increasing amount of real estate where other elements of their identity used to be. As this begins to happen, more of their time also becomes allocated to activities related to their eating disorder rather than activities that fall into the three aforementioned categories. Eating disorder recovery requires increased engagement with activities consistent with a life worth living, both ones that are immediately enjoyable as well as ones that build a sense of accomplishment or purpose. In addition to being consistent with eating disorder recovery, engaging in pleasant activities, values-consistent activities, and activities that build mastery both increases overall positive affect and creates circumstances in which individuals are able to be more resilient in the face of situations likely to evoke negative affect. Another element involved in reducing the likelihood of experiencing unwanted emotions involves teaching patients to cope ahead for challenging situations. When one imagines a challenging situation, plans for intentional skill use, and rehearses coping effectively, there is an increased likelihood that the situation will go better than anticipated and that predicted emotional distress will be lower. Lastly, the Emotion Regulation module covers caring for basic needs, like getting adequate sleep, consuming adequate nutrition, and taking medications as prescribed as methods to reduce vulnerability to unwanted emotions.

Finally, the Emotion Regulation module teaches skills for managing extreme emotions. There are two primary areas of focus with regard to skills from this part of the Emotion Regulation module. First, this part of the module builds upon many of the skills discussed in the Mindfulness module, but with a focus on applying mindfulness to one's emotional experiencing. Patients are taught to mindfully attend to their current emotion, rather than trying to hold onto it or push it away. This process not only prevents a situation in which judgment of one's emotional experiencing results in additional unwanted secondary emotions (e.g. feeling guilty about feeling angry), it also creates a situation in which emotional exposure occurs, which can help in reducing the intensity of emotional experiencing over the course of time. The other area of focus in this section of the Emotion Regulation module involves identifying when a situation has gotten to the point at which Emotion Regulation skills are not likely to be effective and Distress Tolerance skills are what are needed instead.

The Distress Tolerance Module

The Distress Tolerance module is the other acceptance-oriented module and is primarily focused on skills that can help our patients to navigate crises and short-term distressing situations without making them worse and ideally in a way that makes them slightly more bearable. One of the unfortunate realities of life is that pain and distress are inevitable regardless of one's physical and mental health status. Experiencing pain and distress in the context of the early phases of eating disorder treatment and recovery is not only inevitable, but an expected part of a person's day-to-day experience as they work to counteract the impact their eating disorder has had on their biological and neurological makeup. Distress Tolerance skills are necessary not only to help them survive through these moments, but also to open up the possibility of being able to implement change-focused interventions that will help to diminish the overall frequency and intensity of their distress over time.

Many of the Distress Tolerance strategies focus on techniques for diverting one's attention through activities that engage thoughts, emotions, and behaviors in a captivating way. Other Distress Tolerance strategies focus on engaging the five senses or changing one's bodily reactions in response to distress. Of note for patients diagnosed with Anorexia Nervosa, there is some emerging evidence that suggests that distraction focused on motor activities, like knitting or drawing, may be helpful to incorporate as routines prior to eating opportunities to block ruminative worry and decrease anticipatory anxiety (Kaye, et al., 2015). The remainder of the Distress Tolerance skills center around the concept of radical acceptance, which involves acknowledging reality just as it is and figuring out how to navigate this reality as effectively as possible, regardless of one's reactions to it. The analogy I (AHK) like to use when describing radical acceptance harkens back to a time in graduate school when I was first learning to play Texas Hold 'Em. During my first many rounds of playing Texas Hold 'Em, I was a terrible player. My playing philosophy at the time was always to match the big blind, regardless of the likelihood that my initial hand would leave me victorious at the end of a given round. I hated the idea of exiting a round without at least giving it a chance! What I learned over time though was that my desire to remain in a round to at least see the flop was jeopardizing my ability to actually remain in the game over time. Once I learned to embody Kenny Rogers' philosophy of poker outlined in the song "The Gambler," I became a much more successful player. I had to radically accept that sometimes, in fact more often than not, I would be dealt a less than ideal hand, and the best thing I could do was fold in terms of my long-term survival in the context of the game. Translating this to the experience of a patient with an eating disorder, there is simply no getting around the fact that extreme emotional discomfort is part of the process of treatment and moving toward recovery. I've had many patients wish aloud that I could perform the equivalent of a brain transplant or a reboot of their biology as a whole and while I completely share that wish, radical acceptance of the pain of the treatment and recovery process is a necessary step in the service of suffering less over time.

RO DBT Skills

Since the publication of the DBT Skills Manual (Second Edition), the Skills Training Manual for Radically Open Dialectical Behavior Therapy has been published. This skills manual outlines twenty new DBT skills specifically focused on targeting behaviors and symptoms associated with disorders of overcontrol, including behaviors and symptoms that are characteristic in individuals diagnosed with Anorexia Nervosa. There are four core deficits that have been identified in disorders of overcontrol: (1) low receptivity and openness, (2) low flexible control, (3) pervasive inhibited emotional expression and low emotional awareness, and (4) low social connectedness and intimacy with others. Each of these core deficits are targeted by the new skills introduced within the RO DBT skills manual, which are oriented toward increasing receptivity, openness, flexible-control, intimacy, and social connectedness.

DBT Skills From the Skills Modules – A Short Summary

As mentioned earlier, there are a number of texts that provide excellent and comprehensive explanations of each of the DBT skills, so we will not be going into depth with regard to reviewing the DBT skills. That said, we have found that it is helpful for providers to at least have access to a brief summary of key DBT skills, if for no other reason than helping to ensure consistency in language and terminology across providers. Below is a brief review of the most critical DBT skills, separated into their respective DBT modules.

Mindfulness:

- *Wise Mind:* Wise Mind is the synthesis of all ways of knowing. It takes into account our emotions, logic and reason, intuition, and so forth. Wise Mind helps our patients to take a step back and assess how to proceed in a way that honors the wisdom that comes with a holistic rather than myopic perspective. For patients with eating disorders, Wise Mind can be a particularly useful skill in helping to ensure decision-making isn't solely driven by emotions, like fear and shame.
- *Observe:* Observe is a skill that focuses on noticing emotions, thoughts, behaviors, and environmental events, without trying to end, prolong, or change them. For patients with eating disorders who struggle with alexithymia, this is an important skill to develop in terms of being able to notice and subsequently put a label on their emotional experiences.
- *Describe:* Describe involves using nonjudgmental, behaviorally-specific words to describe an experience or personal response. Many individuals with eating disorders struggle with using judgmental language or overly

generalized language to describe themselves and their behavior, which can impede their ability to be effective and to move forward in their recovery process.

- *Participate:* Participate is best described as entering completely into the activity of the current moment and responding with spontaneity. For many patients diagnosed with an eating disorder, self-consciousness is a barrier to using the Participate skill and this skill is one that is a critical part of recovery.
- *Nonjudgmentally:* Nonjudgmentally is a skill that focuses on working to reduce judgments toward oneself and others. This can be done through simply observing and describing when one is making a judgment, or extending this a step further by then trying to shift the judgment to a behaviorally descriptive, nonperjorative statement of facts. Patients diagnosed with eating disorders are often relentless in judgments toward themselves, making Nonjudgmentally an essential skill for them to learn and practice over time.
- *One-Mindfully:* One-mindfully involves focusing the mind and awareness in the current moment's activity. Many individuals struggle with ruminating about the past and/or worrying about the future, and individuals diagnosed with eating disorders are no exception. One-mindfully can help our patients to both increase their effectiveness and reduce their suffering through bringing attention to the present moment.
- *Effectively:* Effectively entails doing what is needed or called for, rather than focusing on what is "right" or "fair," in response to a given situation. For example, the parent of an adolescent patient with an eating disorder, in consultation with the patient's dietitian, may set the boundary that they can't participate in soccer practice unless they are willing to compensate for their energy expenditure through extra exchanges beyond those that are part of their meal plan. While the adolescent patient might not think this is "fair," especially if they know someone else with an eating disorder who does not have similar expectations in place, using Effectively would involve letting go of a focus on "fair" or "unfair" and instead channeling their focus toward coming up with a plan for completing the extra exchanges.
- *Loving Kindness:* Loving Kindness is a specific type of meditation aimed at increasing love and compassion for others. Loving Kindness meditations have been found to have a number of benefits, including increasing social pleasant emotions, decreasing unpleasant emotions, increasing social connectedness, and decreasing self-hate. When patients are willing to practice Loving Kindness meditations, they can serve as a helpful antidote to the disgust, anger, and hatred that patients may express toward themselves.
- *Skillful Means:* Skillful Means is a skill that helps patients to balance Doing Mind, which is a state of mind focused on completing tasks and achieving goals, and Being Mind, which is a state of mind focused on being fully present

in the here and now. Many individuals who are diagnosed with eating disorders often find themselves in Doing Mind and have difficulty understanding the value of Being Mind. Yet Being Mind is critical for both physical and emotional self-care, as well as being a necessary state of mind for building a life worth living. On the side of the dialectic, some patients struggle with figuring out how to translate their goals into actionable items steps and how to follow-through on action steps once they are identified. For these patients, figuring out how to be more in Doing Mind is an important target in building a life worth living.

- *Walking the Middle Path:* Walking the Middle Path is a skill that is focused on helping patients to identify extremes in terms of their thoughts, emotions, and behaviors, and to generate strategies to help with more dialectical approaches. One example that is common in patients who struggle with cycles of restricting, bingeing, and purging is striking a balance between self-denial and self-indulgence. It is common for individuals who struggle with these patterns of behavior to deny themselves access not only to the quantity and array of foods necessary to meet their nutritional needs, but also to foods they find to be enjoyable. For most patients, an inevitable outcome of self-denial is an episode of bingeing that often includes the foods to which they have been denying themselves access. Breaking the restricting, bingeing, and purging cycle involves helping patients to walk the middle path by ensuring their body is adequately nourished with a wide array of foods, including foods they find to be enjoyable.

Interpersonal Effectiveness:

- *Challenging Myths in the Way of Interpersonal Effectiveness:* Challenging Myths in the Way of Interpersonal Effectiveness involves challenging worries and beliefs that interfere with individuals getting their needs met, asserting themselves, improving their relationships, and maintaining their self-respect. For example, many patients with whom we have worked have held the belief that asking for help means that they are a weak or incapable person. Holding this belief often influenced both their behavior (e.g. not asking for help when they needed it) and thinking (e.g. upon not getting the help they needed, having the thought, "I should be able to handle this on my own. What is wrong with me?"). Challenging Myths in the Way of Interpersonal Effectiveness focuses on helping our patients to identify their worries and beliefs and explore whether there are other beliefs or perspectives that could have truth and validity.
- *Clarifying Goals in Interpersonal Situations:* Clarifying Goals in Interpersonal Situations involves determining if the top priority in a situation is getting what you want (Objectives Effectiveness), keeping a positive

relationship (Relationship Effectiveness), or maintaining your self-respect (Self-Respect Effectiveness). Each type of effectiveness is typically relevant in a given interpersonal interaction, so it is important to both have clarity about priorities and a plan for navigating situations in which priorities may be in conflict.

- *DEAR MAN:* DEAR MAN is a skill that is focused on asking for what you want or saying no. The "D" in DEAR MAN stands for "Describe," which involves stating the facts of a situation. The "E" stands for "Express," which entails sharing your emotional reactions or beliefs about the situation. The "A" in DEAR MAN stands for "Assert," which involves clearly and succinctly asking for what you want or saying no. The "R" stands for "Reinforce," which entails identifying and outlining the positive or rewarding consequences that would occur for the other person if they respond the way you would like them to respond. The "M" in DEAR MAN stands for "(Stay) Mindful," which involves two separate strategies. First, (Stay) Mindful involves maintaining your current position through using strategies like the "broken record" technique, where you calmly but repeatedly continue to repeat your request or state your position. Second, (Stay) Mindful also involves ignoring attacks or attempts to change the subject.

    The other "A" in DEAR MAN stands for "Appear Confident," which means focusing on having a confident tone of voice, body posture, and eye contact. Finally, the "N" stands for "Negotiate," which entails being willing to give to get or explore other potential solutions. Many patients with eating disorders struggle with advocating for their needs in a variety of situations related to their eating disorder specifically, like asking a loved one to refrain from diet talk or asking for support in the context of a meal or snack. DEAR MAN gives our patients a framework they can use to be more successful in making requests of others.

- *GIVE:* The GIVE skill is focused on improving and maintaining interpersonal relationships. The "G" in GIVE refers to "(Be) Gentle," which involves being kind and respectful, rather than attacking, threatening, or judging the other person. The "I" in GIVE stands for "(Act) Interested." Actions demonstrating interest include removing distractions (e.g. cell phones), listening patiently without interrupting, and refraining from making assumptions about the other person's thoughts and feelings. The "V" in GIVE stands for "Validate," which refers to actively communicating to the other person that their thoughts, emotions, and actions make sense to you, given either current or historical contexts. Finally, the "E" in GIVE refers to "(Use an) Easy manner." Behaviors that are consistent with using an easy manner include smiling, using humor, and working to identify common ground. Both interpersonal disconnection and interpersonal conflict are struggles that regularly arise for individuals diagnosed with an eating disorder. The GIVE skill can be helpful in that it gives patients a concrete framework for actions they can take to improve their relationships with others.

- *FAST:* The FAST skill is a skill that is focused on maintaining self-respect. The "F" in FAST refers to "(Be) Fair," which means making sure you are not taking advantage of others while also making sure that others are not taking advantage of you, as both these situations are likely to result in diminished self-respect. The "A" in FAST stands for "(No) Apologies," which means apologizing when appropriate (e.g. when you have hurt another person), but refraining from overapologizing, which includes situations like apologizing for your opinion or apologizing for making a request of another person. The "S" in FAST refers to "Stick to Values." This means acting in alignment with your values, morals, or beliefs, rather than compromising these things in the service of keeping someone liking you. Finally, the "T" in FAST stands for "(Be) Truthful." Being truthful in this circumstance involves refraining from both minimizing and exaggerating situations or being dishonest about one's capabilities. For patients who struggle with "people pleasing," the FAST skill can provide them with guidance for how to stick up for themselves.

- *THINK:* THINK is a skill from the DBT Skills Manual for Adolescents specifically. This skill is focused on perspective-taking and challenging assumptions about the motivations of others. The "T" in THINK stands for "Think about it from the other person's perspective," which is an encouragement to make active attempts around perspective-taking. The "H" stands for "Have empathy," which involves making an effort to understand the thoughts and feelings of another person and why those thoughts and feelings make sense. The "I" in THINK stands for "Interpretations," which is focused on generating as many interpretations of a person's behavior as possible, including interpretations that are benign or even positive. The "N" stands for "Notice," which refers to making an effort to notice kind things a person has done or is currently doing, as well as making an effort to recognize struggles that a person may be experiencing. Finally, the "K" in THINK stands for "use Kindness," which is an encouragement to focus on ways you can be kind and gentle in interactions with others. For our child and adolescent clients, the THINK skill can be helpful in gaining a better understanding and perspective around limits that may have been set by their parents or guardians, like limitations placed on physical movement or autonomy around meals and snacks.

- *Mindfulness of Others:* Mindfulness of Others is a skill that focuses on applying the Observe, Describe, and Participate skills described in the previous section in the context of interpersonal interactions, with the goal of maintaining or improving relationships. Examples of application of the Mindfulness of Others skill include eliminating distractions (e.g. putting your cell phone away when having a conversation), listening patiently to what the other person is saying, assuming good intent, and refraining from assumptions and judgments.

- *Thinking and Acting Dialectically:* Thinking and Acting Dialectically is a broad array of skills that focus on helping patients to apply the dialectical worldview in a meaningful way in their day-to-day life. Two aspects of Thinking and Acting Dialectically that are particularly relevant for individuals diagnosed with eating disorders are letting go of extremes in thinking and working toward being more open to change through creating opportunities to practice adapting to and radically accepting change, although there are many other components to this skill that patients may find to be helpful as well.

- *Validation:* Validation is a skill that is focused on making efforts to understand another person's thoughts, opinions, emotions, and behaviors, and actively communicating to that person that their thoughts, opinions, emotions, and behaviors make sense in situations where they are actually valid. For patients for whom interpersonal disconnectedness has been fostered by their eating disorder, focusing on regular use of Validation can help them to connect or reconnect with others.

- *Self-Validation:* Self-Validation involves applying validation yourself exactly the way you would validate someone else. This means that you both acknowledge your emotions, thoughts, and behaviors, as well as reflect on how these emotions, thoughts, and behaviors make sense, given your current context. Self-Validation also involves treating yourself with respect. Individuals diagnosed with eating disorders often internalize invalidating messages they have heard (e.g. "Eating disorders are a choice") and may engage in self-invalidation as a result. Self-Validation as a skill provides an antidote to these negative messages.

- *Shaping:* Shaping involves reinforcing small steps toward a desired behavior. Many patients with eating disorders rely heavily on punishment as a method to attempt to change their behavior or have denied themselves reinforcement for incremental progress toward behavior change on a larger scale. Shaping is a way to break large behavioral changes into more manageable steps that can be reinforced to encourage gradual change.

Emotion Regulation:

- *Challenging Myths About Emotions:* Challenging Myths About Emotions involves having patients examine and challenge faulty beliefs they may hold that impede their ability to effectively regulate their emotions. Many patients diagnosed with eating disorders have internalized messages about emotions, like, "My emotions are stupid" or "Letting others know that I'm hurting is a sign of weakness." As with myths about interpersonal effectiveness, myths about emotions can also influence patient behavior (e.g. refusing to be vulnerable by seeking support or sharing with others what they are experiencing) and thoughts (e.g. engaging in further self-invalidation of emotional experiencing). Challenging Myths about Emotions focuses on helping our patients to explore the beliefs they hold about emotions and whether there are shifts to these beliefs that could assist with emotion regulation and building a life worth living.

- *Check the Facts:* Check the Facts acknowledges that sometimes our interpretation of an event or situation directly impacts the emotion we are experiencing. Check the Facts is a skill that is focused on separating facts from assumptions and judgments and changing appraisals and assumptions to fit the facts. The skill is broken down into six steps. First, in order to use Check the Facts, you must first identify what the specific emotion is that you would like to change. Second, you must then outline the specifics of the event or situation that prompted the emotion, with particular attention paid to sorting out observable facts about the event or situation from your judgments about the situation. Third, you should explore your thoughts, interpretations, and assumptions about the event or situation. As part of this step, consider devising methods to test your interpretations and assumptions or generating other potential interpretations and assumptions. Fourth, you should explore whether you are assuming a threat and if so, what the actual likelihood is of that threatening outcome occurring. Fifth, ask yourself, "What's the catastrophe?" and then imagine the catastrophe actually occurring and coping with the catastrophe in a skillful fashion. Finally, you should explore whether your emotion and/or the intensity of your emotion fits the facts of the event or situation. Many patients hold extreme beliefs about food, weight, relationships, and so forth (e.g. "If I drink this milkshake, I am going to gain five pounds?", "She must be mad at me because she hasn't texted back and it's been three hours"). Check the Facts is an excellent skill for exploring this type of thinking when it arises.

- *Opposite Action:* Opposite Action is a skill that is a core skill embedded within many of the most empirically-supported treatments for a variety of psychiatric diagnoses, including eating disorders, anxiety disorders, and major depressive disorder. In short, Opposite Action involves changing emotions through acting in a way that is inconsistent with the emotion. There are seven steps involved in Opposite Action. First, you need to observe and describe the emotion that you want to change. This is important because identifying the appropriate opposite action is dependent upon accurately labeling the emotion you are experiencing. Second, use the Check the Facts skill to gain an understanding of what prompted the emotion you are experiencing, what interpretations, thoughts, or assumptions you may be having, and any perceived threats or anticipated catastrophic outcomes that may be on your mind. Third, identify what it is that you want to do in response to your emotion. Fourth, ask your Wise Mind whether following through on these action urges is likely to be effective in this situation. Assuming the answer is no, the fifth step of Opposite Action involves identifying other actions that you can take in response to your emotion that are likely to be more effective. Once you've identified at least one action you can take, act opposite all of the way! Finally, the last step of Opposite Action involves continuing to repeat acting opposite all the way until your emotional response changes. Let's take a look at how Opposite Action might work in eating disorders. If I am working with a patient for whom pizza with pepperoni is a fear food and they are wanting to use Opposite Action to decrease their fear response to this food, the first step to doing so would be to have them observe and describe their emotional experience, which in this case would be "intense fear." Next, I would have them use the Check the Facts skill. In doing so, we discover that they hold the following two beliefs about eating pizza with pepperoni: (1) "I will gain five pounds if I eat the pizza" and (2) "My stomach is going to visibly protrude if I eat this pizza." These are assumptions that can be challenged with Wise Mind, as well as hypotheses that can be tested and disconfirmed through the use of Opposite Action. The third step of using Opposite Action in this example would be to have the patient identify action urges they are having. The first action urge that they notice is to restrict entirely, however they note that if this isn't possible, they are also having the urges to peel off the pepperoni and throw it away and to blot off the grease on the pizza with their napkin. The first opposite action the patient identifies is to just get through the meal using Distress Tolerance strategies, like distracting themselves with table conversation. However, this is not consistent with the next step of Opposite Action, which involves acting opposite all the way. They decide instead to radically accept that working on their fear of eating pizza with pepperoni is a necessary part of recovery, then they will need to allow themselves to be present with emotions, thoughts, and body sensations that come up as they eat their pizza, while also refraining from peeling off the pepperoni or blotting off the grease with their napkin. Finally, in recognizing that using Opposite Action once to target their fear of eating pizza with pepperoni is not likely to be sufficient in terms of reducing or eliminating their fear, they commit to working with their dietitian to schedule another time to complete an exposure to pizza with pepperoni.

- *Problem Solving:* Problem Solving is a change-focused skill that helps patients to identify and implement solutions to the problems they encounter in a systematic way. There are seven steps involved in Problem Solving. The first step involves identifying and describing the problem in a nonjudgmental and factual manner. The second step of Problem Solving is checking the facts to make sure you have an accurate understanding of the problem situation.

The third step involves identifying your goal in solving the problem. The fourth step in Problem Solving is brainstorming as many solutions as possible while refraining from rejecting any solutions at this point in the process. The fifth step involves selecting a solution that can be implemented and that has a reasonable likelihood of being effective in achieving your goal. The sixth step in Problem Solving is trying the identified solution. The final step of Problem Solving involves evaluating the results of implementing the solution. If the solution has not been effective in solving the problem, consider revisiting step five of Problem Solving. Patients diagnosed with eating disorders often encounter situations that create challenges for participation in treatment or taking actions consistent with their recovery. Problem Solving offers a helpful framework for examining these situations and identifying potential solutions.

- *ABC PLEASE:* ABC PLEASE is an amalgam of various skills that are all focused on reducing one's vulnerability to unpleasant emotions. The "A" in ABC PLEASE refers to "Accumulate positive emotions." This piece of the broader skill focuses on engaging in short-term pleasant activities, taking steps toward achieving long-term goals, and engaging in activities consistent with one's values. Ideally, all of these actions are also done in a mindful manner. The "B" in ABC PLEASE stands for "Build mastery," which is a skill focused on regularly participating in activities that make one feel competent, confident, and in control. The "C" in ABC PLEASE stands for "Cope ahead of time with emotional situations," which involves planning ahead for challenging situations and using imagery to rehearse successfully coping. The remainder of the ABC PLEASE skill focuses on taking care of your mind by taking care of your body through treating physical illness, balancing eating, avoiding mood-altering substances, balancing sleep, and getting exercise. For individuals diagnosed with an eating disorder, when recommending the use of this skill it is particularly important to clarify what is expected in terms of balanced eating and getting exercise, as recommendations for individuals diagnosed with an eating disorder are likely to vary in comparison to recommendations that might be given to someone without an eating disorder diagnosis. For example, we have often found it helpful to rephrase "balancing eating" as "follow the meal plan prescribed by my team" and "getting exercise" to "engage in joyful movement consistent with physical movement recommendations provided by my team."
- *Mindfulness of Current Emotions:* Mindfulness of Current Emotions involves the following four steps: (1) Observe your emotion, (2) Practice mindfulness of body sensations, (3) Remember, you are not your emotion, and (4) Practice loving your emotion. For many patients with eating disorders, they often feel compelled to act in alignment with action urges associated with their emotions (e.g. bingeing when sad, compulsively exercising when anxious).

The Mindfulness of Current Emotions skill can help them to experience their emotions without acting on them.

Distress Tolerance:

- *STOP:* The STOP skill is a skill that is focused on helping patients refrain from acting impulsively. The "S" in STOP stands for "Stop," which refers to immediately pausing if impulsive urges arise or emotions appear to be taking control. The "T" in STOP refers to "Take a step back," which means temporarily removing oneself from the situation at hand, both physically and mentally. The "O" in STOP stands for "Observe," which refers to taking stock of the situation, both in terms of what is going on in your environment and what is going on for you internally, with a focus on the facts at hand. Finally, the "P" in STOP stands for "Proceed mindfully," which refers to using Wise Mind to evaluate each option you have for responding to the situation at hand, and selecting an option that brings you closer to your goals. For eating disorder behaviors that are more impulsive in nature, like bingeing and purging, the STOP skill can help patients shift from impulsivity to intentionality in terms of responding to their urges to engage in eating disorder behaviors.
- *Pros and Cons:* Pros and cons in the context of Distress Tolerance refers to weighing the benefits and downsides of acting on an impulsive urge versus using skills to resist acting upon an impulsive urge. As discussed in previous chapters, pros and cons can also be applied to non-crisis situations to consider various courses of action in response to a given situation.
- *TIP*: TIP is a grouping of skills that focus on changing body chemistry with the goal of reducing the intensity of an emotion being experienced. The "T" in TIP refers to the phrase "Tip the temperature of your face with cold water," which involves dunking one's head in cold water or putting cold packs on one's face. Of note in working with patients with eating disorders, this skill is not recommended for use for patients for whom restriction is a symptom of their illness, as this skill can cause a person's heart rate to drop. The "I" in TIP stands for "Intense exercise." As with the "T" in TIP, intense exercise is often contraindicated in working with patients diagnosed with an eating disorder, although can be considered on an individual basis depending on the specifics of a patient's clinical presentation. The "P" in TIP stands for two different skills. "Paced breathing" involves slowing one's breath down, particularly through lengthening exhalation. The "P" in TIP also stands for "Paired muscle relaxation," which involves pairing the tensing and releasing of one's muscles with one's inhalation and exhalation.
- *Wise Mind ACCEPTS:* Wise Mind ACCEPTS refers to a set of skills that can be used as temporary distractions from extreme emotional pain or as ways to tolerate an unpleasant situation that cannot be immediately resolved or

improved. Many of these skills can be helpful in weathering intense urges to engage in eating disorder behaviors or other behaviors that are inconsistent with building a life worth living. The "A" in ACCEPTS refers to "Activities," which involves engaging in any distracting activity that does not run the risk of making the situation at hand worse, either through creating additional crises or feeding unpleasant emotions. Examples of activities include doing a puzzle, playing a game, or watching entertaining video clips. The first "C" in ACCEPTS stands for "Contributing," which involves participating in an activity that contributes to the well-being of another person, like helping a friend or doing something nice for a family member, as a way of distracting from one's own distress. The second "C" in ACCEPTS refers to "Comparisons," which focuses on comparing your life situation to others who are less fortunate than you or comparing your current circumstances to a time in your life that was more difficult. Because unhelpful comparisons are a phenomenon that commonly occurs for individuals diagnosed with an eating disorder, this specific skill within ACCEPTS may not be appropriate or helpful for many individuals. The "E" in ACCEPTS stands for "Different Emotions," which refers to engaging in activities that are likely to evoke a different emotion than the one currently being experienced. For example, listening to high energy music or watching a comedy are two activities that are likely to evoke emotions that are different from sadness. Of note with the "E" in ACCEPTS, the goal is not to try to force experiencing a different emotion, but rather to engage in activities that allow the possibility of a different emotion occurring. The "P" in ACCEPTS stands for "Pushing away," which involves mentally or physically leaving the situation that is causing distress. This includes strategies like using mental imagery (e.g. imagining putting your problems in a box on a shelf) or mindfully blocking or redirecting ruminative processes. The "T" in ACCEPTS stands for "Other Thoughts," which focuses on engaging in activities that require thought, like doing puzzles or complex math problems. Finally, the "S" in ACCEPTS stands for "Other Sensations," which involves engaging in activities that create intense physical sensations, like holding an ice pack or taking a hot shower.
- *Self-Soothing:* Self-Soothing is a skill that focuses on using the five senses to create a sense of comfort and nurturing. Examples of specific activities that may fall under the umbrella of Self-Soothing include looking at beautiful pictures, listening to calming music, lighting a scented candle, doing a foot soak, or drinking warm tea. As one might expect, the use of taste as a form of Self-Soothing in the context of working with individuals diagnosed with eating disorders is a complex issue and warrants individualized recommendations depending on a patient's specific clinical presentation.
- *Improving the Moment:* Improving the Moment refers to a set of skills that can help in situations in which stress may be more long-lasting and additional

strategies are needed to help with tolerating urges to engage in eating disorder behaviors or other maladaptive behaviors. The "I" in IMPROVE stands for "Imagery," which involves imagining a relaxing or safe place, or imagining a difficult situation going well. The "M" in IMPROVE stands for "Meaning," which refers to finding positive aspects or purpose in a painful situation. The "P" in IMPROVE stands for "Prayer," which involves using prayer (if one identifies as religious or spiritual) or asking Wise Mind for help, with the goal of making tolerating a difficult situation more bearable. The "R" in IMPROVE refers to "Relaxing actions," which are actions one can take to elicit a sense of calm, like taking a warm bath or engaging in gentle stretching. The "O" in IMPROVE stands for "One thing in the moment," which entails focusing one's attention on the present moment and letting go of ruminating about the past or worrying about the future. The "V" in IMPROVE refers to "brief Vacation," which involves taking a short break from reality (anywhere from an hour to a full day) and engaging in a relaxing or pleasurable activity. Finally, the "E" in IMPROVE stands for "Self-Encouragement and rethinking the situation," which can include cheerleading oneself or reframing thoughts about the situation at hand.

- *Sensory Awareness:* The Sensory Awareness skill is focused on noticing the presence or absence of certain sensations related to the body (e.g. "Can you feel your arms touching your body?") or imagining how one's body might feel in a certain situation (e.g. "Can you imagine what it would feel like to float on a cloud?"), with the goal of creating a sense of calmness or peace. While this skill as described in the DBT Skills Manual is structured as a series of questions, any activity focused on mindfully and nonjudgmentally noticing the aforementioned sensations would be consistent with the overall principle of this skill. If you are familiar with grounding skills, these also closely parallel Sensory Awareness.
- *Radical Acceptance:* Radical Acceptance refers to being completely open to reality as it is, rather than actively fighting with reality or refusing to engage with reality. Metaphorically, Radical Acceptance is like playing a round of poker and playing the hand you've been dealt as best you can, even if you've been dealt a poor one, rather than playing your hand as if you had been given different cards or quitting the game entirely. Radical Acceptance is one of the more challenging skills to learn and it is one of the skills that patients have told us they have found to be most helpful, as it applies to so many aspects of eating disorder recovery. For example, for individuals diagnosed with Anorexia Nervosa, Radical Acceptance can be a useful skill in helping them to tolerate distress associated with weight restoration and body changes.
- *Turning the Mind:* Turning the Mind is a skill that can be utilized in situations in which a person is drifting away from Radical Acceptance to a position of nonacceptance. The first step in Turning the Mind is actually catching

yourself being non-accepting. Signs of non-acceptance include emotions like anger or envy, as well as non-accepting thoughts (e.g. "This isn't fair."). The second step in Turning the Mind is making an inner commitment to accept reality as it is. Because step two is not nearly as easy as it seems, step three involves recommitting to acceptance, over and over again. The final step in Turning the Mind is developing a plan for catching yourself when you drift out of acceptance.

- *Willingness:* Willingness involves radically accepting the world as it is and doing just what is needed to respond to reality as it is in the moment. Willingness is a companion skill to Effectiveness, in that both focus on "doing what works." Examples of Willingness for our patients are endless in the context of eating disorders work and can include things like making the choice to eat non-preferred foods from a rest stop while on a road trip in order to meet their nutritional needs, opting to withdraw from school for a semester in order to seek treatment, or following the recommendations of their multi-disciplinary team even if they don't agree with the recommendations or feel that the recommendations are "fair."
- *Half-Smiling:* Half-Smiling is a skill that is focused on creating a sense of acceptance through changing our facial expression. Half-Smiling involves relaxing your face, neck, and shoulder muscles, and then gently upturning the corners of your lips, in a way that is natural rather than forced. The idea behind Half-Smiling is that our bodies send messages to our brains and that by targeting facial expressions, body posture, and so forth, we can alter how we experience a given situation.
- *Willing Hands:* Willing Hands is a companion skill to Half-Smiling. Willing Hands involves placing your hands palms up and fingers relaxed to increase a sense of acceptance.
- *Mindfulness of Current Thoughts:* The Mindfulness of Current Thoughts skill is focused on changing how we relate to our thoughts. Instead of trying to suppress thoughts or challenge the cognitive content of our thoughts, Mindfulness of Current Thoughts encourages observing our thoughts, labeling them as such, and adopting a curious mind toward our thoughts. Through this process, we learn our thoughts don't last forever, do not define who we are, and do not have to dictate our behavior. For many clients who experience a "loud" eating disorder voice, Mindfulness of Current Thoughts can help to give them distance from these thoughts and help them refrain from engaging in eating disorder behaviors in response to these thoughts.
- *Dialectical Abstinence:* Dialectical Abstinence is a skill that was originally developed for the treatment of substance use disorders, however it has also been applied in the context of eating disorders work. Dialectical Abstinence involves making a strong commitment to refrain from eating disorder behaviors and coming up with a plan for how to refrain from behaviors, while at the

same time making a plan for harm reduction in the event an eating disorder behavior does occur.

- *Clear Mind:* Clear Mind is another skill that was developed specifically for the treatment of substance use disorders, however the themes of the Clear Mind skill can be extrapolated to eating disorders. Clear Mind involves being abstinent from addictive behaviors, while also recognizing that relapse is possible. It is the synthesis between Addict Mind, which is a state in which addictive behavior governs all of one's thoughts, emotions, and behaviors, and Clean Mind, which is a state in which one hasn't engaged in addictive behavior for a period of time, but where one is also oblivious to the risk of relapse. Obviously, the terms "Addict Mind," "Clean Mind," and "Clear Mind" do not apply to states of mind for individuals diagnosed with eating disorders, however the principles behind these states of mind can apply. Many of our patients have experienced times where their eating disorder is all consuming, which parallels "Addict Mind." Many of our patients (and their supports!) have also experienced times where they assume that a period of abstinence from eating disorder behaviors means they are "out of the woods," which parallels "Clean Mind." Neither of these states of mind are helpful in terms of long-term recovery, so the goal becomes to maintain both abstinence from behaviors and vigilance about risks of returning to behaviors.
- *Burning Bridges:* Like the previous two skills, Burning Bridges is a skill that was developed for use in the treatment of substance use disorders, however is also a skill that has relevance in the treatment of eating disorders. Burning Bridges involves actively eliminating potential triggers for maladaptive behaviors and taking actions that make it harder for the maladaptive behaviors to occur. Examples from eating disorders work could include getting rid of one's personal scale, canceling one's gym membership, disposing of laxatives and diuretics, and being truthful with one's support system about eating disorder behaviors.
- *Building New Bridges:* Building New Bridges is a companion skill to Burning Bridges that focuses on helping patients to find physical sensations and mental images that compete with urges to engage in behaviors. Many patients report associating certain places or stimuli with engaging in eating disorder behaviors. As an example, some patients may find it helpful to redecorate rooms or spaces where they regularly engaged in eating disorder behaviors as a way to create new associations with these spaces.
- *Alternate Rebellion:* Alternate Rebellion is another skill that was originally developed for use with individuals diagnosed with substance use disorders, particularly individuals for whom their substance use was one manifestation of a broader "rebellious" personality. The idea behind Alternate Rebellion is to find ways to rebel that are expressive, yet safe, like dyeing your hair an interesting color, participating in cultural events that are out of the

mainstream, or wearing edgy clothing. Alternate Rebellion as applied to eating disorders involves channeling our patients' desire for rebellion into rebelling against their eating disorder. For example, patients could choose to rebel against the rules their eating disorder has set for them or rebel against societal beauty standards by presenting as they would like to be seen in the world.

- *Adaptive Denial:* Adaptive Denial is the last of the skills that was originally developed for individuals diagnosed with substance use disorders, although it can be adapted for application with eating disorder behaviors as well. Adaptive Denial involves patients adamantly convincing themselves that engaging in a maladaptive behavior is not possible or convincing themselves that even if they are having urges to engage in a behavior that they don't actually want to do so. One common form of Adaptive Denial is the "one day at a time" concept from Alcoholics Anonymous/Narcotics Anonymous. When using this approach to Adaptive Denial, a person convinces themselves they only need to refrain from engaging in maladaptive behavior for a set period of time. However, when they reach the end of the set period of time, they recommit to refraining from the behavior for another set period of time. The reality is that the set period of time that they are refraining from the behavior is not the ultimate goal – indefinite abstinence from the behavior is – however for many people, a shorter set period of time can feel more tolerable.

RO DBT Skills:

- *Radical Openness:* Radical Openness is the core skill in RO DBT and involves openness to new information and/or disconfirming feedback, as well as actively seeking out things that you are avoiding or that make you uncomfortable, all in the service of learning.
- *Flexible Mind DEFinitely:* Flexible Mind DEFinitely is a critical skill in RO DBT that is focused on helping patients to engage in radical openness. The "D" stands for "Acknowledge Distress or unwanted emotion," and involves focusing on simply observing one's emotion, rather than trying to regulate, control, accept, or avoid it. The "E" stands for "Use self-Enquiry to learn from the distress rather than automatically attempting to regulate, distract, change, deny, or accept," and involves using self-inquiry to ask what you might learn from the situation. Finally, "F" stands for "Flexibly respond with humility by doing what's needed in the moment, in a manner that accounts for the needs of others," which involves taking personal responsibility for your reactions, while also not overthinking what to do next.
- *The Big Three + 1:* The Big Three + 1 skill is designed to activate the social safety system. The skill begins with "+1," which is only relevant if the person is sitting down. If they are sitting down, "+1" simply involves leaning back

in one's chair. One can then use the Big Three skills simultaneously, which include taking a slow, deep breath, engaging in a closed-mouth cooperative smile, and using an eyebrow wag (raising both eyebrows). This skill communicates to the individual using it that all is well and that there are no threats present.

• *Flexible Mind VARIEs:* Flexible Mind VARIEs is a skill that is focused on helping patients engage in novel behavior and evaluate their experiences. The "V" stands for "Verify one's willingness to experience something new" and is focused on enhancing willingness to engage in novel behavior by connecting the practice of engaging in novel behavior to valued goals, while also exploring and targeting fears that may be present. The "A" stands for "check the Accuracy of hesitancy, aversion, or urges to avoid engaging in the new behavior in order to determine whether your emotions are warranted" and is particularly focused on whether the person is in Fixed Mind or Fatalistic Mind. The "R" stands for "Relinquish compulsive planning, rehearsal, or preparation prior to trying out the new behavior" and is focused on trying to reduce unnecessary planning and preparation, which can result in exhaustion and burnout. The "I" stands for "activate one's social safety system and Initiate the new behavior" and is focused on using the Big Three + 1, coupled with mindful participation in the novel behavior. Finally, "E" stands for "look back over what happened, and nonjudgmentally Evaluate the outcome" and is focused on honing in on objective evidence from the experience, including acknowledging what went well about the experience.

• *Flexible Mind SAGE:* Flexible Mind SAGE is a skill that can be utilized to help individuals effectively navigate situations in which they feel shame or embarrassment, or where they feel rejected or excluded. The "S" in Flexible Mind SAGE stands for "use Self-enquiry to determine if shame is warranted." This component of the skill encourages individuals to practice self-enquiry during and after the shame-evoking event, with an emphasis on pausing to ask what they need to learn from their shame before reacting to it. The "A" stands for "If shame is warranted to partially warranted, then Appease." This part of the skill is relevant only in situations in which shame is justified and involves taking responsibility for wrongdoing, taking steps to repair the transgression, and using social signaling that is consistent with the severity of the transgression. The "G" stands for "If shame is unwarranted, then Go opposite to urges to hide." This component of the skill is only appropriate in situations in which shame is not justified and involves refraining from apologies and signaling confidence, in addition to exploring whether the social environment is toxic and if so, considering appropriate subsequent actions. Finally, the "E" stands for "show Embarrassment to enhance trust and socially connect." This part of the skill is focused on encouraging individuals to show embarrassment rather than masking it, since embarrassment shows you care about others and because expressing embarrassment is actually appealing to others.

- *Flexible Mind is DEEP:* Flexible Mind is DEEP is a skill that is focused on teaching patients to express emotions in a way that enhances interpersonal relationships and brings them closer to their valued goals. The "D" stands for "Determine your valued goal and the emotion you wish to express" and is focused on identifying valued goals for an interpersonal relationship, connecting emotional expression to those valued goals, and determining what channel of expression is most appropriate for the emotion. The first "E" stands for "Effectively Express by matching nonverbal signals with valued goals" and involves using facial expressions, body language, and physical touch that is consistent with a valued goal while interacting with the other person. The second "E" stands for "use self-Enquiry to Examine the outcome and learn" and is focused on reflecting on interpersonal interaction and lessons to be learned, as well as radically accepting and honoring differences in expression. Finally, the "P" stands for "Practice open expression, again and again" and is centered on the importance of making a commitment to continuing to practice open expression.
- *Flexible Mind:* Flexible Mind is the synthesis between Fixed Mind and Fatalistic Mind. It is characterized by openness to change, to feedback or criticism, and to different perspectives. It involves self-enquiry and exploration, taking ownership of one's emotions and reactions, and doing what is needed in any given moment.
- *With Self-Enquiry:* With Self-Enquiry is a RO DBT-specific Mindfulness "how" skill that represents the approach one takes when applying the Mindfulness "what" skills. With Self-Enquiry is focused on openness to learning, willingness to challenge core beliefs, the pursuit of truth, and taking ownership of one's beliefs and choices.
- *With Awareness of Harsh Judgements:* RO DBT normalizes the experience of judging, while simultaneously acknowledging that certain types of judgments can be problematic, like those that decrease openness to new information or judgments that impact social signaling in an unhelpful manner. With Awareness of Harsh Judgments focuses on helping individuals become aware of unhelpful judgments, out themselves when they are having unhelpful judgments, and practice self-enquiry around judgmental thinking.
- *With One-Mindful Awareness:* With One-Mindful Awareness is similar to the One-Mindfully skill, with a twist. One-Mindful Awareness not only involves intentional focus on the present moment, it also involves doing so with humility. This means acknowledging that what one is aware of in the present moment is a version that is edited by what information one's brain has taken in, rather than a "true" representation of reality. With One-Mindful Awareness also encourages individuals to enjoy the moment they

are in, rather than focusing on immediately moving on to the next task or goal.

- *Effectively and With Humility:* Effectively and With Humility is also similar to the Effectively skill, but with a twist. Effectively and With Humility still focuses on doing what is needed to achieve goals and/or live in closer alignment with one's values, while also taking into account the needs and desires of other people. This may mean having to let go of rigidly held beliefs or rules or focusing less on winning and achievement in order to take all aspects of the Effectively and With Humility skill into account.

- *Flexible Mind REVEALs:* Flexible Mind REVEALs is a skill that is focused on helping individuals let go of "don't hurt me" responses, which are responses that convey the message that the person with whom the individual is communicating should stop giving feedback and/or stop asking them to change because it is painful, and "pushback" responses, which are responses that convey the message that the person with whom the individual is communicating should stop challenging them and/or giving them feedback or otherwise that individual will act such that the person will wish they had. The "R" stands for "Recognize secret desires for control" and is focused on helping the individual identify indicators that they have a secret desire for control in a given moment. The "E" stands for "Examine your social signaling and label what you find" and expands upon the previous component in this skill by helping the individual to identify body language, cognitive content, and emotions that might be signaling "don't hurt me" or "pushback" responses. The "V" stands for "Remember your core Values" and is focused on helping the person identify core values that are inconsistent with desires to manipulate or control others and utilize the Opposite Action skill to engage in social signaling that is inconsistent with "don't hurt me" and "pushback" responses. The second "E" stands for "Engage with integrity by outing yourself" and involves the individual being honest about their desires for control, desires for the person to change, or desires for the person to be soothing, while at the same time also being clear that in sharing this, you are not implying that they need to change their behavior. The "A" stands for "Practice Flexible Mind ADOPTS" and simply involves practicing the steps of this skill. Finally, the "L" stands for "Learn through self-enquiry" and focuses on the individual reflecting on a question related to this experience in order to enhance learning.

- *Flexible Mind ROCKs ON:* Flexible Mind ROCKs ON is a skill that helps patients plan for interpersonal interactions, with a focus on their interpersonal effectiveness goals, and subsequently interact with others in a way that places kindness at the forefront and takes into account the other person's needs. The "R" stands for "Resist the urge to control other people" and is focused on letting go of control and rigidity in the service of maintaining and improving interpersonal relationships. The "O" stands for "identify your interpersonal effectiveness goals and degree of Openness," which involves identifying goals the patient may have with regard to objectiveness effectiveness, relationship effectiveness, self-respect effectiveness, and self-enquiry effectiveness and exploring the extent to which they are open to questioning beliefs or assumptions they may have about the person with whom they will be interacting. The "C" stands for "Clarify the interpersonal effectiveness goal that is your priority" and is focused on identifying which of the four types of effectiveness is most important in the interaction and using that information to guide their behavior. The "K" stands for "practice Kindness first and foremost" and involves helping the person learn to default to kindness toward self and others as both an initial response and a response to try when they are unsure how to proceed in a social interaction. Finally, the "ON" stands for "take into account the Other person's Needs" and is focused on helping the other person to achieve their goals and objectives when possible, while also honoring one's own goals and objectives, and slowing the pace or taking a break if there is tension or if an impasse is reached.

- *Flexible Mind PROVEs:* Flexible Mind PROVEs is a skill that helps individuals to balance being assertive with being open-minded and humble in order to achieve success when asking someone for something or turning down a request that is being made. The "P" stands for "Provide a brief description of the underlying circumstances," which involves outlining the circumstances around why you are making or turning down a request, but in a way that uses language that reflects open-mindedness and non defensiveness. The "R" stands for "Reveal your emotions about the circumstances, without blaming." This entails openly sharing one's emotional experience while also taking responsibility for one's emotions, rather than making statements that imply the other person is responsible for having caused them. The "O" stands for "Acknowledge the Other Person's needs, wants, and desires," which involves the individual letting the other person know that they want to take their needs, wants, and desires into account and directly asking them about their needs, wants, and desires. The "V" stands for "Using your Valued Goals to guide how you socially signal your needs." This is focused on signaling non-dominance and being polite, while also avoiding disguised demands and insincere expressions of admiration as methods to achieve one's objective. Finally, the "E" stands for "Practice self-Enquiry to decide whether (or not) to repeat your assertion," which involves sensing how intense or repetitive to be in asking for what you want or turning a request down, as well as pausing at times when things may not be going well to engage in self-enquiry to assist in learning before proceeding forward in the interaction. It can also involve using self-enquiry to explore the situation and relationship at a broader level.

- *Flexible Mind ALLOWs:* Flexible Mind ALLOWs is focused on strategies for enhancing the quality and intimacy of interpersonal relationships. The "A" stands for "Assess with you are committed to improving the relationship and are willing to let go of mistrust" and is focused on exploring reasons for potentially enhancing the intimacy of the relationship, as well as fears and reservations one might have about being more open. The first "L" stands for "Look for concrete evidence that mistrust is justified or the relationship is toxic" and involves looking for Fixed Mind thinking, Fatalistic Mind thinking, and potential misperceptions about the relationship. The second "L" stands for "Loosen your grip on past hurts and fears" and is focused on giving people the benefit of the doubt and allowing for the possibility you misjudged them, or in circumstances where genuine hurts did occur, exploring the possibility of forgiveness. The "O" stands for "Out yourself by revealing inner feelings" which involves taking the lead when it comes to self-disclosure and not giving up if the person does not reciprocate in making efforts toward an improved relationship. Finally, the "W" stands for "Welcome feedback and continue to dialogue" which is focused on genuinely listening to the other person, remaining engaged if things don't go as planned, and taking a temporary break from discussion if needed if emotions become too intense.
- *Match + 1:* Match + 1 is a skill that is focused on creating or enhancing interpersonal connectedness through revealing personal information that is appropriate for how well you know a given individual. Overcontrolled individuals have a tendency not to share personal information, and yet the sharing of personal information is important in enhancing intimacy and conveying trust. The Match + 1 skill provides a structure for transitioning from "chit-chat" to a more intimate conversation by encouraging a person to share something about themselves, mindfully listen to the person's response, and to then not only match that person's level of self-disclosure, but actually go slightly deeper in terms of information shared. The Match + 1 skill also encourages self-enquiry after the interaction, where the person reflects on information shared and the level of intimacy they felt they experienced.
- *Flexible Mind ADOPTS:* Flexible Mind ADOPTS is a skill that is focused on helping individuals to increase their openness to feedback and/or information and to alter their behavior in response to this feedback, if needed. The "A" stands for "Acknowledge that painful feedback is occurring" and is focused on enhancing one's ability to be aware of verbal, nonverbal, and situational information that suggests feedback is occurring. The "D" stands for "Describe and observe emotions, bodily sensations, and thoughts," and involves attending to rather than ignoring or dismissing one's emotions, bodily sensations, and thoughts. The "O" stands for "Open to new information by cheerleading and fully listening" and entails activating one's social safety system and letting go of rebutting or explaining and instead

focusing on fully listening to the feedback being provided. The "P" stands for "Pinpoint what new behavior is being recommended by the feedback" and involves identifying, clarifying, and verifying what specific changes are being suggested. The "T" stands for "Try out the new behavior," although before doing this, one should consider whether to accept or decline the feedback, based on factors like the reason for making the change and the impact the change will have on relationships and/or long-term goals. If one decides to accept the feedback, the next step is either to try out the new behavior fully and without judgment or if the behavior cannot be used immediately, to practice imaginal rehearsal of the behavior. Finally, the "S" stands for "Self-soothe and reward yourself for being open and trying something new" which involves letting go of judgment and rumination and focusing on rewarding oneself instead.

- *Flexible Mind DARES (to Let Go):* Flexible Mind DARES (to Let Go) is a skill that is focused on letting go of unhelpful envy. The "D" stands for "Determine if you are experiencing unhelpful envy" and involves the individual reflecting on their thoughts, behaviors, and urges as a way to determine whether they are experiencing unhelpful envy. The "A" stands for "Admit your envy and decide whether you want to change it" and is focused on observing and describing the emotion of envy, as well as weighing the pros and cons of taking action to decrease the emotion of envy versus maintaining the current state of affairs. The "R" stands for "Recognize envious thoughts and action urges" and involves noticing action urges for revenge, for shame, and for seeking validation from others. The "E" stands for "Go opposite to Envious anger" and is focused on identifying one's specific action urges associated with envious anger (e.g. fantasizing about the other person failing, engaging in gossip about the other person) and utilizing opposite action instead (e.g. practicing gratitude for what one does have, refraining from gossip). Finally, the "S" stands for "Go opposite to Shameful envy" and involves utilizing opposite action by being honest with oneself and others about one's feelings of envy.

- *Flexible Mind is LIGHT:* Flexible Mind is LIGHT is a skill that is focused on targeting bitterness. The "L" stands for "Label your bitterness, using self-enquiry" and involves asking a series of self-enquiry questions (e.g. "Do I feel my efforts often go unrecognized?") to explore how bitterness might manifest for that individual. The "I" stands for "Notice bitter Intentions by examining action urges" and is focused on exploring whether one is experiencing bitter emotions or engaging in bitter actions or thinking, like being judgmental toward optimistic people or holding the belief that considering progress is possible is naïve. The "G" stands for "Go opposite to bitter beliefs" and involves using Opposite Action to address behaviors, thoughts, and emotions associated with bitterness that were identified. For example, instead of being judgmental toward optimistic people, an opposite action might be actively and nonjudgmentally listening to an optimistic person. The "H" stands for "Help others, and allow others to Help" and is focused on both soliciting and providing help, while also letting go of unhelpful beliefs one holds about giving and receiving help. Finally, the "T" stands for "Practice kindness and being Thankful" and involves prioritizing and regularly engaging in kind thinking and kind behaviors.

- *Flexible Mind Has HEART:* Flexible Mind Has HEART is a skill that is focused on healthy forgiveness. The "H" stands for "Identify the past Hurt" and involves asking oneself a variety of questions to explore whether there are past hurts one is holding onto. The "E" stands for "Locate your Edge that's keeping you stuck in the past" and is focused on noticing desires to explain, justify, or blame, coupled with using self-enquiry to locate one's edge. The "A" stands for "Acknowledge forgiveness is a choice" and involves the individual thinking through whether or not they would like to practice forgiveness. The "R" stands for "Reclaim your life by grieving your loss and practicing forgiveness" and is focused on allowing oneself to experience emotions associated with a loss, while at the same time not holding onto these emotions when they occur, as well as practicing forgiveness, over and over again. Finally, the "T" stands for "Practice Thankfulness and then pass it on" and involves being thankful for the opportunity to practice forgiveness, coupled with practicing kindness.

Self-Management Skills

Although not explicitly taught as part of DBT skills training for the most part, self-management skills are an additional set of skills that can be useful for a patient to learn. The bulk of self-management skills focus on helping patients to establish reasonable and achievable goals and to structure contingencies and the environment to make it more likely that the identified goals can be realized.

Self-management skills also include relapse prevention planning. Relapse prevention planning should be individualized and we would encourage the creation of a written, living document as part of this process. Topics that may be helpful to cover when engaging in relapse prevention planning include the pros and cons of engaging in eating disorder behaviors versus the pros and cons of engaging in recovery-oriented behaviors, your patient's values and goals and how these relate to reasons for pursuing recovery, positive changes your patient has made since entering treatment and their plan for sustaining these changes, useful skills and information your patient has learned about in treatment, goals your patient has for the upcoming weeks and steps they plan to take to achieve these goals, structure your patient would like to put in place, challenges and high-risk situations your patient anticipates encountering and how they will navigate these challenges and high-risk situations, warning signs of a slip, lapse, or relapse, helpful challenges to eating disorder thoughts, your patient's support system and how they can utilize this support system in their recovery process, and their plan for getting back on track in the event of a lapse or a relapse. In addition to having a copy for themselves that they reference and update on an ongoing basis, we would also recommend that patients share their relapse prevention plans with all members of their multidisciplinary team, as well as with key natural supports.

Bringing DBT to Life – Exploring Skills Megan Needs to Acquire to Help Her Build a Life Worth Living

As with many patients who present with longstanding eating disorders and multiple complex comorbidities, each of the skills modules within DBT has skills that are relevant for Megan's care. Additionally, the aforementioned self-management skills as well as skills outside of the psychotherapeutic realm are also applicable in Megan's treatment.

Although Megan is someone who experiences negative affect, both frequently and intensely, she has difficulty accurately labeling her emotional experiences and responding to them effectively. All of the skills within the Mindfulness module could be of benefit for Megan. Enhancing her application of the Observe and Describe skills as they relate to her emotional experiencing would help Megan to be able to more accurately label her emotions, in turn increasing the likelihood of her ability to regulate them. Megan would also benefit from further work on accessing Wise Mind and using this skill to guide her decision-making in the moment. Increased focus on the Effectively skill would also supplement Wise Mind nicely.

Megan is someone who tends to struggle with asking for support effectively. Additionally, she experiences difficulty in cultivating and enhancing her interpersonal relationships. Targeted skills practice focused on the use of DEAR MAN could help to enhance Megan's ability to advocate for her needs. Intentional use of both the GIVE skill and the Mindfulness of Others skill provide two options for increasing Megan's connectedness to others. Although not explicitly mentioned as a skill, guidance is provided within the DBT skills manual around responding to invalidation and Megan would likely benefit from learning to respond to invalidation more effectively, in addition to applying the Self-Validation skill at those times.

Pervasive emotion dysregulation and the problems associated with it are core maintaining factors in Megan's eating disorder. While some of the work for Megan would be focused on tolerating emotional distress, which we will speak to shortly in a review of Distress Tolerance skills she may find to be useful, Megan will also need to learn how to regulate her emotions in order to achieve a sustained recovery. Opposite Action is a skill that could assist Megan in reducing the frequency and intensity of the anxiety, sadness, and unjustified shame she experiences. Mindfulness of Current Emotions is another skill from which Megan could benefit, in that it will be important for her to learn to be present with her emotional experiences without always taking action, either adaptive or maladaptive, to try to cause an immediate shift in her emotional experiencing. Check the Facts is an additional skill that is critical for Megan to put into practice, as applied to both her complex and entrenched eating disorder thinking, as well as to a variety of unhelpful beliefs she holds about herself as a person. Lastly, Megan is someone who does not have a fully formed identity outside of her eating disorder, which impedes her ability to experience pleasant emotions. The ABC PLEASE skill is one that could help Megan experience more frequent pleasant emotions by helping her to engage in short-term pleasant activities, in addition to activities consistent with her values and long-term goals.

Skills from the Distress Tolerance module of DBT are also highly relevant to the challenges Megan experiences. Skills like STOP and Pros and Cons could be useful in targeting Megan's impulsivity specifically, and Wise Mind ACCEPTS, Self-Soothing, and Improve the Moment are all options of skills that Megan could use to tolerate distress associated with resisting urges to engage in impulsive behaviors. Sensory Awareness could also be used for this purpose and additionally is a skill that Megan could use as a form of grounding in the event of experiencing heightened trauma-related symptoms. Megan is also someone who struggles with ambivalence around recovery, so Radical Acceptance, Turning the Mind, and Willingness are all skills she may find to be helpful in staying on track with wise minded, recovery-oriented behaviors. Eating disorder thinking is another pervasive challenge for Megan. Mindfulness of Current Thoughts is a skill that could assist her in beginning to observe and describe these thoughts, as well as beginning to create distance from her thoughts through various strategies that parallel cognitive defusion strategies from Acceptance and Commitment Therapy. Megan is someone who is also prone to black-and-white thinking when it comes to situations in which she experiences a lapse or relapse. Dialectical Abstinence is likely to be a critical skill for Megan to learn and put into practice, particularly early on in her recovery. Lastly, Megan's impulsivity and ambivalence make it risky for her to leave any option for engaging in disordered behaviors open. Burning Bridges is a skill that Megan could apply to ensure that she has limited her access as much as possible to items associated with her eating disorder (e.g. a scale, fitness watches), her alcohol use disorder (e.g. glasses specifically used to drink alcohol), and her self-harm behaviors (e.g. items that she might use specifically for self-harm purposes).

There are also a number of skills from RO DBT that Megan is likely to find beneficial. The core skill of Radical Openness coupled with Flexible Mind DEFinitely are skills that could assist Megan in being more flexible, less avoidant, and more open to new information. Megan also struggles with interpersonal relationships, both in terms of finding social interactions outside of her closest social circle to be anxiety-provoking, as well as in terms of knowing how to go about enhancing social connectedness and interpersonal intimacy. Skills like the The Big Three + 1, Flexible Mind is DEEP, Flexible Mind ALLOWs, and Match + 1 may all be of help in this area. Lastly, Megan struggles with openness around novel experiences and may benefit from Flexible Mind VARIEs.

While Megan's therapist and Megan's DBT skills group facilitators would be the ones primarily responsible for teaching Megan each of these skills, the other members of Megan's team each play a role in skills strengthening and skills generalization. Megan's art therapist finds she is able to use a variety of art therapy directives to assist Megan in observing and describing her emotions, connecting with her values, and challenging perfectionism through the use of Opposite Action. As mentioned earlier, Megan's dietitian and culinary staff are working with her around enhancing her cooking skills. Megan's psychiatric provider and medical provider, as well as nursing staff, are assisting her with medication compliance. The psychiatric technicians with whom Megan interacts are helping her to apply the skills she is learning in the moments that she needs them the most. Lastly, Megan's case manager is assisting her with basic life skills, like effectively structuring her day and managing her finances. The key point here is that everyone on Megan's treatment team has a responsibility for helping her acquire, strengthen, and generalize skills within their scope of practice.

Provider Exercise – What Skills Does My Patient Need?

Think about a patient with whom you are currently working. Based on the information you learned above, make notes about the following questions below. Which skills do you think your patient would most benefit from? How do you envision your patient using these skills in the context of their eating disorder treatment and recovery process? Are there skills that were not mentioned above that might also benefit your patient? Which skills fall within your scope of practice and which skills might fall within the scope of practice of other members of your patient's treatment team?

Chapter 19

The Third Mode of DBT

In-the-Moment Coaching

When DBT was initially created, in-the-moment coaching referred only to tele-phone contacts between the patient and therapist in between therapy sessions, with the overarching purpose of teaching the patient how to apply the skills they are learning in treatment to situations in their day-to-day lives. As we will discuss in more detail below, there are additional strategies now available to providers that honor the intent of in-the-moment coaching, yet go beyond what was described in the initial DBT text.

Purposes of In-the-Moment Coaching

There are three primary purposes that in-the-moment coaching serves (Linehan, 1993). As mentioned above, the primary purpose of in-the-moment coaching is helping patients to translate what they are learning in the context of treat-ment into moments in their day-to-day lives, known in DBT as skills general-ization. For those of you who are providing treatment at an outpatient level of care, you are probably only seeing your patients for an hour or so each week. While your patients are likely fairly skillful during the hour they are in session with you, they have 167 additional hours each week during which they have to remember to use their skills, find the willingness to apply them, and use them effectively! In-the-moment coaching is intended to help make sure that patients have targeted support in between sessions at times when they need that sup-port the most. The key with in-the-moment coaching is that it should be brief and skills-focused, rather than functioning as an additional provider session in between scheduled sessions. Although you certainly should endeavor to help your patient solve the problem that led to them seeking in-the-moment coaching in the first place if this can be done with relative ease and brevity, the reality is that many in-the-moment coaching contacts will likely lean toward helping your patient tolerate their distress skillfully with the intent of taking a closer look at the problem that led them to seek help in a future scheduled individual session. Metaphorically, I think of in-the-moment coaching like the time I (AHK) called

DOI: 10.4324/9781003495604-19

my mother to help me with a flat tire I had gotten on an onramp to the highway. After gathering information about the situation at hand, it became clear to her she would not be able to guide me in solving the problem of putting on my spare tire over the phone. Instead, the focus of her support became helping me with ideas for tolerating my distress until assistance arrived. What her support didn't focus on were the factors leading up to why I had gotten a flat tire in the first place, which is a longer list than I would like to publicly admit, nor what I was going to do in the future to prevent a similar situation. The sole focus was on tolerating the current moment, knowing additional discussions could come later.

The second purpose of in-the-moment coaching is relationship repair. Interpersonal difficulties are often one of the challenges that patients with eating disorders face and the context of the therapeutic relationship is fertile ground for helping our patients to learn how to navigate interpersonal relationships more effectively within a context that is also a safe space. I (AHK) can think of only a few examples of interpersonal situations where a timeframe beyond a day or two would exist that a person would have to wait in order to address an interpersonal concern that had arisen. By allowing for patients to reach out to briefly check-in in situations where a relationship rupture has occurred, we not only prevent situations in which feelings of hurt, resentment, alienation, shame, and so forth are allowed to fester for an extended period of time, we also provide our patients with an opportunity to initiate a more naturalistic way of approaching and resolving interpersonal discord when it occurs. As with in-the-moment coaching focused on skills use, in-the-moment coaching focused on relationship repair should also be targeted and brief in nature. The patient should be given space to express their feelings and concerns and the provider should do their best to provide support in the moment, however more extended discussions around the therapeutic relationship should be tabled until the next scheduled section with the provider. This approach strikes a balance between being compassionate while also being able to maintain reasonable boundaries.

The final purpose of in-the-moment coaching is sharing good news. As with relationship repair, there are few instances we can think of where two individuals in an authentic interpersonal relationship would have to wait for an extended period of time to share something positive that happened in their life. Allowing in-the-moment coaching to focus on the patient briefly sharing good news again helps to mimic more socially normative interpersonal interactions. It also has the added benefit of preventing situations in which the only way a patient can have in-between session contact with a provider is when something "bad" has happened or is happening. If interpersonal interactions with a provider are indeed reinforcing to a patient, this prevents establishing situations in which crises and relationship ruptures become paired with a reinforcing consequence, whereas positive situations do not.

Steps of In-the-Moment Coaching

In-the-moment coaching as it relates to helping patients apply skills in their day-to-day life is intended to be a brief intervention, lasting no more than 10–15 minutes in most circumstances. In order to ensure that in-the-moment coaching remains brief, many providers with whom I (AHK) have worked have found it to be helpful to have step-by-step guidance for how to go about in-the-moment coaching. The recommended steps are as follows:

1. *Assess the problem situation.* The first step in providing in-the-moment coaching is to get an understanding of the problem situation. Remember, most errors in treatment are errors of assessment, not errors of intervention. As such, it is important to get information about the patient's understanding of what caused the problem situation, what is contributing to it continuing to remain a problem situation, and what they have done so far to try to address the problem situation, which may include both change-focused and acceptance-focused skills. It is important to note that your assessment of the problem situation should not necessarily go into the same level of depth as you might during an individual provider session. Rather, you are aiming for a succinct, yet accurate summary.
2. *Summarize your understanding of the problem situation.* Once you believe you have an understanding of the problem situation, you will want to summarize your understanding of the situation aloud. This gives your patient the opportunity to confirm the accuracy of your summary or to provide corrective feedback if elements of your summary are inaccurate.
3. *Generate potential skills the patient can use to navigate the situation effectively.* After you have an accurate assessment of the situation that has been confirmed by the patient, you will then want to make recommendations about specific skills the patient can use to navigate the situation effectively. If your assessment is that the patient may be able to solve or at least improve the problem situation, you may want to focus on change-oriented skills from the Interpersonal Effectiveness and Emotion Regulation module. If your assessment is that your patient cannot solve the situation, at least not at the present moment, then you will likely want to provide acceptance-oriented skills from the Mindfulness and Distress Tolerance modules.
4. *Determine a plan of action and obtain commitment to the plan of action.* Once you have brainstormed skills that a patient may be able to use to navigate the problem situation effectively, you will then want to solicit their input about which skill or skills they are willing to try. Once the skill or skills have been identified, you will want to help the patient develop a plan for when, where, and how they will implement the skill or skills identified. It is helpful in most circumstances to ask the patient to write the plan down,

such that they have a visual cue they are able to reference rather than relying on memory alone.

5. *Reassess the problem situation.* Once you have a plan of action outlined, you will want to reassess the problem situation. If the problem situation is one involving potential safety-related concerns, you will want to ensure that the patient believes the plan that has been determined sufficiently addresses the problem situation, such that the risk of an adverse event (e.g. suicide attempt, self-injurious behavior) is sufficiently diminished. If the problem situation does not involve safety-related concerns, you will still want to check with the patient to make sure the plan in place adequately addresses the factors, like urges, emotions, or thoughts, that prompted them to reach out to you for assistance in the first place.

6. *Outline a plan for follow-up.* The final step of in-the-moment coaching is outlining a plan for follow-up. This plan should be twofold. First, you and your patient should come up with a plan for what they will do if the situation gets worse again, a related or new problem situation emerges, or if the plan you have outlined isn't working. Second, you should review the plan for follow-up, such as making a plan to discuss the problem situation in further detail during an upcoming provider session, making a plan to check-in with the patient prior to their next appointment, and/or reminding the patient of the day and time of your next appointment.

In-the-Moment Coaching Adaptations in an Outpatient Environment

If you are a therapist who is providing full-model DBT, offering in-the-moment coaching is a required element of the services you provide. However, if you are an outpatient provider who wants to take advantage of the benefits of in-the-moment coaching and you are not providing full-model DBT, there are a number of actions you could consider taking to weave this element of DBT into your practice. The original DBT text was written before the time of smartphones and apps, which have drastically changed the ways in which we can communicate with others. The original intent was for in-the-moment coaching to be provided via in-between session telephone calls. The use of e-mail and text messages have become methods that some providers are using to provide in-the-moment coaching, although with newer methods of communication, it is important to take ethics codes, recommended best practices for your discipline, HIPAA, and policies and procedures of organizations where you may work into consideration when it comes to patient communication. Smartphone apps are a newer method of in-between session communication that we have found particularly helpful in our work. As an example, one app we have used has the ability for patients to provide photographic documentation of meal and snack completion, in addition to providing detailed information about their experience with any given meal or snack in terms of context, emotions experienced, urges to engage in behaviors, and hunger and fullness ratings. The app also enables the patient to communicate with providers through a secure messaging function, and allows providers to provide encouragement to their patients, offer suggestions of skills, and so forth. Finally, having the patient bring the situation where they need coaching the most to you through having them bring a meal or snack into session and providing meal support and meal coaching is another creative way to allow in-the-moment coaching to serve the function it was intended to serve.

In-the-Moment Coaching Adaptations in Higher Levels of Care

There are two ways in which in-the-moment coaching can be adapted at higher levels of care that are worth consideration when working in these settings. At inpatient and residential levels of care, frontline staff members like nurses and mental health technicians are present all day, every day. If frontline staff members are trained about each of the DBT skills and about how to provide in-the-moment coaching, this creates the opportunity for patients to be provided with guidance around skill use at the exact moment where assistance is needed. The other way in which in-the-moment coaching can be adapted to higher levels of care is through creativity on the part of the patient's multidisciplinary team as a whole. When a patient is at a higher level of care, many experiences where a patient would need support can easily be replicated as part of the overall treatment experience. Rather than talking about how a patient might navigate a restaurant, the grocery store, or a cooking experience, the patient's multidisciplinary team can actually allocate their time to accompany patients in these experiences. This is useful both from an assessment standpoint, in that you can witness directly where a patient is experiencing challenges, as well as from a treatment standpoint, in that you can provide in-the-moment coaching to assist them in these specific contexts.

Meal Coaching – A Contextually-Specific Adaptation of In-the-Moment Coaching

Meal coaching is a contextually-specific form of in-the-moment coaching that is relevant in the treatment of patients diagnosed with eating disorders. While meal coaching is most commonly implemented by providers at higher levels of care, it can be utilized at any level of care if you ascertain that it would be clinically beneficial.

Although meal coaching does not follow the steps of in-the-moment coaching, the principles underlying in-the-moment coaching and meal coaching are quite similar. Both involve providing in-the-moment support that is focused on helping patients apply the skills they have learned in treatment in the situations where these skills are needed the most. The approach of individuals providing meal coaching and in-the-moment coaching is also nonjudgmental and calm, weaving validation throughout, while also being concrete and directive.

There are three main differences between meal coaching and in-the-moment coaching that are worth noting. First, less time is spent on information gathering when providing meal coaching, since this can actually serve to distract from the meal or snack on hand. Instead, the person providing meal coaching searches for opportunities to provide validation and guidance around the use of specific skills with the information that presents itself in the moment, without extensive probing. Second, with in-the-moment coaching, the provider and patient are usually working to come up with a plan that the patient will implement independently, rather than the patient implementing the plan as they are speaking with the provider. With meal coaching, the provider is actively helping the patient implement skills throughout the meal or snack. Finally, meal coaching tends to include more firm directives (e.g. "Take a bite of the chicken," "Please stop blotting your pizza") than is typical with in-the-moment coaching, where the patient is given a bit more autonomy around choices they make.

Bringing DBT to Life – Providing In-the-Moment Coaching and Meal Coaching to Megan

In order to illustrate the similarities and differences between in-the-moment coaching and meal coaching, we thought it could be helpful to provide examples of each being used with Megan.

In-the-Moment Coaching

In this specific vignette, Megan has recently transitioned to an IOP level of care and she has reached out to her therapist (Serena) for support in between sessions.

Serena: "Hey Megan, I saw you called. What's up?"

Megan: "I just got home from the grocery store, and…well, nevermind. It's fine."

Serena: "Megan, I know that you called me for a reason and I suspect it's an important one. How can I help?"

Megan: "So yesterday, I went in for my nurse visit for my weekly weights and vitals. The nurse was new to the practice, or I didn't recognize her, and must've missed my eating disorder diagnosis. She commented that I had put on a lot of weight in the past six months and actually suggested I try to increase my body movement. Of course I heard that I need to lose weight. Her comment definitely sent me spiraling for a minute. I tried to push it out of my mind, but I guess it must not have worked because when I was at the grocery store today, I bought a box of diet pills and I'm having a really hard time not taking them."

Serena: "First off, I'm so glad you called me, Megan. I know it's not always easy to reach out for help. What a crappy situation! I'm so sorry that happened. I definitely think you and I can work through this and as a starting point, are you willing to take the diet pills out to the dumpster while we chat?"

Megan: "They were expensive. I'll probably just return them to the store if I don't end up taking them tonight."

Serena: "Gotcha, I understand. I wonder if we can still get some distance between you and the pills. Are you willing to put them in the trunk of your car for now instead?"

Megan: "I think I can do that." (Serena hears a door opening, footsteps, and a trunk opening and shutting) "Okay, they're in the trunk."

Serena: "Thanks for doing that, Megan. I think that will help to make it a bit easier to access Wise Mind. I have a good handle on why you purchased the diet pills, but what's making it so difficult at this moment not to take the pills?"

Megan: "I can't stop thinking about that nurses' comment. She was clearly trying to encourage me to lose weight. My eating disorder found it validating, but on some level, I know that's not true...I know I need to be at this weight. [sigh] I do look so gross and I definitely feel gross."

Serena: "If I'm hearing you correctly, it really sounds like your ED voice is pretty loud at the moment and that your body image distress is also pretty high. Is that accurate?"

Megan: "Yup."

Serena: "Are there any skills you have tried so far?"

Megan: (laughs) "Well, I called you!"

Serena: "And I'm so glad you did! I'm getting the sense that perhaps you've been too overwhelmed to even think through what skills you might be able to try."

Megan: "Yeah."

Serena: "Well, there are a few skills that come to mind for me that you might find to be helpful. It seems like you've been doing a good job trying to Check the Facts, and that the facts you've come up with have been hard to hold on to. I wonder about actually writing down some of the facts you've come up with, in addition to trying to come up with more. I also wonder about doing a Pros and Cons list of taking the pills versus using Distress Tolerance skills to get through this tough moment. You've come so far in your treatment and recovery process, and I wonder if that might help you to better access Wise Mind."

Megan: "I like the idea about writing down Check the Facts stuff, and trying to come up with other statements that also feel true. I think if I did the Pros and Cons list it might get me more focused on the pills, so I don't know if I want to do that."

Serena: "I gotcha, that makes total sense. I wonder about the next steps after working on the Check the Facts piece? It seems like this could be a night where focusing on some self-soothing and distraction could be really helpful."

Megan: "Yeah, I guess I could take a shower since that usually calms me down a bit, and then maybe get into some comfortable clothes and watch some episodes of Parks and Rec. I usually find those to be pretty distracting."

Serena: "I like that as an idea and I think the key to all of this is that if you find your mind getting focused on what the nurse said and all the ED thoughts that cascade from that, it's going to be important to reference what you came up with as part of Check the Facts and then mindfully bring yourself back to the moment you're in. Okay, you want to reflect back to me what we've talked about and maybe write it down as we review?"

Megan: "Sure...so after we get off the phone, I'm going to work on Check the Facts. Then I'm going to take a shower, get into some comfortable clothes, and put on Parks and Rec. And if I find my mind wandering to unhelpful places, Check the Facts and then focus back on my show."

Serena: "Exactly. So where are you now in terms of urges to take the pills, on a scale of 0 to 10?"

Megan: "I was at a 7 or 8, but I'd say I'm more at a 4 now. The urge is still there, but it's helpful to have them out of my sight, and I feel like I have a plan for now."

Serena: "That's great, Megan. So last thing...what are you going to do if your urges get worse again?"

Megan: "I think if they get really, really bad, I can ask my mom to come over and take the pills. I just really don't want to do that because I don't want her to get mad at me or get worried that I'm backsliding. I feel like it will be a whole conversation, and I really don't want that. I guess if it also gets really bad, I could just go to bed and call it a day. I'm honestly pretty exhausted."

Serena: "I can understand not wanting to have your mom come over to get the pills, and if you end up in a bind, I do really think that is the better of the two options. I know we're still working on you being more open with your mom about when you're struggling and your mom responding in a way that makes you more willing to be open when you're struggling in the future, and I think this is a serious enough situation that it's important to prioritize you not taking those pills over the discomfort that might come with being honest with your mom. Also, you're welcome to give me a call tomorrow if you need to check in. Otherwise, I've got our individual session on the calendar for Thursday and we can dig into all of this in more detail then if we need to. Does that sound like an okay plan?"

Megan: "That works. Thanks, Serena."

Meal Coaching

In this example, Megan is early on in her residential treatment stay. She's seated at the meal table with her dietitian, Claire. Megan has been dreading this meal, which consists of a fast food cheeseburger and fries, for weeks. Claire agreed to share the meal with Megan and engage Megan in meal coaching.

Megan: [staring at the cheeseburger, still in wrapper] "...yeah this is not going to happen."

Claire: "Let's get that cheeseburger unwrapped."

Megan: [continues to stare] "I... don't think I can. I'm too anxious."

Claire: "I get it. I'm not asking you to commit to anything else at this time aside from taking the burger out of the wrapper."

Megan: [sighs]. "Okay…. here. Look, it's out of the wrapper."

Claire: "Great! Now pick up the burger and see if you can take a bite."

Megan: "Heck no. Not happening."

Claire: "Okay. How about a french fry then?"

Megan: "Look, just stop. I appreciate you trying to support me, but you know this is the top of my fear food hierarchy and I'm not ready for it."

Claire: "I know this is a challenging meal for you, and that's why I'm here to support you! Okay, how about we shift gears. Can you start with your soda? Bring your cup closer to you. Go ahead and take a sip."

Megan: [takes a sip] "Ugh. Regular Coke. I really prefer Diet Coke…"

Claire: "Now I want you to grab that small french fry. I've seen you do a lot of difficult things in our time working together, and I believe you can complete this meal. Take a bite."

Megan: [takes a bite] "Okay, I did it. Are you happy now?"

Claire: "I'm proud of you. And let's keep going. This time, I want you to pick up the burger, and hold it for a moment. I'm going to take a bite of my cheeseburger, and then I'd like to see you take a bite of yours."

Megan: "Fine…one bite. And then we're done here!"

Claire: "You know I'm going to keep pushing you for the next twenty five minutes. I believe you can do it! Time to pick up another fry."

Provider Exercise – In-the-Moment Coaching

In the space below, write about your initial reactions to incorporating in-the-moment coaching into your work. Consider discussing your reactions with a trusted peer for feedback.

If you are open to incorporating some form of in-the-moment coaching into your work, if this is not part of your work already, write initial thoughts about what form of in-the-moment coaching you might use and why.

If you've decided that you'd like to incorporate in-the-moment coaching into your work, write out the action steps you will need to take in order to do so. Examples of potential action steps could include updating paperwork you provide to patients to include information about in-the-moment coaching, setting up methods of contact for in-the-moment coaching, informing your patients that you will now be offering in-the-moment coaching, and so forth.

Chapter 20

The Fourth Mode of DBT

Case Consultation Meetings

The following chapter is operating under the assumption that the reader does not have the capacity to be part of a full-model DBT program and rather is seeking to utilize principles and strategies from the case consultation mode of treatment. In the event that this assumption is not accurate, the reader is encouraged to review DBT Teams: Development and Practice by Sayrs and Linehan (2019) as a comprehensive resource for creating and sustaining a DBT team in the context of a full-model DBT program.

Functions of the Case Consultation Mode of Treatment

There are two primary functions of the case consultation mode of treatment. The first function is to increase providers' motivation. While working with patients diagnosed with eating disorders is incredibly rewarding work, it can also be emotionally taxing, particularly when working at higher levels of care. The focus on motivation as one of the two primary functions of the case consultation mode of treatment recognizes that providers need support. As we will discuss in more detail later, support can mean a variety of things, including validation of a provider's experience, problem-solving around patient- and provider-related factors leading to an increase in burnout, cheerleading and encouragement, and simply having a space where providers can be vulnerable with one another. The general idea here is that case consultation teams function as a form of "therapy for the provider."

The second function of the case consultation mode of treatment is to increase capability. There is a high degree of specialized knowledge that is needed to conduct effective eating disorders care, particularly treatment at higher levels of care. Furthermore, DBT as a treatment approach is highly complex and nuanced. The second function of case consultation ensures that providers have a space to continuously learn and refine their craft, as well as a space to increase the extent to which providers are implementing treatment with fidelity.

DOI: 10.4324/9781003495604-20

DBT Provider Consultation Agreements

No matter what framework you are using in terms of patient care, when you have a case consultation meeting, it can be helpful to have a foundational set of agreements as providers that help you to honor the "spirit" of the treatment approach and stay within the frame of your treatment approach. The DBT provider consultation agreements were created with these aims in mind. There are lots of ways in which you can weave the DBT provider consultation agreements into case consultation team meetings. A couple of the ways that we have found to be most effective are having the DBT provider consultation agreements clearly posted in the room where case consultation meetings occur, in addition to having an agenda item on the case consultation meeting agenda where one of the DBT provider consultation agreements is read aloud and reflected upon. Let's take a peek at each of the DBT provider consultation agreements, originally outlined in Linehan (1993).

Dialectical Agreement. The teams with which we have worked have summarized the Dialectical Agreement as follows: "We agree to accept a dialectical philosophy. There is no absolute truth. When caught between two conflicting opinions, we agree to look for the truth in both positions and to search for a synthesis by asking such questions as, 'What is being left out?'" The reality in working with psychiatric illnesses in general, let alone psychiatric illnesses that are as complex and challenging as eating disorders, is that there is no singular, "right" way to approach treatment of these disorders. Yet if you've ever sat in on morning rounds or peer supervision meetings, you'll find that treatment team members often have very strong opinions about what should be done in the treatment of a patient. The Dialectical Agreement reminds us of the value of stepping back as individuals and as a collective to consider what other options exist. What we have found when these discussions occur is that it is quite rare that the exact original course of action is the one that the team ultimately selects. Rather, we have found that teams may end up choosing an entirely different course of action, or even if they have chosen to go in the general direction of their original course of action, there are nuanced ways in which the plan shifts. The times where we have found the Dialectical Agreement to be most helpful are situations in which there is a high degree of emotional intensity associated with the decision at hand, for example, when a team is trying to decide whether to transfer a patient to a different facility due to lack of progress in treatment or to stay the course of treatment in the hopes that progress will eventually be perceptible. I (AHK) have both been involved in these discussions as the provider, as well as participated in them in situations where I was not a member of the patient's treating team. It can be helpful when passionate debate is occurring for others to step back, summarize the options that have been discussed, and then ask what options may not yet have been considered.

Consultation-to-the-Patient Agreement. The Consultation-to-the-Patient Agreement can be summarized as follows: "We agree that the primary goal of this group is to improve our own skills as DBT providers, and not to serve as a go-between for patients to each other. We agree not to treat patients or each other as fragile. We agree to treat other group members with the belief that they can speak on their own behalf." Many patients who are diagnosed with an eating disorder will also struggle with difficulties in interpersonal relationships, including deficits in skill sets necessary to be appropriately assertive with others. When providers serve as go-betweens for patients or attempt to solve our patients' problems on their behalf, this reinforces active passivity and denies our patients the opportunity to develop the skills they need to assert themselves and get their needs met. For example, I've (AHK) worked with patients who have wanted me as their therapist to speak to their dietitian about making changes to their meal plan. My approach in these situations is to help the patient figure out how to effectively utilize interpersonal effectiveness skills to make their request directly. Refraining from fragilizing patients or each other as providers is also another key piece of this agreement. Our patients often have both more skills and more resilience than we give them credit for and providers are no different in this regard. While I (AHK) think that fragilizing is often done from a well-meaning place (e.g. not wanting to hurt someone's feelings), by fragilizing others, we stymie their ability to grow.

Consistency Agreement. The Consistency Agreement can be summarized as follows: "Because change is a natural life occurrence, we agree to accept diversity and change as they naturally come about. This means that we do not have to agree with each others' positions about how to respond to specific patients nor do we have to tailor our own behavior to be consistent with everyone else's." Both inconsistency and change are challenging for a subset of patients diagnosed with eating disorders and learning to navigate inconsistency and change effectively when they occur is a necessary skill set for our patients to learn. We are doing our patients no favors when we attempt to shield them from natural change and natural inconsistency, since we live in a world that is constantly in flux and where inconsistency is often far more common than predictability. For example, our patients need to have the capacity to navigate situations like picking a different restaurant when the one they planned to go to was closed, meeting their nutritional needs at a party where they couldn't have anticipated what foods would be available, or being willing to have a piece of cake that is outside of their exchanges in the service of normative, social eating. The key with the Consistency Agreement is allowing for natural change to occur while refraining from instituting arbitrary change for change's sake. It is also important to note that the Consistency Agreement refers more to consistency from therapist-to-therapist, dietitian-to-dietitian, and so forth. In circumstances in which you are a professional functioning within a hospital or facility and things like unit rules exist, it is important to make one's best effort to adhere to and hold patients accountable to unit rules, while also recognizing that errors are inevitable and are opportunities for patients to practice using skills.

Observing-Limits Agreement. The Observing-Limits Agreement can be summarized as follows: "We agree to observe our own limits. As providers and group members, we agree not to judge or criticize other members for having different limits from our own (e.g. too broad, too narrow, "just right")." Earlier in this text you had an opportunity to learn about what Observing Limits is and the importance of Observing Limits in enhancing patient care and preventing provider burnout. One way in which case consultation meetings can be useful are in supporting providers in identifying their personal limits and addressing barriers that get in their way when it comes to adhering to their personal limits, like judgments about their limits or comparisons to the limits of others. Because personal limits can also shift temporarily due to contextual factors, like physical illness or the death of a family member, or shift more permanently as natural change occurs, case consultation meetings can also be a space where providers continue to explore their personal limits over time. The key is that case consultation meetings need to be a safe and nonjudgmental space where providers can examine their personal limits and receive support around them. This doesn't mean that the other side of the dialectic isn't explored when appropriate (e.g. "Is there a way to adhere to your personal limit while also finding a creative way to be flexible in the service of..."), and ensuring that case consultation meetings remain a space that providers find to be supportive is critical.

Phenomenological Empathy Agreement. The Phenomenological Empathy agreement can be summarized as follows: "All things being equal, we agree to search for non-pejorative or phenomenologically empathic interpretations of our patients', our own, and other members' behavior. We agree to assume we and our patients are trying our best, and want to improve. We agree to strive to see the world through our patients' eyes and through one another's eyes. We agree to practice a non-judgmental stance with our patients and one another." Although we hope you take a lot from this text, if you take nothing else from reading this book, please make an intentional effort to eliminate the word "manipulative" from the list of words you use to describe your patients. Not only does the word "manipulative" fail to be an accurate description of our patients' behaviors, it also comes loaded with associated judgmental connotations and it hinders gaining an accurate understanding of the function of our patients' behaviors, which could help to inform effective treatment interventions. If you are willing, take a moment to pause and think of a time when you felt a patient was being "manipulative" and instead ask yourself, what purpose was my patient's behavior serving? How was this behavior helping them in getting a need met? Asking these questions can help you to begin to make the shift from a stance of judgment toward your patient to one in which you are able to have a more behaviorally specific, non-judgmental understanding of their behavior. For example, I've (AHK) worked with a subset of patients whose support system provided them with more attention and support when they were incredibly ill than when they were abstinent from behaviors. For many of these patients (though not all), this created a situation in which eating disorder behaviors were reinforced. Putting myself in my patients' shoes, I could understand why I would engage in eating disorder behaviors if this was the only way I knew how to get attention and caring from my support system. Another key element of the Phenomenological Empathy agreement is that we take the same empathic and nonjudgmental stance toward each other as providers. Instead of viewing each other through lenses like "too sensitive," "no boundaries," "too rigid," "not motivated," and so forth, we try to deeply and genuinely understand the perspective of our peers and use more specific language in describing the behaviors of our peers that we have observed.

Fallibility Agreement. Finally, the Fallibility Agreement can be summarized as follows: "We agree ahead of time that we are each fallible and make mistakes. We agree that we have probably either done whatever problematic things we're being accused of, or some part of it, so that we can let go of assuming a defensive stance to prove our virtue or competence. Because we are fallible, it is agreed that we will inevitably violate all of these agreements, and when this is done we will rely on each other to point out the polarity and move to a synthesis." The Fallibility Agreement is critical in helping to create a space where it is not only okay to have made a mistake, but also to be able to discuss that mistake without the fear of judgment or criticism. Patient care is such a messy art and science and no amount of education, training, or preparation can create a situation in which a provider will never make a mistake. When we radically accept that mistakes are an inevitable part of the process in doing this brave work and let go of our judgment toward ourselves and others for mistakes that have been and will be made, we create an opportunity for mistakes to be used to enhance our growth as providers.

Roles in the Case Consultation Team

Because DBT is implemented in a wide variety of settings, many of which will have unique needs, there are no rigid rules about the roles needed to accomplish the functions listed above. Teams may find they can combine roles or need to create new ones in order to accomplish what is intended by the case consultation mode of treatment. With this in mind, there are three roles that are fairly common across case consultation teams: the team leader, the observer, and the note taker.

The team leader has three primary roles in the case consultation team. First, they are responsible for managing the process of setting the agenda. I (AHK) have been a member of five case consultation teams to date, and each team went about setting the session agenda in different ways. One team had every member of the team come prepared with a written list of their agenda items such that all the team leader did with regard to agenda setting was compile their lists into a master agenda. Other teams I have been a part of set their agenda at the beginning of the team meeting, either verbally or through having team members write agenda items on a large whiteboard. Some teams I have been part of have chosen to include the amount of time they need for each agenda item, whereas other teams have relied more heavily on the team leader to determine the point at which sufficient discussion of each agenda item has occurred. As with many aspects of DBT, there is no specific way that agenda setting must be done. Individual teams should determine what works best in terms of efficiently and effectively setting a session agenda. The second role of the team leader is to remind the team of the DBT provider consultation agreements. This is typically done through the team leader selecting an agreement to read, ideally one that is particularly relevant to the team at that present time, and then reading it aloud to the team. This is done each week to reinforce the desired culture of the team and to prevent provider drift to cultures of other types of teams they may have been part of historically. We have found that it can also be helpful to occasionally (e.g. every six months) give space for all DBT provider consultation agreements to be reviewed, particularly if the team is experiencing challenges with regard to team culture. Finally, the team leader is responsible for managing time. This includes starting the meeting on time, ensuring that the amount of time spent on each agenda item is effectively managed, and ending the meeting on time. The size of the majority of case consultation teams we have been part of has not allowed for every agenda item to be covered. In these circumstances, it can be helpful to receive periodic feedback from the team as a whole about how they feel time management is going, such that team leaders can better calibrate their approach to time management to optimally meet the needs of the group.

The observer is responsible for monitoring team process, noting when deviations from the intended process occur, and initiating team members in making change as needed. What the observer monitors includes adherence to the DBT provider consultation agreements, as well as the extent to which the team is living into the "spirit" of DBT. Some examples of behavior that would be inconsistent with the principles of DBT include taking a defensive stance, using judgmental language, avoiding discussion of an uncomfortable topic, coming to team late or unprepared, or making a decision about a course of action without considering the other side of the dialectic. The behaviors that the observer attends to will vary across teams and should be driven by what is in the best interests of the patients treated by the team, individual providers who make up the team, and the team itself as a whole. It is important that each team outline the behaviors that they feel should be targeted to assist in creating an effective group process and this list should periodically be revisited and modified over time based on what the team feels is needed to create an effective team culture consistent with the "spirit" of DBT. What you may have noticed is that the observer role is something that is quite unique to DBT when compared to common roles in other provider group meetings, like patient rounds or peer supervision. When individuals serving in the role of observer make their best efforts to follow through on what is intended for the role, many of the challenges that are encountered in other group meetings are significantly reduced as attention is drawn to them in a nonjudgmental manner.

The note taker documents key information covered in each case consultation team. This typically includes the agenda items discussed, team contributions to discussion, and what was decided as course of action or follow-up, if relevant. The note taker role helps to bridge one week's team to the next and ensure that follow-ups occur and that team members are receiving the ongoing support they may need. Finally, each patient is viewed not as a patient of their specific team of individual providers, but rather as a patient of the case consultation team as a whole. Tracking how a patient's care is progressing and having an opportunity to provide input is consistent with the psychological ownership that goes along with each patient being a patient of the team.

As a final note about team roles, there is benefit in rotating team roles amongst all team members. We have found that this helps to create a more egalitarian team environment, empowers all team members to take ownership in the team as a whole, and can help to block patterns of avoidance. The frequency with which roles are rotated is somewhat arbitrary, although most teams we have been part of rotate roles no less frequently than a monthly basis.

Agenda of the Case Consultation Team

Each of the case consultation teams that I (AHK) have been part of have had both common agenda items as well as agenda items that have been distinct to a specific organization or type of treatment environment. When determining what items to include on an agenda versus what items should be left off, the two primary deciding factors are whether or not the agenda item facilitates the process of members of the team receiving the support they need and whether or not the agenda item is consistent with or fosters the "spirit" of DBT.

The majority of teams we have been a part of start team meetings with a short mindfulness exercise, typically lasting no longer than five minutes. There are a number of reasons why most teams choose to include a mindfulness exercise as part of the case consultation team agenda. First, having the case consultation team begin with a mindfulness exercise gives space for team members to transition to fully focusing their attention on the case consultation team. Second, there is value in practicing the skills we are teaching our patients and encouraging them to use. Our patients are quite adept at sensing whether a provider knows skills through having memorized them versus knows skills through having actively used them. Third, mindfulness exercises can increase team cohesion. In fact, one of my (AHK) most salient memories from a case consultation meeting is a mindfulness exercise that did not go as planned, yet got a hearty laugh out of all team members present. I still chuckle about that mindfulness exercise with others who were part of that team to this day. Finally, having the opportunity to participate in at least one mindfulness exercise on a weekly basis can help to keep ideas of mindfulness activities to do with our patients fresh and varied. I have found this to be particularly helpful when working with child and adolescent patients, where creativity with mindfulness activities can be an asset in terms of getting buy-in and increasing engagement. Once providers have completed the mindfulness exercise, space should be given for brief reflections about the experience.

The mindfulness exercise is usually then followed by the team leader reading one of the DBT provider consultation agreements and the note taker reading notes from the previous meeting. Some teams that we have been a part of have tended toward more detailed notes, depending on the individual serving in the note taker role in a given week. When this is the case, it can sometimes be beneficial to have the note taker focus on highlighting key topics and action items, rather than reading notes in exhaustive detail.

Once notes have been read, the team then sets the agenda for the remainder of the meeting. How the agenda setting process has been approached from a process standpoint has varied across the various teams I (AHK) have been part of, with some teams specifically prompting for each level of target behaviors (e.g. "Does anyone have any level one target behaviors they would like to discuss?") and other teams simply prompting team members for agenda items and asking them to share how urgent their agenda item is using a Likert scale (e.g. 0–10) that takes into account the DBT treatment target hierarchy and other important factors, like the impact of the agenda item on the provider or whether the agenda item is time-sensitive in nature. While the process by which a team sets a meeting agenda may vary, the principle of using the DBT treatment target hierarchy to guide the order of the agenda is an important one.

The majority of team is then spent moving through the session agenda. The last component of the agenda is closing team. Some teams I (AHK) have worked with have chosen to end team with a celebration of good news, which I think has had a positive impact on staff morale and cohesion. Other teams have simply chosen to end at the scheduled end of team with the ringing of a mindfulness bell or the team leader indicating that it is time for the meeting to end.

Process Within the Case Consultation Team

The process of case consultation team is arguably the primary element that differentiates case consultation teams from other forms of peer consultation. The overall process of case consultation team can be summarized as "therapy for the provider" (originally "therapy for the therapist," expanded here to account for the multidisciplinary nature of eating disorders work), which involves applying the principles and strategies of DBT to challenges that providers are experiencing. There are four common targets a provider may have in seeking support from the case consultation team: validation from the team, help increasing empathy toward their patient, assistance with assessment of their patient, and problem-solving suggestions that draw from the four core CBT change strategies within DBT. Let's take a look at how each of these things might look in the context of a case consultation team.

Validation from the team. Working with individuals diagnosed with eating disorders is incredibly challenging work. Even without an explicit request from a team member for validation from the team, validation should be woven throughout interactions amongst team members. That said, it is not uncommon for a team member to make a request specifically for validation from others on the case consultation team. Let's see how this might look:

In this specific scenario, a therapist is working with an adolescent patient who has been admitted to treatment against their will by their parents. The therapist has experienced difficulty connecting with the patient, who presents as either angry or withdrawn during their sessions. The patient's parents have also been contacting the therapist multiple times per week, asking what the treatment plan is for their child and expressing concern and frustration that their child's intake has actually worsened rather than improved since entering treatment.

Team Leader: "Dominique, I see you wanted to talk a bit about Maria. How can we help?"

Therapist: "I feel like I have a good plan in place for this patient from a treatment standpoint. I'm honestly just looking for validation from the team. How she is presenting in sessions coupled with the pressure from her parents has just been a lot, I guess."

Dietitian: "I can imagine if I was in your shoes, I'd be feeling both a sense of urgency and a sense of powerlessness."

Therapist: "That summarizes it pretty well, actually. I'm genuinely working as hard as I can and I've articulated my treatment plan on multiple occasions to her parents, and it still feels like I'm not being heard."

Medical Provider: "That has to be awfully frustrating. And I know this is coming on the heels of that really challenging admission you had recently where it felt like the patient's family was asking a lot of you."

Therapist: "Yeah, I think my brain has been going to, 'Oh, great. Here we go again.' And I know that I'm still fairly early into this admission, so who's to really say, and that's a thought that I've been noticing is coming up for me."

Therapist #2: "I know that thought would be coming up for me too, if I was working directly with this family. For what it's worth, I think you're doing good work and have really shown this patient and family compassion, even though you're feeling frustrated."

Therapist: "Thanks, Sam. And thanks, y'all. It's helpful to feel understood. I think I got what I needed."

Help increasing empathy toward a patient. Difficulty with empathy toward a patient is another theme that emerges regularly in the context of eating disorders work. In the following example, the provider presenting on the patient did not originally ask for assistance in increasing empathy toward their patient, however another team member notices that it appears like empathy is a challenge for them at the present time and that difficulties with empathy might be contributing to the challenges that they have verbalized. Let's take a peek at this scenario:

Therapist: "So I just kind of wanted to get input from the team about putting together a treatment agreement for Sarah, since I think we're at the point where we may not be the best treatment setting for her. Today she told nursing that I had given her permission to skip all of her morning groups because she didn't sleep well last night, and so apparently she had just been sleeping in her room until I found out about it and told her that she needed to go to group. Yesterday, she managed to convince staff to let her choose one of her safe foods in lieu of dessert for her snack. Over the weekend, she told staff that her team had given her permission to do her PT exercises multiple times per day, instead of just once, so she was exercising in her room all weekend. The list goes on and on...so anyway, what are folks thinking about contingencies for her treatment agreement?"

Medical Provider: "Rachel, I know that you're asking the team for feedback about specific contingencies to put in place for this treatment agreement, but I'm actually wondering if that's what

	you're needing. I'd be curious to hear what others think, but moving to a treatment agreement this early in the game feels a bit premature. Sarah only got here a couple of weeks ago and she's pretty profoundly malnourished."
Dietitian:	"I agree with Rachel on this one. I think we've given her a lot of chances and she's continuing to find ways to get around doing what's needed to stay in treatment."
Medical Provider:	"I totally hear you, Michael. I know that both you and Rachel have often been identified as the people who supposedly gave her special permission to do various things and that this has caused some relationship strains with staff. It's really, really frustrating. And I wonder if that frustration is leading you both to want to put contingencies in place where she either gets in line or gets out of here."
Therapist:	"I am really frustrated and I don't see any other way to get Sarah to do what it is she needs to do in order to stay in our program."
Medical Provider:	"I'd be happy to help brainstorm with you all around that, and I'm sure the rest of the team would be too, and I wonder if working on trying to put yourself in Sarah's shoes a bit might help you to feel less frustrated and maybe more able to generate some other ideas of things to try with her? Like, I'm imagining if I was as malnourished and cognitively compromised and afraid as she is, I would be doing all sorts of things to try to hold onto whatever parts of my eating disorder I could. What Sarah's being asked to do in treatment is vastly different from how she was living her life outside of here."
Therapist:	"What you're saying makes sense and that does help me feel a bit less frustrated. I think I'm just tired of feeling blamed when she gets around rules and expectations, and I worry about the impact that her behavior is having on the milieu as a whole."
Medical Provider:	"Both those things are totally valid and I have some ideas of things we could try as a team to better support Sarah. Want to talk through them a bit?"

Assistance with assessment of a patient. There are a couple of ways in which providers might need assistance with assessment of a patient. First, a provider may not know how to go about assessing a certain problem (e.g. suicide risk), utilizing assessment tools to determine if a patient meets criteria for a specific diagnosis (e.g. ADHD), or may not know other specific assessment strategies relevant to eating disorders (e.g. what laboratory tests to get for certain eating disorder diagnoses presenting with specific comorbid medical or psychiatric conditions). Other providers can serve as excellent resources for providing information about these concrete areas of interest. In other circumstances, the assessment that a provider may need assistance with may be more broad. In these cases, utilizing dialectical assessment to ask, "What is being left out?" can assist in considering new angles. For example, I (AHK) was working with a patient who was reporting significant restricting behaviors in the absence of bingeing behaviors, yet this patient's weight was trending in a direction that suggested there might be more to the picture than what my patient was reporting. Taking the approach of dialectical assessment helped myself and the other members of the treatment team consider other areas to explore and angles to consider.

Problem-solving suggestions. Before we jump into how the four core CBT change strategies embedded within DBT can be offered as solutions to the various challenges that arise for providers, it is important to remember to be sure that you have an accurate understanding of the problem at hand before making suggestions about solutions. This includes having clarity about the specific target behavior for a provider, as well as an understanding of the antecedents and consequences associated with this target behavior. Missing links analysis can also be a helpful tool in examining situations in which an adaptive provider behavior did not occur. Once the provider and team have a sufficient understanding of the problem, they can then move to solutions, many of which will draw from the same four core CBT change strategies embedded within DBT.

Behavioral Skills Training. Behavioral skills training as applied to providers focuses on identifying potential Mindfulness, Interpersonal Effectiveness, Emotion Regulation, and Distress Tolerance skills that could help the provider to address the problem at hand. For the following example, a dietitian has identified that they are feeling intense frustration with a patient. In discussion with the team, they have been able to identify that their frustration has led them to avoid their patient outside of session times when they see them in the milieu and schedule shorter appointments right before meals and snacks in order to ensure their meetings are brief, in addition to recognizing that their body posture during sessions is likely more tense and that their tone of voice is probably more curt. Here is a snippet of the team discussing the possibility of using Opposite Action to decrease frustration:

Medical Provider:	"Let me make sure that I've heard you correctly…I hear that you are trying to avoid spending time with your patient as much as possible, and that even though your words aren't necessarily reflecting it, you think your body language and tone of voice might be letting on that you're feeling pretty frustrated."
Dietitian:	"Yeah, that sounds about right."
Medical Provider:	"I know this isn't probably going to be your favorite idea, but I wonder if this is a good time for some Opposite Action?"

Dietitian:	"You're right – my knee jerk reaction is to say no, and I'm curious to hear more about what you have in mind."
Medical Provider:	"I wonder about seeing them first thing Monday morning next week and making a longer session. Maybe taking a moment before the session to do an emotional temperature check and perhaps mindfully observing your body posture and tone of voice on occasion. And stopping to chat with them periodically in the milieu like I've seen you do with other patients."
Dietitian:	"I really want to hear you out and this sounds hard. I'm dreading it already, even just thinking about it."
Medical Provider:	"I totally get it! I think Opposite Action is one of the hardest skills to practice, honestly. And I also think it's one of the skills that helps most with changing the intensity of your emotions! I also recognize that what I'm suggesting is a lot. But I'm really thinking about all of this as doing Opposite Action all the way, you know? Plus I'm wondering if there are other skills that could help in making Opposite Action a more feasible solution? I'm thinking maybe ABC PLEASE or something along those lines…"
Therapist:	"I'd throw some Self-Validation in there, too."
Medical Provider:	"Good call. I don't know, what do you think?"
Dietitian:	"I think the point about trying some other skills in conjunction with Opposite Action makes a lot of sense. I'm not sold 100% and I'm also willing to try what you're suggesting and see how it goes. I really am tired of feeling so frustrated."
Medical Provider:	"I'm glad you're willing to try. This is coming from a place of compassion and wanting you to feel better! I hope that's been clear."
Dietitian:	"It has. I know that you do really have my best interests at heart."

Contingency Management. If you recall the DBT assumptions reviewed earlier in this text, assumption number twelve states, "Behavioral principles are universal, affecting providers no less than patients." Contingency management applied in the context of case consultation teams involves drawing awareness to contingencies at play and strategically applying behavioral principles to increase the likelihood of desirable provider behaviors and decrease the likelihood of maladaptive provider behaviors, both in the context of patient care as well as in the context of the team itself. As was discussed previously, reinforcement is the most effective way to change behavior and as such, should generally be the first behavioral principle considered when shaping provider behaviors. For example, if a provider follows-through on a challenging conversation with a patient they had been avoiding or if a provider who typically doesn't share about their emotional reactions to patients discloses a strong reaction they are having to the team, these are opportunities for team members to reinforce these desirable behaviors. It is important to keep in mind that what one provider finds to be reinforcing, like praise, may actually be experienced as aversive by another provider, so it is important to ensure that reinforcement is something that is highly individualized. Punishment should be used sparingly, if at all, as a method of behavior change. However, it is important for team members to stay attuned to how punishment may be functioning in the context of patient care or case consultation team. For example, if a patient becomes angry with a provider any time they attempt to do a chain analysis of a behavior, this may decrease the likelihood that a provider will attempt to do a chain analysis in the future. Similarly, if a team member becomes angry or defensive in response to feedback provided by the case consultation team, this may decrease the likelihood that team members will provide feedback to each other in the future, unless this response is actively addressed by the observer and targeted by the team. The key here is for individual team members and the team as a whole to be aware of contingencies at play and to adjust these contingencies as necessary to shape provider behaviors.

Exposure-Based Procedures. Exposure-based procedures as applied to providers involves targeting maladaptive avoidance on the part of a provider by having the provider repeatedly expose themselves to avoided situations. One of the most common examples of avoided situations that we have encountered is reluctance on the part of providers to eat with patients and provide meal coaching within the context of meals and snacks. Given the many potential benefits of meal coaching as a therapeutic intervention, targeting provider avoidance is critical, particularly at higher levels of care. If provider emotions, like unjustified fear, are the primary barrier to providing meal coaching, exposure-based procedures are an excellent intervention to target these emotions. Exposures that could be conducted include role-played meal coaching scenarios or planned meal coaching opportunities with patients, with gradations of difficulty if needed (e.g. starting by providing meal coaching to a patient who is likely to be receptive, then working up to providing meal coaching for more challenging patients).

Cognitive Modification Procedures. Cognitive modification procedures as applied to providers involves exploring cognitions that may be interfering with treatment in some way and targeting them through either acceptance-based (e.g. observing and describing thoughts) or change-based (e.g. challenging maladaptive cognitions) approaches. For the following example, a therapist on the team is struggling with judgments toward themselves because a parent of a patient recently expressed being frustrated with them for not responding fast enough to their phone calls and emails about their child. Let's see how the team navigates this discussion:

Therapist:	"The email that my patient's father sent was pretty long and intense! It's too much. He accused me of not being

quick enough in my responses to them, but I responded yesterday to another email. What does he actually expect of me?"

Dietitian: "For what it's worth, I think it's possible for there to be some validity to your patient's dad behaving in an anxious way. I mean, his child is ill and currently hospitalized. And at the same time, it's not factually accurate that you aren't being quick enough in your responses to them. Give yourself some compassion."

Therapist: "Can you say more?"

Dietitian: "Well, I've been trying to imagine being in that dad's shoes and I imagine he's probably feeling terrified. He has a child who is really, really ill at the moment. Dad seems like kind of a facts and logic sort of guy and I wonder for him if feeling like he has the most up-to-date information helps to quell some of his anxiety in some way, even if it's just momentarily. So I can imagine it being hard to want the most up-to-date information and for there to be a delay in receiving it. But on the other side of things, how could you reasonably be any quicker than you have been in communication? Between all of the groups you run, the patients and families who you have appointments with, and the staff meetings on your schedule, I don't think it's a reasonable expectation that you respond any more rapidly. Even if you do have a few moments of downtime throughout your day, it doesn't mean that you should have to use it to respond to an email or phone call. You need a break on occasion, too! Also, I feel like there might be more going on for you with this situation than feeling like you're not responding fast enough to phone calls and emails..."

Therapist: "I guess this situation has made me start to wonder... like, maybe I'm a bad therapist somehow?"

Medical Provider: "Can you say more?"

Therapist: "I just feel like I'm falling short. I know this started with me talking about feeling like I'm not quick enough in my responses to my patient's father, but I think what this really boils down to is me feeling like I'm totally ineffective with this patient and her family."

Medical Provider: "Whoa, whoa...I wonder if this could be a good time to use Check the Facts? I can't speak for others, but that's not my perspective in this situation. This is a totally challenging patient and family and they've just barely gotten started in treatment. Everything you've shared with the team about what you've done with them so far sounds totally reasonable for this point in treatment."

Psychiatric Provider: "I agree. I think you've done a really good job working to build rapport with a kiddo who really doesn't want to be in treatment and I think you've done a great job engaging her parents in treatment. Even if dad is perhaps more engaged than you would like him to be at the moment!"

Therapist: (chuckles) "Thanks, y'all. Those are some helpful perspectives. I do think I need to do a bit more reminding myself that I really am doing the best that I can."

The last thing to note about the process within a case consultation team is that the observer plays a critical role in helping the process remain consistent with the "spirit" of DBT. This includes addressing the multitude of challenges mentioned previously that can arise with individual team members (e.g. defensiveness) as well as team dynamics (e.g. failing to address the "elephant in the room"). The scope of discussing the specifics of team-interfering behaviors is beyond what is intended for this specific text, however interested readers are encouraged to read the aforementioned text by Sayrs and Linehan (2019) for a more in-depth exploration of this topic.

Adaptations of the Case Consultation Team

There are a couple of adaptations of the case consultation team mode of DBT that we think are worth mentioning. Particularly inpatient and residential levels of care, frontline staff like nurses and mental health technicians are heavily involved in patient care. We would furthermore argue that in some ways, their patient care experiences are more physically and emotionally taxing than those of the rest of the patient's treatment team. Frontline staff are often the individuals who are responding to self-injurious behavior, enforcing facility rules, managing patient crises, and so forth. Yet they also tend to be the staff with the least clinical training and regular supervisory support. With this in mind, just like all of the other members of a patient's treatment team, they need a space where they can receive support as well.

Unfortunately, the nature of the work of frontline staff does not easily lend itself to allowing for staff to be involved in the same case consultation team attended by the rest of the patient's treatment team. Some inpatient and residential facilities have managed this dilemma by providing "chalk talks," which are a substantially briefer variation on case consultation teams. "Chalk talks" are meetings for frontline staff lasting no more than 15 minutes or so and facilitated by a therapist or psychiatric provider well-versed in DBT. During these meetings, frontline staff are given space to bring up challenging patient scenarios from their day and receive specific suggestions of strategies to try. These meetings can also serve as a space for frontline staff to participate in brief training relevant to DBT. For example, some facilities where we have worked have had a DBT Skill of the Week for patients, and "chalk talks" would be an excellent space to review the Skill of the Week to assist frontline staff members in reinforcing the patients' use of the selected skill over the course of the week. Finally, "chalk talks" provide a venue to conduct brief role-plays, which can help staff to practice what they have learned and receive feedback in the moment that can help them to further the development of their skills in providing patient care.

Establishing formal or informal mentorship opportunities for frontline staff is another way to provide frontline staff with support. While serving in leadership roles previously, I (AHK) made it known to frontline staff that they were welcome to ask for guidance around patient care at any time. On the units where I worked, it wasn't uncommon for staff to pull me aside to ask for suggestions of strategies to try to address challenging patient situations they were encountering. It also wasn't unusual for them to ask for my assistance in intervening directly with patients. These situations provided an excellent opportunity to help staff learn through modeling the very strategies we would like them to learn. To help staff get the most benefit from learning through modeling, it's also important to find time for them to reflect on and ask questions about what they observed.

Finally, we recognize that not every environment where individuals reading this book work may lend themselves to implementation of a case consultation team or a variation of it. If you find yourself in this position, we'd encourage you to explore other options available in your community that may incorporate some of the "spirit" of what the case consultation mode of DBT offers. For example, as we established our first case consultation team together, we learned from one of our family medicine practitioners about Balint Groups, which were groups that were originally created to give space for primary care providers to discuss feelings they have about the provider-patient relationship. This parallels the "therapy for the provider" function that case consultation offers. So if you are in a position where implementation of the case consultation mode of treatment is not feasible, consider other options that you may have within your community that could provide you with support and continued clinical growth as you do this challenging work!

Bringing DBT to Life – Discussing Megan's Care During Case Consultation Team

The following example shows the value of case consultation teams in action. In this situation, Megan is a number of weeks into her stay at a residential level of care and she is having significant difficulties with her intake. Her therapist asks to add Megan to the agenda for discussion. Here is how that conversation transpires:

Vivian (Art Therapist, functioning as Team Leader for case consultation team today):	"Alright, looks like we have Megan next on the list for discussion. Serena, how can the team help?"
Serena (Therapist):	(sighs) "Oh, Megan. What to do about Megan? So, I think everyone is aware that her intake has been terrible the past few weeks. I think it's time to put her on a behavioral contract, so I guess what I was wanting was input from the team about the parameters of the contract."
Terri (Case Manager):	"I think a contract is a good idea. She's just not putting in the work. I think we set the contract so that the next time she restricts, we start facilitating a transfer. I already have a list of places that take her insurance and I can have her sign some ROIs (releases of information) for them when we present her with the contract."
Serena (Therapist):	"...I guess I wasn't thinking something quite that extreme, but maybe if she restricts more than three times in a week, that starts the transfer process. I mean, I think the outcome is still going to be the same, but I don't want to totally set her up to fail, you know?"
Carlos (Medical Provider):	"That's fine by me. Probably going to want to get the gears in motion for the transfer process after she signs those ROIs, Terri."
Terri (Case Manager):	(laughs) "On it!"
Claire (Dietitian, functioning as Observer for case consultation team today):	(rings observer bell) "Hey, y'all...I'm noticing a couple of things going on. This conversation is taking on a bit of a judgmental tone from my perspective. Is there a way we can cultivate a bit more compassion and pull back from predicting the worst for Megan? I'm also sitting here wondering what's being left out? It could

be that putting Megan on a behavioral contract is the best intervention we've got and I'm wondering what we haven't considered or tried?"

Serena (Therapist): "I feel like I've tried everything with Megan. We've talked about values and I've tried commitment strategies and we've done chain analyses. I really feel at a loss."

Terri (Case Manager): "I really don't think she wants to get better. I think she likes being in treatment but still getting to keep her eating disorder."

Ayesha (Psychiatric Provider): "I'm hearing that folks are feeling a bit hopeless about Megan and perhaps like they've been working harder than she has in treatment." (numerous team members nod) "You all really have tried a lot! I can see why it might feel like you're at the end of the track with Megan, and I wonder if I could offer an alternative perspective here?" (team appears interested) "Given Megan's history, if I put myself in her shoes, I would feel ambivalent or even fairly willful about making change. She's stopped drinking, hasn't engaged in self-harm since she's been here, and now we're pushing, hard, for her to make a whole-scale change around her eating disorder behaviors? Not saying that's not the right thing to do, and I can see how this could be potentially pretty overwhelming to her. I mean, I think about how hard it was for me to get in the habit of meditating on a regular basis, and that was something I actually wanted to do! I guess I say all this just to see if it can help us to have a bit more compassion for Megan."

Serena (Therapist): "I think you make a good point, Ayesha. I think with clients like Megan, I sometimes forget that their pace of change may not look how I want it to look, and that doesn't mean that change isn't still possible."

Ayesha (Psychiatric Provider): "For what it's worth, I think the dialectical worldview helps me here. I think a lot about the principle of interrelatedness and wholeness coupled with the principle of continuous change. There are an infinite number of variables interacting with our clients on a day-to-day basis and in turn meaning that change is happening, even if it may be slow, non-linear, or invisible to us. Remember Camille who we worked with last year?" (Serena nods) "I remember feeling so hopeless at a point in working with her and then all of a sudden, she started putting one foot in front of the other in terms of her path to recovery."

Serena (Therapist): "I totally see what you're saying and I still really feel at a loss. I landed on a behavioral contract for Megan because I seriously feel tapped out when it comes to other solutions. It feels like I'm trying the same thing over and over again, to no good effect."

Claire (Dietitian): "I don't know if it's to no good effect? I think sometimes it takes a while for interventions to click. I mean, I'd be inclined to keep doing chain analyses with Megan, for example. I am hearing that you do want some other things to try, though?"

Serena (Therapist): "Yeah. I mean, I'm willing to keep doing chain analyses and such, and I genuinely feel like I'm spinning my wheels a bit."

Vivian (Art Therapist): "I have an idea."

Serena (Therapist): "Let's hear it!"

Vivian (Art Therapist): "So, I know you don't feel like you're getting anywhere with Megan and I think you two have good therapeutic rapport. Like, if she was asked, I think she would say that she enjoys her time with you. Would you agree?" (Serena nods) "So I wonder if we set up the contingency that all of your therapy sessions will be coached meals until her intake improves?"

Serena (Therapist): "Not gonna lie, I can't say I'm thrilled about that idea."

Vivian (Art Therapist):	"I didn't necessarily think that you would be. I am definitely getting the sense that you are feeling pretty cashed in your work with Megan. And I believe that this intervention could be very effective and that you genuinely care about Megan and want to see her improve. I wonder if your reluctance is coming from a place of not actually thinking this will be an effective intervention or from a place of feeling like it's going to be an exhausting one to implement? Or maybe some other place entirely?"
Serena (Therapist):	"I think it has the possibility to be effective. I'm just already tired just thinking about doing full on meal coaching for an entire meal with Megan."
Ayesha (Psychiatric Provider):	"If I were in your shoes, I'd feel tired thinking about it, too. You've put in a lot of hard work. And I'm hearing you think it has the possibility of being an effective intervention. I wonder if there is some way to help it more tolerable?"
Serena (Therapist):	"As I'm thinking about it, timing matters. This is definitely something I should schedule on the same days I have sessions with patients who are doing a bit better in treatment. I think if I can approach it with an attitude of curiosity, that might help, too. Claire, that was a suggestion you gave me around meal coaching a while back and it's really stuck with me."
Claire (Dietitian):	"I'm glad! That's been a helpful lens for me, too. As we're talking about it, I'm thinking it may be helpful for me to shift my individual sessions to coached meals, too. I think it would help to underscore just how important we feel this aspect of her treatment is. And hey, maybe a bit of solidarity?"
Serena (Therapist):	"Solidarity, indeed! I'll take it. Thanks, y'all. This has been helpful."
Vivian (Art Therapist):	"I'm glad it was helpful, Serena. Is there other support you're wanting at the moment?"

Serena (Therapist):   "Thanks for asking. I think I'm good for now!"
Vivian (Art Therapist): "Alright, looks like James is next on our list. Claire, how can the team help?"

Provider Exercise – Incorporating the Principles of Case Consultation Teams

For this provider exercise, if you participate in any type of meeting involving a team of providers, or if you plan on joining a meeting of providers in the future, reflect on the information you reviewed about case consultation teams. Use the prompts below to guide you through determining whether to implement aspects of case consultation teams in your work and how to go about implementing these elements, should you choose to do so. Once you have completed the below, consider discussing your reflections with a trusted colleague for feedback.

Which elements of case consultation teams would you like to consider implementing, either from a principle-driven standpoint (e.g. extracting the principles of the components of case consultation teams and adapting them to my theoretical orientation, practice setting, etc.) or as described within DBT?

- ☐ Functions of case consultation teams (e.g. ensuring that my existing team adjusts such that there is a focus on enhancing provider motivation and/or capabilities)
- ☐ DBT provider consultation agreements (e.g. adopting the DBT provider consultation agreements or creating your own agreements)
- ☐ Roles in the case consultation team (e.g. creating an observer role to assist in managing team process)
- ☐ Agenda of the case consultation team (e.g. incorporating a mindfulness activity into team)
- ☐ Process of case consultation team (e.g. focusing more on provider support in team)
- ☐ Other:

What specifically would you like to implement based on the above?

What is my step-by-step plan for implementation?

What barriers do you anticipate encountering in implementation?

What strategies might assist in addressing these barriers?

Chapter 21

Case Management Strategies

What Are Case Management Strategies?

Case management strategies focus on how you as a patient's provider interact with individuals other than the patient. These individuals can include the other members of a patient's current treatment team, members of the treatment team to which you are referring the patient after treatment with you at a different level of care, the patient's family, friends, and other supports, or other individuals or entities in the patient's life, like employers, universities, or insurance companies. The goal behind case management is to empower our patients in effectively navigating their lives outside of their interactions with us as providers. It is important to note that DBT takes a different perspective on case management than more traditional case management approaches, in that the goal is to avoid intervening on the patient's behalf and instead help the patient to apply skills they have learned to serve as their own case manager of sorts. The following chapter provides a brief overview of case management strategies, however readers are encouraged to reference Linehan, 1993, pp. 401–423 for more in-depth coverage.

Consultation-to-the-Patient Strategies

Consultation-to-the-patient strategies embody the spirit of the case management strategies. These strategies focus on consulting with the patient about how to navigate their environment effectively, rather than intervening in the environment on their behalf. In doing so, we teach patients the skills they will need long-term to navigate their day-to-day lives, avoid the "splitting" that can occur with other providers and family members of a patient, and demonstrate that we believe our patients have the capability to intervene on their own behalf. Let's take a look at an example of how consultation-to-the-patient strategies work:

DOI: 10.4324/9781003495604-21

Patient: "My dietitian gave me another meal card increase and I don't think I can eat all of this food. Can you talk to them and tell them they need to decrease me to where I was before?"

Therapist: "I trust that your dietitian had a good reason behind the increase and if you're wanting a decrease, I don't think I'm the best person to have that conversation with her. Maybe you and I could spend part of our session today scripting out and role-playing a DEAR MAN you could use to have that discussion with her?"

Patient: "But she won't listen to me! And I know she will listen to you!"

Therapist: "Hmmm…this seems like all the more reason to work on a DEAR MAN in our session today! I want you to have the ability to have these tough conversations, especially because I won't always be around to have them, even in situations where it might make sense. What do you say we get started on a DEAR MAN and go from there?"

Patient: (sighs) "Okay, we can put one together."

As you're reading this example, you may be wondering why the therapist is seemingly setting the patient up for a conversation that is highly unlikely to result in the patient's desired outcome of getting a meal card decrease. The rationale for this approach in this circumstance is threefold. First, in going through the process of completing a DEAR MAN, it is possible the patient may start to see the disordered thinking underlying their request to have a meal card decrease. Second, even in the event the patient is not able to recognize their disordered thinking, it is important for them to develop the ability not only to use interpersonal effectiveness skills independently, but also to be able to tolerate when they use their skills as effectively as possible and still do not achieve a desired outcome from their perspective. Finally, this approach prevents "splitting" among the patient's multidisciplinary treatment team members by preventing the therapist from becoming a "go-between" for the patient with her dietitian.

Environmental Intervention Strategies

On the other side of the dialectic from consultation-to-the-patient strategies are environmental intervention strategies. As you likely gleaned from the section above, a critical goal in DBT is to help patients actively participate in solving their own problems, to the extent this is possible. There are four types of situations, however, where environmental intervention is appropriate.

The first of these circumstances are any situations in which the outcome is essential, which refers mostly to situations in which a patient's life or well-being is at risk. If intervening with regard to suicidal ideation is within your scope of practice as a provider and you have made your best effort to create a workable safety plan with your patient and your patient is still unwilling to do what is needed to maintain safety, this is a situation where environmental intervention is not only permissible but required. Since outcomes of environmental intervention when a patient is experiencing suicidal ideation can be potentially reinforcing, it is critical that you have made efforts to the best of your ability to avoid resorting to environmental intervention as a course of action. As with situations where your patient's life or well-being are at risk, it is also required that you intervene if you have reason to believe that your patient is a significant risk to the life or well-being of another individual.

The second of these circumstances are situations in which the patient lacks the skill necessary to achieve a desired outcome and such outcome is important to their treatment and building a life worth living. With adolescents, young adults, and couples, especially early on in treatment, it is common for these types of situations to arise with family members. For example, an adolescent patient may not yet have the Interpersonal Effectiveness skills to speak to their parents about what is helpful and unhelpful to them in the context of meal support. In this case, it might be appropriate for the therapist to intervene and provide guidance around the "do's" and "don'ts" of meal support.

The third of these circumstances are situations in which the patient lacks the authority or power necessary to achieve a desired outcome and such outcome is important to their treatment and building a life worth living. For example, a psychiatric provider may think an adolescent patient would benefit from the use of medications as part of their treatment, however the adolescent has expressed that their parents are not on board. In this case, it would make sense for the psychiatric provider to initiate a discussion with the adolescent's parents about the recommendation to incorporate the use of medications in their treatment, rather than expecting the adolescent to have this conversation themselves. With an adult collegiate athlete, they may find themselves in a situation where a coach is insisting they do something that is contraindicated for their recovery (e.g. follow a certain diet or engage in a certain workout routine, participate in regular weigh-ins where they are exposed to their current weight) and that despite the patient's efforts to discuss this with their coach, they have been unsuccessful in convincing them to allow for appropriate adjustments. In this case, it may be clinically indicated for the patient's dietitian to contact the coach directly to discuss the needed accommodations.

Finally, environmental intervention strategies may be appropriate in situations where intervening is the humane thing to do and intervening does not cause harm in any fashion. For example, if a patient is experiencing significant financial problems that are impeding both their ability and willingness to engage in a food-related exposure, you may choose to purchase that specific food and conduct an in-session food exposure during your next session. While ultimately the patient's financial problems will need to be addressed, temporarily removing a barrier to addressing an important treatment target is a humane action, the benefits of which are likely to outweigh the downsides.

Bringing DBT to Life – Balancing Environmental Intervention vs. Consultation-to-the-Patient With Megan

In this particular example, we find Megan at an IOP level of care. She started a job as a pharmacy technician a couple of weeks ago and her therapist notices that she has been either skipping afternoon snack or combining the exchanges from afternoon snack with her lunch on days that she works. Megan's therapist decides to explore this pattern further. The following is the dialogue between Megan and her therapist:

Serena: "In looking at your diary card, it seems like afternoon snack is still really posing some challenges with your work schedule. I know you mentioned that you hadn't had your one-on-one with your new boss yet and that you planned to talk with him about your needs. How did that go?"

Megan: "Well, I told him that sometimes I need to have a snack in the afternoon and I was wondering if it would be possible for me to maybe have a few minutes in the afternoon to eat a quick snack on occasion. He said that afternoons are usually their busiest time and unless it's a slow day, I'll just have to power through. It's really nice to be working again, so I decided not to push the issue further. Maybe once I'm settled in a bit more I can revisit things with him. I think I'll just do my best to try to combine my exchanges with lunch for now."

Serena: "On one hand, I can totally appreciate having some reservations about being super-assertive with your new boss at a new job. On the other hand, I see you slipping back into patterns of restriction, and you and I both know how this has worked out historically. Also, in hearing you describe the interaction with your boss, I'm not sure if I was in his shoes that I would have gotten just how important it is for you to have afternoon snack each day."

Megan: "What do you mean?"

Serena: "Well, the way I heard things framed was that you sometimes need a snack and that you were hoping that would be a possibility, but that if you weren't able to have one on occasion that would be okay. To me that's really different than disclosing that you have a medical condition that necessitates that you be allowed a few minutes to have an afternoon snack each day. If I was in his shoes, I might have interpreted your request as wanting special privileges to have an extra break to have a snack if you're hungry, rather than needing accommodations for a medical condition that requires that you nourish yourself at a certain time each afternoon. Does that make sense?"

Megan: "Okay, I see what you're saying."

Serena: "I'm wondering if it would be helpful to draft up a DEAR MAN for your boss about afternoon snack and we can see how things go?"

Megan: "I really don't want to, and I understand why I need to. I can do that for homework."

In the dialogue above, you see Serena functioning as a consultant to Megan, rather than a person intervening on her behalf. Megan tends to have a more passive approach in interpersonal interactions and a more passive approach when in terms of problem-solving more broadly, so Serena recognized that it was important for her to coach and support Megan in using Interpersonal Effectiveness skills, rather than taking steps to intervene on Megan's behalf. Let's see how Megan's conversation went:

Serena: "It looks like you're back on track with meeting all of your exchanges this week, although I'm seeing that it still looks like you're combining your afternoon snack exchanges with your lunch. How'd that conversation with your boss go?"

Megan: "Well, I did the DEAR MAN with him like we talked about, which was really hard. He didn't seem thrilled by my request and he told me that the only way he could provide medical accommodation is if he had a letter from my treatment team outlining why the accommodation is necessary. Honestly, I think we can just drop it. I'll keep meeting all of my exchanges by combining afternoon snack with lunch and it will be fine."

Serena: "Okay, first off I'm so proud of you for following through on using DEAR MAN. I totally know that wasn't an easy thing for you, so I want to give kudos where kudos are due! Nice work."

Megan: "Thanks."

Serena: "Okay, now I want to talk about this letter. I know that you're trying not to 'rock the boat' so to speak because you're a new employee and you really like your new job *and* I think this is one of those times where it is important to advocate for your needs even if it feels uncomfortable. I'm wondering if there is more getting in the way of you being willing to submit a letter for a medical accommodation than what you're sharing?"

Megan: "I guess I don't want the other employees to think that I'm lazy and trying to get out of work or weird for having to eat a snack when they don't need to."

Serena: "Can we Check the Facts and explore that a little bit?"

What you see in this second piece of dialogue is that Serena and Megan have encountered a situation where environmental intervention is appropriate, in addition to being an approach that will help to block Megan's passive approach in interpersonal interactions. After Checking the Facts with Megan, she ultimately agrees to allow her team to provide a letter to her boss stating that a medical accommodation to allow time for her to complete an afternoon snack is necessary for her physical and psychological health. The take-home point here is that it is important to err on the side of acting as a consultant to our patients, rather than opting to intervene on their behalf, particularly before we have had a chance to see if environmental intervention is necessary.

Provider Exercise – Environmental Intervention vs. Consultation-to-the-Patient

It is common for providers to tend to lean toward one side of the dialectic when it comes to environmental intervention versus consultation-to-the-patient strategies. It is also often the case that individual patient characteristics may influence the extent to which a provider utilizes environmental intervention versus consultation-to-the-patient strategies. This may be helpful in certain circumstances (e.g. having a conversation with an adolescent's parents early in treatment about refraining from diet culture talk that has been pervasive within the home) and potentially problematic in others (e.g. treating an adult patient as fragile by communicating information to their partner on their behalf, rather than having them use their Interpersonal Effectiveness skills to communicate about their needs and preferences). For this provider exercise, consider each patient on your caseload and whether you need to increase your use of either of these strategies to help them make progress toward their treatment goals. For patients for whom you think these strategies could be helpful, make some notes about your rationale for using them. Once you have completed the below, consider discussing your reflections with a trusted colleague for feedback.

Patients With Whom Increased Use of Environmental Intervention Strategies May Be Helpful

Patient Identifier	How These Strategies May Be Helpful

Patients With Whom Consultation-to-the-Patient Strategies May Be Helpful

Patient Identifier	How These Strategies May Be Helpful

The Involvement of Families and Supports in Eating Disorder Treatment and Revisiting Your Initial Thoughts About Megan

We have alluded to the involvement of families and supports at various points throughout this book, however thought it could be useful to have a more explicit discussion on this particular topic, from the standpoint of both prevailing opinions within the DBT community as well as what is recommended based on the existing research literature.

The Involvement of Families and Supports for Preadolescent Children

The variation of DBT developed for preadolescent children (DBT-C) explicitly states caregiver commitment to treatment is necessary, and views caregiver behavior as the driving force behind changes in the child's behavior. The creator of DBT-C goes as far as to state that a child's behavior is irrelevant until the child's environment is able to consistently and effectively promote progress. In order for the child to be able to make change, caregivers must model skill use, reinforce adaptive behaviors, ignore dysfunctional behaviors, suppress dangerous behaviors, validate their child's distress, and create a change-ready environment (Perepletchikova, 2017). As such, caregiver training is a significant and essential component of DBT-C.

It is important to note that DBT-C was not created for the treatment of pre-adolescent children diagnosed with an eating disorder, so let's take a look at what the literature on eating disorders says about the involvement of family in the treatment of children diagnosed with an eating disorder. The recently released Canadian practice guidelines for the treatment of children and adolescents with eating disorders states that Family-Based Treatment (FBT) has substantial evidence supporting its use in the treatment of children and adolescents diagnosed with Anorexia Nervosa, and also notes that Parent-Focused Family Therapy (a form of FBT in which most therapy sessions are spent with parents alone) may be just as effective as standard FBT. Additionally, the practice guideline notes emerging evidence for the effectiveness of FBT in the treatment of children

DOI: 10.4324/9781003495604-22

and adolescents with Bulimia Nervosa, Atypical Anorexia Nervosa, and ARFID. This guideline echoes the sentiment from DBT-C that caregiver involvement in the treatment of children with eating disorders is critical (Couturier, et al., 2020).

The Involvement of Families and Supports for Adolescents

Although DBT-A does not require family work as part of treatment, family work is strongly encouraged for two primary reasons. First, family work allows for providers to more directly assess dysfunctional patterns in interactions between family members and intervene accordingly. Second, family work provides a venue for family members to learn about the same skills that the patient is learning about, which both helps them to coach the patient in the use of skills, in addition to using these skills to navigate their own lives in a more effective manner. The involvement of families is encouraged in a variety of ways in DBT-A, including family therapy sessions, multifamily DBT skills groups, and telephone coaching (Miller, Rathus, & Linehan, 2007).

As discussed previously, the Canadian practice guidelines for the treatment of children and adolescents with eating disorders strongly recommends the involvement of caregivers of adolescents in treatment.

The Involvement of Families and Supports for Adults

The original text on DBT, Cognitive-Behavioral Treatment of Borderline Personality Disorder (Linehan, 1993) touches on the involvement of families and supports of adults receiving DBT, although does not elaborate substantially on this topic. It is noted that families and supports can be important allies in treatment, and that family therapy and couples' therapy sessions are not inconsistent with DBT and may actually be prescribed at times. It is also noted that sessions with family members or supports of the patient without the patient present are inconsistent with DBT, which focuses on the approach of consultation-to-the-patient whenever possible. Potential targets of family therapy sessions are not elaborated upon, other than to note that one goal within these sessions should be to increase family members' capacities to validate the patient. Since the release of the original text on DBT, other authors have expanded upon ideas for the involvement of families and supports of adult patients in treatment. Fruzzetti (2019) suggests that the involvement of families and supports in treatment can augment treatment outcomes for patients by helping the patient and their family and supports learn skills to interact with each other more effectively, practicing these skills in the moment with each other during treatment sessions, and ascertaining ways in which interactions with family members individually or the family environment more broadly can be altered to enhance patient motivation and reinforce skillful behavior. As such, he strongly encourages family and support involvement that focuses on psychoeducation, skills acquisition and generalization, strategic application of behavioral principles, and decreasing invalidating responses while increasing validating responses.

The research literature based on the involvement of families and supports in the treatment of adult patients diagnosed with eating disorders is an emerging, yet promising area of inquiry. Some studies have explored adaptations of FBT (e.g. FBT-TAY, FBT-Y) for young adults and preliminary results suggest positive outcomes for both patients (Chen, et al., 2016; Dimitropoulos, Landers, Freeman, Novick, Garber, & Le Grange, 2018) and caregivers (Dimitropoulos, et al., 2018). Other studies have started to explore interventions that involve carers and supports for patients who are beyond the age of young adults (e.g. the New Maudsley Model for Collaborative Care, MANTRA) and preliminary evidence suggests these interventions may enhance caregiver skills and reduce the amount of time carers spend caring without compromising patient outcomes (Adamson, Cardi, Kan, Harrison, Macdonald, & Treasure, 2019; Treasure, Parker, Oyelele, & Harrison, 2021). Finally, although only a pilot study has been completed to date, there is some evidence that suggests that couples' therapy in the context of eating disorders work may result in reductions in eating disorder symptoms and improvements in psychological and relationship functioning (Kirby, Runfola, Fischer, Baucom, & Bulik, 2015).

Additional Comments on the Involvement of Families and Supports

Beyond what the DBT and eating disorders research literature has to say about the involvement of families and supports in treatment, we can also turn to what clinical wisdom might suggest. It is important to remember that all of our patients come from a context and will return to a context. If we have the opportunity to support our patients in impacting their context in such a way that is more conducive to their recovery, we are likely setting them up for a more favorable outcome. Elaborating substantially on the involvement of families and supports is beyond the scope of this particular text, however readers are encouraged to learn more about this aspect of eating disorders care.

Provider Exercise – Revisiting Your Initial Thoughts About Megan

Let's revisit your initial thoughts about Megan's case, which you can find in the provider exercise you completed in Chapter 3. Having read through this text, what would you change and what would remain as it is in terms of your recommendations for treatment, case conceptualization, and treatment interventions?

Chapter 23

Tips for Administrators and Supervisors

I (AHK) have had the privilege of being involved in starting two DBT programs from scratch in my professional career to date and thought it could be useful to share some of the lessons learned from these experiences for those of you who are in roles where you are overseeing teams who you would like to see integrate the principles and strategies we have discussed. It's only more recently that people have begun writing on this topic, however a number of recent book chapters have touched nicely on this area (e.g. Best & Lyng, 2018; Comtois & Landes, 2018; Gaglia, 2018; Sayrs & Linehan, 2019; Schmidt III & Russo, 2018; Swales & Dunkley, 2018). If this is a topic of interest to you, I would strongly encourage reviewing these resources as well.

Actions to Consider Prior to Systemic Integration of DBT Principles and Strategies

If you are attempting to create a new program or adapt an existing program to include the use of DBT principles and strategies or are working to create an adherent program, a helpful starting place can be to ask yourself where you fall in terms of desiring to adhere as closely as possible to DBT as outlined in the original DBT texts versus adapting DBT to fit within your specific treatment environment. Once you have a sense of this, it can be helpful to think about a high-level view of what you hope to accomplish and what you'll need in order to get there. Particularly with the second program I (AHK) had a hand in creating, the very first step that I took in this process was asking myself where I hoped to see the program in five years, after which I brainstormed a comprehensive, detailed "to do" list of all the actions that would be necessary and things that would need to be in place to achieve this goal. If you are in a role where you are currently working with a team that would have shared responsibility for achieving this goal, I would strongly encourage approaching this process collaboratively from the very beginning, as there is benefit in collective wisdom as well

DOI: 10.4324/9781003495604-23

as benefit in increasing the likelihood of buy-in from all parties involved. Some examples of areas to explore include:

1. *Programming.* Depending on your level of care, patient population served, and disciplines included as part of your program, this might impact a host of actions you might take with regard to programming. For example, an inpatient unit staffed with multiple therapists might choose to offer a DBT-focused group, like a DBT Skills Group or a Chain Analysis group, each day. An outpatient practice with only dietitians may choose not to change existing programming offered at their practice in any way, but may elect to partner with an outpatient psychotherapy practice that offers DBT skills groups. Changes to the interventions and therapeutic process in your individual sessions with patients should also be considered when thinking about programming. For example, we have found that many dietitians have chosen to incorporate DBT diary cards into their practice after having heard us speak about them at conferences. It can be helpful to look at each component of DBT we discussed in this book and consider whether it is something you want to incorporate into the individual services provided in your practice setting.

2. *Staffing.* Another area to consider is whether what you hope to achieve in terms of changes in your practice setting requires hiring new staff. For example, you may be a therapist who owns a group private practice who sees value in hiring dietitians in order to help live into the vision of applying DBT principles in an integrated, multidisciplinary fashion. Or perhaps you are a dietitian who owns a group private practice where you would like to offer DBT skills groups, while also recognizing that providing these groups with your current staff of dietitians would be outside of your scope of practice. Depending on the extent of changes you are considering making, changes to staff schedules may also need to be considered.

3. *Systems.* Systems are another area that warrant consideration when exploring the possibility of making changes to your practice that incorporate DBT principles and strategies. One area to consider that falls under the umbrella of systems is documentation. The structure and prompts within documentation templates can help to support changes you are aiming to make to align more closely with a DBT framework. For example, if you would like all members of your professional staff to utilize DBT diary cards as part of their individual sessions, having a prompt built into their documentation that asks them to share information they obtained from their patient's DBT diary card during their sessions can help to reinforce them reviewing patient DBT diary cards in session. Another area to consider that falls under the umbrella of systems is the logistics associated with making changes to staff meetings or clinical services. For example, if you decide that you would like to initiate

a case consultation team, staff schedules and physical space availability become important considerations. If you decide that you would like to offer in-the-moment coaching, thought has to be given as to the communication method or methods that will be used, parameters around providing in-the-moment coaching, and policies and procedures that may require updating.

4. *Materials.* Materials are typically another area that must be considered when implementing elements of DBT. On the patient-focused side of things, you might consider updates to existing patient orientation packets or handbooks, making DBT skills handouts available, or updating the décor in your workspace to provide visual reinforcement of DBT skills and concepts. On the staff-focused side of things, you may want to consider purchasing books or making available journal articles that staff can reference as they further incorporate DBT into their work.

5. *Training and Supervision.* Training and supervision must also be considered when weaving elements of DBT into clinical care. If you are hoping to incorporate all or the majority of principles and strategies reviewed in this text, a more robust initial training for all individuals who will be involved in providing clinical care is worth consideration. If you only plan on implementing very specific strategies or principles, briefer training on these topics will likely suffice. Changes you will need to make to supervision content and structure in order to reinforce the use of DBT principles and strategies should also be considered. In our experience, finding a way to incorporate an ongoing focus on DBT principles and strategies on a weekly basis, either in the form of training, supervision, or both, is necessary in order to create sustainable change in staff clinical practice.

6. *Outcomes Measurement.* If you are going to make changes to your clinical approach, it can also be helpful to have a plan for quantitative and qualitative outcomes measurement. It can be difficult to have an accurate picture as to the impact of changes you implement without data to draw from. Data can also help to inform changes beyond those that you implement initially. Thankfully, implementation science provides us with some guidance around the categories of outcomes that may be of interest to you, as well as more specific variables you might want to measure that fall within these categories. Implementation outcomes that may be of interest include acceptability, adoption, appropriateness, costs, feasibility, fidelity, penetration, and sustainability. Service outcomes include efficiency, safety, effectiveness, equity, patient-centeredness, and timeliness. Finally, patient outcomes include satisfaction, function, and symptomatology (Comtois & Landes, 2018).

7. *Consultation.* Consultation is the last area to consider prior to making efforts to incorporate DBT principles and strategies in your workplace setting. Particularly if you are newer to DBT as a treatment or program development

and implementation as a process, you may consider whether outside consultation could be helpful initially or even on an ongoing basis.

Once you have clarity around your vision, the next potential step is somewhat dependent on your current context. If you are truly building a program from scratch and the process of creating this program is solely within your scope of control, excellent! Take your first step toward your vision and consider reviewing some of the points below about ongoing implementation. Odds are this is a smaller subset of individuals reading this book. Most readers likely report to additional individuals above you in your organizational chart and have a team of supervisees they oversee as well. This is where the issue of buy-in across the organization is critical. In the implementation literature, pre-implementation buy-in is considered from a couple of angles – acceptability and appropriateness. Acceptability refers to the extent to which individuals who would be impacted by any changes are on board with the elements of DBT that will be implemented. Appropriateness refers to whether the changes that are being considered are helpful to and compatible with the environment in which they would be made. If either acceptability or appropriateness are absent or only partially present, changes that are being considered for implementation either will not be put in place or if they are, are not likely to remain in place long-term.

Actions to Consider Ongoing With Regard to Systemic Integration of DBT Principles and Strategies

Once the initial implementation of changes has begun, implementation science points to two areas that can be helpful to explore ongoing – feasibility and fidelity. Considering appropriateness prior to implementation of changes is a form of exploring feasibility. However, even if one gives careful consideration to appropriateness, this doesn't always mean that changes will be found to be feasible once they are actually in place. Once changes are made, it is important to assess and reassess whether changes are doable, giving consideration to things like time investment, cost, and so forth.

Fidelity refers to the extent to which the changes implemented have actually taken hold as they were intended. Maintaining fidelity is arguably the most difficult piece of implementing DBT principles and strategies, as it requires disciplined, ongoing focus and action. For the remainder of this chapter, we will explore strategies that we have found to be helpful in terms of improving and sustaining fidelity.

While one may have the aspirational aim of all staff involved in implementation of DBT principles and strategies committing to the shared responsibility of holding themselves and each other accountable to fidelity, a different approach is almost always needed from a pragmatic standpoint in order for change to take hold. We have found that identifying a person to have psychic ownership of the implementation and maintenance of changes is crucial for the purpose of fidelity. Having one individual identified as the person to hold psychic ownership prevents diffusion of responsibility and lack of clarity in terms of vision. Ideally, other team members involved in implementation also strive to hold themselves and other members of the team accountable for change and having someone with psychic ownership helps to ensure that if other team members aren't focused on fidelity, at least one individual is. So what qualities are helpful in an individual who wants to assume the role of holding psychic ownership? First, the individual must be wholeheartedly and enthusiastically committed to the changes being implemented. Second, they must be willing to address drifts and deviations from fidelity consistently. While not all conversations about drifts and deviations from fidelity will be uncomfortable or challenging, many of them will be. As such, another quality that is helpful in a psychic owner is the ability to tolerate negative affect and unpleasant thoughts that may arise in the context of difficult discussions and in the context of slow, incremental change. It is inevitable that one will encounter situations in which "holding the frame" as a psychic owner is met with resistance and that team members will experience emotions like anger or anxiety in response to efforts aimed at moving toward or maintaining fidelity. Finally, it is important that the individual who is holding psychic ownership has the ability to take a long-term vision that will likely require years to successfully implement and determine what day-to-day actions are necessary to move the team closer to this vision as time passes.

Another strategy that is helpful in terms of moving toward and maintaining fidelity is to have ongoing, regularly scheduled points where all individuals involved in implementing the vision that has been decided upon have a chance to reflect on the changes that have been made to date. This includes providing input about what has and has not been working well, discussing areas of resistance around change, and collaboratively determining next steps that both individuals and the team are willing to take to continue to move forward in further aligning with the vision that has been outlined. The recommended frequency of these conversations will vary depending on a variety of factors, including the extent of changes being made, the number of team members impacted by the change, and so forth. It is typically helpful for these discussions to occur more frequently initially and then gradually taper in frequency over the course of time.

Finally, ongoing clinical supervision is another mechanism that can be utilized to help staff move toward and maintain fidelity. When we think about clinical supervision as it pertains to treatment fidelity, the first thing that we consider is how to bring the spirit and principles of DBT into the supervisory space. Approaching your supervision from that framework widens the possibilities of specific supervisory interventions that may be helpful in working toward enhanced fidelity, rather than being more prescriptive with regard to the types of approaches and strategies you might use. That being said, there are a number of specific strategies we have found to be helpful. First, if you have an opportunity to do something in supervision, rather than just talk about something, take advantage of this opportunity! While many people shy away from doing role-plays, they are also an invaluable teaching tool. Role-plays can also be conducted in such a way that pushes supervisees to enhance their clinical skills, while also honoring where they are in terms of their development as professionals. For example, I might start by having a supervisee play the role of the professional in the role-play, with me playing the role of the patient, however if they find themselves stuck, I might swap in as the professional to model clinical skills that I would want them to develop. After seeing some of the skills modeled, I might then ask the supervisee to pick back up as the professional in order to get further practice. Second, in settings where consent has been obtained for audio and video recordings to be used in the context of supervision or where live observation is feasible and permissible, getting to see your supervisee providing actual clinical care can be incredibly helpful in terms of identifying areas of focus for supervision and providing timely and behaviorally-specific feedback. Third, incorporating permanent products, like diary cards or chain analyses completed by patients, is another way to help with enhanced fidelity. For example, when supervisees have shared diary cards that either they or their patients have found to be ineffective or unhelpful, we have been able to adjust things like formatting or scale in such a way that has made them a more useful tool. In turn, patients have been more likely to complete them and providers have been more likely to use them. Finally, consider how you can model the spirit of DBT within your dialogue in supervision. This can look like balancing validation and pushing for change with your supervisees, modeling dialectical thinking and consideration of "what is being left out," and using nonjudgmental and behaviorally-descriptive language. What we hope to have emphasized here is that unlike with projects or goals one may have, which have starting points and ending points, fidelity is all about how you endeavor to adhere to a model day-to-day in your interactions with clients, their families and supports, and your work colleagues.

Provider Exercise – Translating Learning into Practice

Congratulations! You have reached the final provider exercise in our book. We want to leave you with an exercise that encourages you to consider how you can take what you have learned in this book and translate it into meaningful change in your clinical practice. With this in mind, there are a number of questions we believe are worth reflecting upon.

1. What are the most challenging situations you face in terms of your practice where information you have learned from this book could be potentially beneficial? How specifically will you implement what you have learned in the context of those clinical situations? What will you do to evaluate if the changes you have made have been beneficial?

2. What other strategies did you learn about in this book that you would like to incorporate into your practice? What is your specific plan for implementing these strategies? How will you assess if the use of these strategies has been beneficial?

3. What next steps do you think could be helpful in terms of your continued growth and development with regard to the material we covered? You may wish to consider self-study, online and in-person training, targeted supervision, and professional consultation as potential options.

References

Adamson, J., Cardi, V., Kan, C., Harrison, A., Macdonald, P., & Treasure, J. (2019). Evaluation of a novel transition support intervention in an adult eating disorders service: ECHOMANTRA. *International Review of Psychiatry*, *31*(4), 382–390. https://doi.org/10.1080/09540261.2019.1573721

Algars, M., Alanko, K., Santtila, P., & Sandnabba, N. K. (2012). Disordered eating and gender identity disorder: A qualitative study. *Eating Disorders*, *20*(4), 300–311. https://doi.org/10.1080/10640266.2012.668482

Baker, J. H., Mazzeo, S. E., & Kendler, K. S. (2007). Association between broadly defined bulimia nervosa and drug use disorders: Common genetic and environmental influences. *International Journal of Eating Disorders, 40*(8), 673–678. https://doi.org/10.1002/eat.20472

Bankoff, S. M., Karpel, M. G., Forbes, H. E., & Pantalone, D. W. (2012). A systematic review of dialectical behavior therapy for the treatment of eating disorders. *Eating Disorders*, *20*(3), 196–215. https://doi.org/10.1080/10640266.2012.668478

Barbarich, N. C. (2002). Lifetime prevalence of eating disorders among professionals in the field. *Eating Disorders*, *10*(4), 305–312.

Baudinet, J., Simic, M., Griffiths, H., Donnelly, C., Stewart, C., & Goddard, E. (2020). Targeting maladaptive overcontrol with radically open dialectical behaviour therapy in a day programme for adolescents with restrictive eating disorders: An uncontrolled case series. *Journal of Eating Disorders*, *8*(1), 68. https://doi.org/10.1186/s40337-020-00338-9

Becker, C. B., Farrell, N. R., & Waller, G. (2019). *Exposure therapy for eating disorders.* New York, NY: Oxford University Press.

Best, H. & Lyng, J. (2018). The dialectical dilemmas of implementation. In M. A. Swales (Ed.). *The Oxford Handbook of Dialectical Behaviour Therapy* (pp. 831–844). New York, NY: Oxford University Press.

Buerger, A., Vloet, T. D., Haber, L., & Geissler, J. M. (2021). Third-wave interventions for eating disorders in adolescence – Systematic review with meta-analysis. *Borderline Personality Disorder and Emotion Dysregulation, 8*(20). https://doi.org/10.1186/s40479-021-00158-6

Calero-Elvira, A., Krug, I., Davis, K., López, C., Fernández-Aranda, F. & Treasure, J. (2009). Meta-analysis on drugs in people with eating disorders. *European Eating Disorders Review, 17*, 243–259. https://doi.org/10.1002/erv.936

Carter, J. C., Kelly, A. C., & Norwood, S. J. (2012). Interpersonal problems in anorexia nervosa: Social inhibition as defining and detrimental. *Personality and Individual Differences, 53*(3), 169–174. https://doi.org/10.1016/j.paid.2012.02.020

Cassin, S. E., & von Ranson, K. M. (2005). Personality and eating disorders: A decade in review. *Clinical Psychology Review, 25*, 895e916.

Cassin, S. E., von Ranson, K. M., Heng, K., Brar, J., & Wojtowicz, A. E. (2008). Adapted motivational interviewing for women with binge eating disorder: A randomized controlled trial. *Psychology of Addictive Behaviors, 22*(3), 417–425. https://doi.org/10.1037/0893-164X.22.3.417

Chen, E. Y., Matthews, L., Allen, C., Kuo, J. R., & Linehan, M. M. (2008). Dialectical behavior therapy for clients with binge-eating disorder or bulimia nervosa and borderline personality disorder. *International Journal of Eating Disorders, 41*(6), 505–512.

Chen, E. Y., Segal, K., Weissman, J., Zeffiro, T. A., Gallop, R., Linehan, M. M., Bohus, M., & Lynch, T. R. (2015). Adapting dialectical behavior therapy for outpatient adult anorexia nervosa--A pilot study. *The International Journal of Eating Disorders, 48*(1), 123–132. https://doi.org/10.1002/eat.22360

Chen, E. Y., Weissman, J. A., Zeffiro, T. A., Yiu, A., Eneva, K. T., Arlt, J. M. & Swantek, M. J. (2016). Family-based therapy for young adults with Anorexia Nervosa restores weight. *International Journal of Eating Disorders, 49*, 701–707. https://doi.org/10.1002/eat.22513

Claes, L. & Muehlenkamp, J. J. (2014). Non-suicidal self-injury and eating disorders: Dimensions of self-harm. In Muehlenkamp, J. J. & Claes, L. (Eds.). *Non-Suicidal Self-Injury in Eating Disorders* (pp. 3–18). Springer-Verlag Publishing. https://doi.org/10.1007/978-3-642-40107-7_1

Comtois, K. A. & Landes, S. J. (2018). Implementing DBT: An implementation science perspective. In M. A. Swales (Ed.). *The Oxford Handbook of Dialectical Behaviour Therapy* (pp. 831–844). New York, NY: Oxford University Press.

Couturier, J., Isserlin, L., Norris, M., Spettigue, W., Brouwers, M., Kimber, M., McVey, G., Webb, C., Findlay, S., Bhatnagar, N., Snelgrove, N., Ritsma, A., Preskow, W., Miller, C., Coelho, J., Boachie, A., Steinegger, C., Loewen, R., Loewen, T., Waite, E., … Pilon, D. (2020). Canadian practice guidelines for the treatment of children and adolescents with eating disorders. *Journal of Eating Disorders, 8*, 4. https://doi.org/10.1186/s40337-020-0277-8

Crow, S. J., Peterson, C. B., Swanson, S. A., Raymond, N. C., Specker, S., Eckert, E. D., & Mitchell, J. E. (2009). Increased mortality in bulimia nervosa and other eating disorders. *American Journal of Psychiatry, 166*(12), 1342–1346. https://doi.org/10.1176/appi.ajp.2009.09020247

Dawe, S. & Loxton, N. J. (2004). The role of impulsivity in the development of substance use and eating disorders. *Neuroscience and Biobehavioral Reviews, 28*(3), 343–351. https://doi.org/10.1016/j.neubiorev.2004.03.007

Diemer, E. W., Grant, J. D., Munn-Chernoff, M. A., Patterson, D. A., & Duncan, A. E. (2015). Gender identity, sexual orientation, and eating-related pathology in a national sample of college students. *Journal of Adolescent Health, 57*(2), 144–149. https://doi.org/10.1016/j.jadohealth.2015.03.003

Diemer, E. W., White Hughto, J. M., Gordon, A. R., Guss, C., Austin, S. B., & Reisner, S. L. (2018). Beyond the binary: differences in eating disorder prevalence by gender identity in a transgender sample. *Transgender Health, 3*(1), 17–23. https://doi.org/10.1089/trgh.2017.0043

Dimitropoulos, G., Landers, A. L., Freeman, V. E., Novick, J., Cullen, O., Engelberg, M., Steinegger, C., & Le Grange, D. (2018). Family-based treatment for transition age youth: Parental self-efficacy and caregiver accommodation. *Journal of Eating Disorders, 6*, 13. https://doi.org/10.1186/s40337-018-0196-0

Dimitropoulos, G., Landers, A. L., Freeman, V., Novick, J., Garber, A., & Le Grange, D. (2018). Open trial of family-based treatment of anorexia nervosa for transition age youth. *Journal of the Canadian Academy of Child and Adolescent Psychiatry, 27*(1), 50–61.

Eldredge, K. L., Locke, K. D., & Horowitz, L. M. (1998). Patterns of interpersonal problems associated with binge eating disorder. *International Journal of Eating Disorders, 23*(4), 383–389. https://doi.org/10.1002/(sici)1098-108x(199805)23:4<383::aid-eat5>3.0.co;2-e

Eubanks, C. F., Burckell, L. A., & Goldfried, M. R. (2018). Clinical consensus strategies to repair ruptures in the therapeutic alliance. *Journal of Psychotherapy Integration, 28*(1), 60–76. https://doi.org/10.1037/int0000097

Farrell, N. R., Bowie, O. R., Cimperman, M. M., Smith, B. E. R., Riemann, B. C., & Levinson, C. A. (2019). Exploring the preliminary effectiveness and acceptability of food-based exposure therapy for eating disorders: A case series of adult inpatients. *Journal of Experimental Psychopathology, 10*(1). https://doi.org/10.1177/2043808718824886

Fischer, S., & Peterson, C. (2015). Dialectical behavior therapy for adolescent binge eating, purging, suicidal behavior, and non-suicidal self-injury: A pilot study. *Psychotherapy, 52*(1), 78–92. https://doi.org/10.1037/a0036065

Fruzzetti, A. E. (2019). Dialectical behaviour therapy with parents, couples, and families to augment Stage 1 outcome. In M. A. Swales (Ed.), *The Oxford Handbook of Dialectical Behaviour Therapy* (pp. 389–411). New York, NY: Oxford University Press.

Fruzzetti, A. E., & Payne, L. (2015). Couple therapy and borderline personality disorder. In A. S. Gurman, J. L. Lebow, & D. K. Snyder (Eds.). *Clinical Handbook of Couple Therapy* (pp. 606–634). New York, NY: The Guilford Press.

Gaglia, A. (2018). Shaping therapists towards adherence: A how-to guide. In M. A. Swales (Ed.). *The Oxford Handbook of Dialectical Behaviour Therapy* (pp. 831–844). New York, NY: Oxford University Press.

Garner, D. M., & Bemis, K. M. (1982). A cognitive-behavioral approach to anorexia nervosa. *Cognitive Therapy and Research, 6*, 123–150.

Gordon, A. R., Austin, S. B., Krieger, N., White Hughto, J. M., & Reisner, S. L. (2016). "I have to constantly prove to myself, to people, that I fit the bill": Perspectives on weight and shape control behaviors among low-income, ethnically diverse young transgender women. *Social Science & Medicine, 165*, 141–149. https://doi.org/10.1016/j.socscimed.2016.07.038

Graves, L. L. & Kalata, A. H. (2021). *Not today ED! Cultivating resilience through multidisciplinary exposure-based interventions.* 2021 IAEDP Symposium, Virtual.

Gregorowski, C., Seedat, S. & Jordaan, G. P. (2013). A clinical approach to the assessment and management of co-morbid eating disorders and substance use disorders. *BMC Psychiatry, 13*, 289. https://doi.org/10.1186/1471-244X-13-289

Guan, K., Fox, K. R., & Prinstein, M. J. (2012). Nonsuicidal self-injury as a time-invariant predictor of adolescent suicide ideation and attempts in a diverse community sample. *Journal of Consulting and Clinical Psychology, 80*(5), 842–849. https://doi.org/10.1037/a0029429

Harned, M. (2020, November 19). *Annual update on DBT research.* 25th Annual ISITDBT Conference, Presented Virtually.

Henretty, J. R., Currier, J. M., Berman, J. S., & Levitt, H. M. (2014). The impact of counselor self-disclosure on clients: A meta-analytic review of experimental and quasi-experimental research. *Journal of Counseling Psychology, 61*(2), 191–207. https://doi.org/10.1037/a0036189

Heruc, G., Hart, S., Stiles, G., Fleming, K., Casey, A., Sutherland, F., Jeffrey, S., Roberton, M., & Hurst, K. (2020). ANZAED practice and training standards for dietitians providing eating disorder treatment. *Journal of Eating Disorders, 8*(77). https://doi.org/10.1186/s40337-020-00334-z

Hill, D. M., Craighead, L. W., & Safer, D. L. (2011). Appetite-focused dialectical behavior therapy for the treatment of binge eating with purging: A preliminary trial. The *International Journal of Eating Disorders, 44*(3), 249–261. https://doi.org/10.1002/eat.20812

Isaksson, M., Ghaderi, A., Ramklint, M., & Wolf-Arehult, M. (2021). Radically open dialectical behavior therapy for anorexia nervosa: A multiple baseline single-case experimental design study across 13 cases. *Journal of Behavior Therapy and Experimental Psychiatry, 71,* https://doi.org/10.1016/j.jbtep.2021.101637.

Johnston, J. A., O'Gara, J. S., Koman, S. L., Baker, C. W., & Anderson, D. A. (2015). A pilot study of Maudsley family therapy with group dialectical behavior therapy skills training in an intensive outpatient program for adolescent eating disorders. *Journal of Clinical Psychology, 71*(6), 527–543. https://doi.org/10.1002/jclp.22176

Kaye, W. H., Wierenga, C. E., Knatz, S., Liang, J., Boutelle, K., Hill, L., & Eisler, I. (2015). Temperament-based treatment for anorexia nervosa. *European Eating Disorders Review, 23(1),* 12–8. https://doi.org/10.1002/erv.2330. PMID: 25377622.

Kirby, J. S., Runfola, C. D., Fischer, M. S., Baucom, D. H., & Bulik, C. M. (2015). Couple-based interventions for adults with eating disorders. *Eating Disorders, 23*(4), 356–365. https://doi.org/10.1080/10640266.2015.1044349

Kröger, C., Schweiger, U., Sipos, V., Kliem, S., Arnold, R., Schunert, T., & Reinecker, H. (2010). Dialectical behaviour therapy and an added cognitive behavioural treatment module for eating disorders in women with borderline personality disorder and anorexia nervosa or bulimia nervosa who failed to respond to previous treatments. An open trial with a 15-month follow-up. *Journal of Behavior Therapy and Experimental Psychiatry, 41*(4), 381–388.

Lammers, M. W., Vroling, M. S., Crosby, R. D., & van Strien, T. (2020). Dialectical behavior therapy adapted for binge eating compared to cognitive behavior therapy in obese adults with binge eating disorder: A controlled study. *Journal of Eating Disorders, 8,* 27. https://doi.org/10.1186/s40337-020-00299-z

Lenz, A. S., Taylor, R., Fleming, M., & Serman, N. (2014). Effectiveness of dialectical behavior therapy for treating eating disorders. *Journal of Counseling & Development, 92*(1), 26–35.

Linehan, M. M. (2015). *DBT® skills training manual* (2nd ed.). New York, NY: Guilford Press.

Linehan, M. M. (1993). *Cognitive-behavioral treatment of borderline personality disorder.* New York, NY: Guilford Press.

Linehan, M. M., Armstrong, H. E., Suarez, A., Allmon, D., & Heard, H. L. (1991). Cognitive-behavioral treatment of chronically parasuicidal borderline patients. *Archives of General Psychiatry, 48*(12), 1060–1064.

Lynch, T. R. (2018). *Radically open dialectical behavior therapy: Theory and practice for treating disorders of overcontrol.* Oakland, CA: New Harbinger Publications, Inc.

Lynch, T. R. (2018). *The skills training manual for radically open dialectical behavior therapy: A clinician's guide for treating disorders of overcontrol.* Reno, NV: Context Press.

Lynch, T. R., Gray, K. L., Hempel, R. J., Titley, M., Chen, E. Y., & O'Mahen, H. A. (2013). Radically open-dialectical behavior therapy for adult anorexia nervosa: Feasibility and outcomes from an inpatient program. *BMC Psychiatry, 13*, 293. https://doi.org/10.1186/1471-244X-13-293

Lynch, T. R., Hempel, R. J., & Dunkey, C. (2015). Radically open-dialetical behavior therapy for disorders of over-control: Signalling matters. *American Journal of Psychotherapy, 69*(2), 141–162.

Masson, P. C., von Ranson, K. M., Wallace, L. M., & Safer, D. L. (2013). A randomized wait-list controlled pilot study of dialectical behaviour therapy guided self-help for binge eating disorder. *Behaviour Research and Therapy, 51*(11), 723–728. https://doi.org/10.1016/j.brat.2013.08.001

Miller, A. L., Rathus, J. H., & Linehan, M. M. (2007). *Dialectical behavior therapy with suicidal adolescents.* New York, NY: The Guilford Press.

Murray, S. B., Anderson, L. K., Cusack, A., Nakamura, T., Rockwell, R., Griffiths, S. & Kaye, W. H. (2015). Integrating family-based treatment and dialectical behavior therapy for adolescent bulimia nervosa: Preliminary outcomes of an open pilot trial. *Eating Disorders, 23*(4), 336–344. https://doi.org/10.1080/10640266.2015.1044345

Nagy, A., McMahon, A., Tapsell, L., & Deane, F. (2021). How is the client-dietitian relationship embedded in the professional education of dietitians? An analysis of curriculum documentation and program coordinators' perspectives in Australia. *Nutrition & Dietetics, 78*, 218–231. https://doi.org/10.1111/1747-0080.12657

National Center on Addiction and Substance Use (CASA). (2003). *Food for thought: Substance abuse and eating disorders.* Columbia University. www.casacolumbia.org/templates/Publications_Reports.aspx

Nordbø, R. H., Espeset, E. M., Gulliksen, K. S., Skårderud, F., & Holte, A. (2006). The meaning of self-starvation: Qualitative study of patients' perception of anorexia nervosa. *International Journal of Eating Disorders, 39*(7), 556–564. https://doi.org/10.1002/eat.20276

Papadopoulos, F. C., Ekbom, A., Brandt, L., & Ekselius, L. (2009). Excess mortality, causes of death and prognostic factors in anorexia nervosa. *British Journal of Psychiatry: The Journal of Mental Science, 194*(1), 10–17. https://doi.org/10.1192/bjp.bp.108.054742

Pennell, A., Webb, C., Agar, P., Federici, A., & Couturier, J. (2019). Implementation of dialectical behavior therapy in a day hospital setting for adolescents with eating disorders. *Journal of the Canadian Academy of Child and Adolescent Psychiatry,* *28*(1), 21–29.

Perepletchikova, F. (2017, December). Dialectical behavior therapy for pre-adolescent children: Helping parents help their kids [Webinar]. *National Education Alliance for Borderline Personality Disorder.* www.borderlinepersonalitydisorder.org/wp-content/uploads/2017/12/ DBT-C_NEABPD_Webinar_Dec-2017.pdf

Perepletchikova, F. (2020, August 24). Understanding dialectical behavior therapy for children (part 3). *BTech Blog.* https://behavioraltech.org/understanding-dbt-c-part-3/

Peterson, C. M., Van Diest, A. M. K., Mara, C. A., & Matthews, A. (2020). Dialectical behavioral therapy skills group as an adjunct to family-based therapy in adolescents with restrictive eating disorders. *Eating Disorders, 28*(1), 67–79. https://doi.org/10.1080/10640266.2019.1568101

Rahmani, M., Omidi, A., Asemi, Z., & Akbari, H. (2018). The effect of dialectical behaviour therapy on binge eating, difficulties in emotion regulation and BMI in overweight patients with binge-eating disorder: A randomized controlled trial. *Mental Health & Prevention, 9*, 13–18.

Root, T., Pinheiro, A. P., Thornton, L., Strober, M., Fernandez-Aranda, F., Brandt, H., Crawford, S., Fichter, M. M., Halmi, K. A., Johnson, C., Kaplan, A. S., Klump, K. L., La Vie, M., Mitchell, J. E., Woodside, D. B., Rotondo, A, Berrettini, W. H., Kaye, W. H., & Bulik, C.M. (2010). Substance use disorders in women with anorexia nervosa. *International Journal of Eating Disorders, 43*, 14–21.

Rozakou-Soumalia, N., Dârvariu, Ş., & Sjögren, J. M. (2021). Dialectical behaviour therapy improves emotion dysregulation mainly in binge eating disorder and bulimia nervosa: A systematic review and meta-analysis. *Journal of Personalized Medicine, 11*(9), 931. https://doi.org/10.3390/jpm11090931

Safer, D. L., Robinson, A. H., & Jo, B. (2010). Outcome from a randomized controlled trial of group therapy for binge eating disorder: Comparing dialectical behavior therapy adapted for binge eating to an active comparison group therapy. *Behavior Therapy, 41*(1), 106–120. https://doi.org/10.1016/j.beth.2009.01.006

Safer, D. L., Telch, C. F., & Agras, W. S. (2001). Dialectical behavior therapy for bulimia nervosa. *The American Journal of Psychiatry, 158*(4), 632–634. https://doi.org/10.1176/appi.ajp.158.4.632

Safer, D. L., Telch, C. F., & Chen, E. Y. (2009). *Dialectical behavior therapy for binge eating and bulimia.* New York, NY: Guilford Press.

Safran, J. D., Muran, J. C., & Eubanks-Carter, C. (2011). Repairing alliance ruptures. *Psychotherapy, 48(1),* 80–87.

Salbach-Andrae, H., Bohnekamp, I., Pfeiffer, E., Lehmkuhl, U., & Miller, A. L. (2008). Dialectical behavior therapy of anorexia and bulimia nervosa among adolescents: A case series. *Cognitive and Behavioral Practice, 15*(4), 415–425. https://doi.org/10.1016/j.cbpra.2008.04.001.

Sayrs, J. H. R. & Linehan, M. M. (2019). *DBT teams: Development and practice.* New York, NY: The Guilford Press.

Schaumberg, K., Welch, E., Breithaupt, L., Hübel, C., Baker, J. H., Munn-Chernoff, M. A., Yilmaz, Z., Ehrlich, S., Mustelin, L., Ghaderi, A., Hardaway, A. J., Bulik-Sullivan, E. C., Hedman, A. M., Jangmo, A., Nilsson, I., Wiklund, C., Yao, S., Seidel, M., & Bulik, C. M. (2017). The science behind the Academy for eating disorders' nine truths about eating disorders. *European Eating Disorders Review, 25*(6), 432–450. https://doi.org/10.1002/erv.255

Schmidt III, H. & Russo, J. C. (2018). The structure of DBT programmes. In M. A. Swales (Ed.). *The Oxford Handbook of Dialectical Behaviour Therapy* (pp. 831–844). New York, NY: Oxford University Press.

Serpell, L., Treasure, J., Teasdale, J., & Sullivan, V. (1999). Anorexia nervosa: Friend or foe? *The International Journal of Eating Disorders, 25*(2), 177–186. https://doi.org/10.1002/(sici)1098-108x(199903)25:2<177::aid-eat7>3.0.co;2-d

Sladdin, I., Ball, L., Bull, C., & Chaboyer, W. (2017). Patient-centred care to improve dietetic practice: An integrative review. *Journal of Human Nutrition and Dietetics, 30*, 453–470. https://doi.org/10.1111/jhn.12444

Smart, H., Clifford, D., & Morris, M. N. (2014). Nutrition students gain skills from motivational interviewing curriculum. *Journal of the Academy of Nutrition and Dietetics, 114*(11), 1712–1713.

Swales, M. A. & Dunkley, C. (2018). Structuring the wider environment and the DBT team: Skills for DBT team leads. In M. A. Swales (Ed.). *The Oxford Handbook of Dialectical Behaviour Therapy* (pp. 831–844). New York, NY: Oxford University Press.

Swenson, C. R. (2016). *DBT® principles in action: Acceptance, change, and dialectics.* New York, NY: The Guilford Press.

Tagay, S., Schlottbohm, E., Reyes-Rodriguez, M. L., Repic, N., & Senf, W. (2014). Eating disorders, trauma, PTSD, and psychosocial resources. *Eating Disorders, 22*(1), 33–49. https://doi.org/10.1080/10640266.2014.857517

Telch, C. F., Agras, W. S., & Linehan, M. M. (2001). Dialectical behavior therapy for binge eating disorder. *Journal of Consulting and Clinical Psychology, 69*(6), 1061–1065. https://doi.org/10.1037//0022-006x.69.6.1061

Testa, R. J., Rider, G. N., Haug, N. A., & Balsam, K. F. (2017). Gender confirming medical interventions and eating disorder symptoms among transgender individuals. *Health Psychology, 36*(10), 927–936. https://doi.org/10.1037/hea0000497

Tiggemann, M. (2011). Sociocultural perspectives on human appearance and body image. In Cash, T. F. & Smolak, L. (Eds.). *Body Image: A Handbook of Science, Practice, and Prevention* (pp. 12–19). New York, NY: The Guilford Press.

Treasure, J., Parker, S., Oyeleye, O., & Harrison, A. (2021). The value of including families in the treatment of anorexia nervosa. *European Eating Disorders Review, 29*, 393–401. https://doi.org/10.1002/erv.2816

Udo, T., Bitley, S., & Grilo, C.M. (2019). Suicide attempts in US adults with lifetime DSM-5 eating disorders. *BMC Medicine, 17*, 120. https://doi.org/10.1186/s12916-019-1352-3

Ung, E. M., Erichsen, C. B., Poulsen, S. Lau, M. E., Simonsen, S., & Davidsen, A. H. (2017). The association between interpersonal problems and treatment outcome in patients with eating disorders. *Journal of Eating Disorders, 5*(53). https://doi.org/10.1186/s40337-017-0179-6

Wampold, B. (2015). How important are the common factors in psychotherapy? An update. *World Psychiatry, 14*(3), 270–277. doi:10.1002/wps.20238

Watson, R. J., Veale, J. F., & Saewyc, E. M. (2016). Disordered eating behaviors among transgender youth: Probability profiles from risk and protective factors. *International Journal of Eating Disorders*. https://doi.org/10.1002/eat.22627

Wisniewski, L., & Ben-Porath, D. D. (2015). Dialectical behavior therapy and eating disorders: The use of contingency management procedures to manage dialectical dilemmas. *American Journal of Psychotherapy, 69*(2), 129–140. https://doi.org/10.1176/appi.psychotherapy.2015.69.2.129

Wisniewski, L. & Kelly, E. (2003). The application of dialectical behavior therapy in the treatment of eating disorders. *Cognitive and Behavioral Practice, 10,* 131–138.

Wisniewski, L. (2018, September 13–15). *The role of DBT in the treatment of complex eating disorders*. The Veritas Collaborative Symposium on Eating Disorders, Atlanta, GA, United States.

Witterholt, S. T. (2020, November 19). *Applying principles of DBT to the practice of pharmacotherapy*. 25th Annual ISITDBT Conference, presented virtually.

Zanarini, M. C., Frankenburg, F. R., Hennen, J., Reich, D. B., & Silk, K. R. (2004). Axis I comorbidity in patients with borderline personality disorder: 6-year follow-up and prediction of time to remission. *American Journal of Psychiatry, 161*(11), 2108–2114.

Index